AF510448

Gastrointestinal Tract Disorders: Diagnosis and Treatment

Gastrointestinal Tract Disorders: Diagnosis and Treatment

Editor: Ivana Hall

MURPHY & MOORE
www.murphy-moorepublishing.com

www.murphy-moorepublishing.com

MURPHY & MOORE

Cataloging-in-Publication Data

Gastrointestinal tract disorders : diagnosis and treatment / edited by Ivana Hall.
p. cm.
Includes bibliographical references and index.
ISBN 978-1-63987-253-4
1. Gastrointestinal system--Diseases. 2. Gastrointestinal system--Diseases--Diagnosis.
3. Gastrointestinal system--Diseases--Treatment. 4. Digestive organs--Diseases. I. Hall, Ivana.
RC816 .G37 2022
616.33--dc23

© Murphy & Moore Publishing, 2022

Murphy & Moore Publishing,
1 Rockefeller Plaza,
New York City, NY 10020, USA

ISBN 978-1-63987-253-4 (Hardback)

This book contains information obtained from authentic and highly regarded sources. Copyright for all individual chapters remain with the respective authors as indicated. All chapters are published with permission under the Creative Commons Attribution License or equivalent. A wide variety of references are listed. Permission and sources are indicated; for detailed attributions, please refer to the permissions page and list of contributors. Reasonable efforts have been made to publish reliable data and information, but the authors, editors and publisher cannot assume any responsibility for the validity of all materials or the consequences of their use.

Trademark Notice: Registered trademark of products or corporate names are used only for explanation and identification without intent to infringe.

Contents

Preface

The purpose of the book is to provide a glimpse into the dynamics and to present opinions and studies of some of the scientists engaged in the development of new ideas in the field from very different standpoints. This book will prove useful to students and researchers owing to its high content quality.

The gastrointestinal tract extends from the mouth to the anus. The diseases and disorders which affect the gastrointestinal tract are termed as gastrointestinal diseases. These can be classified into two categories, functional and structural. The diseases wherein the gastrointestinal tract appears to be normal but does not function properly are termed as functional gastrointestinal diseases. Structural gastrointestinal diseases are the disorders of the gastrointestinal tract in which the bowel does not function properly and appears to be abnormal upon examination. A few disorders of the gastrointestinal tract are constipation, irritable bowel syndrome, hemorrhoids, anal fissures and anal fistula. This book discusses the fundamentals as well as modern approaches to the research on gastrointestinal disorders. Also included herein is a detailed explanation of the clinical management of these disorders. This book includes contributions of experts and scientists which will provide innovative insights into this field.

At the end, I would like to appreciate all the efforts made by the authors in completing their chapters professionally. I express my deepest gratitude to all of them for contributing to this book by sharing their valuable works. A special thanks to my family and friends for their constant support in this journey.

Editor

1

Neurological Manifestations of Inflammatory Bowel Disease

Julio Plata-Bello and Silvia Acosta-López

Abstract

The inflammatory bowel disease (IBD) is associated with different neurological and psychiatric disorders, which are integrated among the extra-intestinal manifestation of this disease. The physiopathology of neurological manifestations of IBD varies among the different kind of complications. The origin and the significance of these manifestations must be understood by clinicians who manage IBD patients. Some of them are related to therapeutic agents. The present chapter consists of a review of the most prevalent neurological and psychiatric disorders associated with IBD. The physiopathology of those entities will also be discussed, as well as the appropriate management for their prevention and treatment.

Keywords: neurological disorders, psychiatric disorders, thrombosis, demyelination, peripheral neuropathy, extra-intestinal manifestations

1. Introduction

Inflammatory bowel disease (IBD) is a chronic disease of the gastrointestinal tract with an unknown etiology, which alternates between periods of symptoms relapse and remission [1, 2]. IBD involves various entities. Crohn's disease (CD) and ulcerative colitis (UC) are the most common, but other inflammatory conditions of the gastrointestinal tract are also included under this term, such as the indeterminate colitis, microscopic colitis and pouchitis [3]. In the present chapter, only CD and UC are discussed.

The incidence of IBD is different depending on its two main forms. CD is diagnosed in 0.5–10.6 patients/100,000 inhabitants/year, while the global incidence of UC is estimated at 0.9–24.3 patients/100,000 inhabitants/year. There is some evidence about the increase of these incidence figures in the past 10 years [2]. On the other hand, the prevalence of CD in European countries ranges from 1.5 to 213 cases per 100,000 people and the prevalence of UC ranges from 2.4 to 294 cases per 100,000 people [2].

IBD consists of an inflammation of the bowel, with different extension and histological features between CD and UC. However, this disease does not only involve the gastrointestinal tract, but there is also a long list of extraintestinal manifestations that can emerge prior to or during the disease. The most frequent ones are those involving the skin (dermatological), the joints (rheumatological), the eyes (ophthalmological), the liver and/or the biliary tract and the genitourinary area (gynecological and/or urological). The prevalence of at least one extraintestinal manifestation varies from 6.2 to 46.6% [4].

Neurological manifestations of IBD are unusual, but they are potentially harmful, leading to severe and irreversible consequences if they are not detected and managed early and properly. The prevalence of neurological manifestations has not been appropriately established, but some authors have reported a prevalence of 20–30%, although there is a general belief that subclinical or unrecognized neurological impairment may be present in IBD patients [4–6].

The aim of the present chapter is to briefly review the main neurological manifestations associated with IBD, with a special focus on their physiopathological mechanisms.

2. General pathophysiological considerations of IBD and its neurological manifestations

Although a specific etiological agent in the development of IBD has not been established, it is widely accepted that some scenarios may be associated with the development of this disease [4]:

- An inflammatory reaction to a persistent bowel infection.
- The presence of defects in the barrier of the intestinal mucosa to act against certain antigens.
- The presence of disturbances in the immune response to certain antigens.

In this regard, a dysfunction of the immune system and a chronic inflammatory response appear both in the context of a specific environmental situation and in a genetically predisposed patient [1]. However, bearing in mind the physiopathology of neurological manifestations, there are different mechanisms that may specifically be involved in their development [4]:

- Malabsorption and secondary deficit of vitamins (mainly vitamin B12), which are essential for myelin maintenance and regeneration [7].
- Hypercoagulability state, related to a chronic inflammatory response that may lead to ischemic events.
- Formation of metabolic toxic agents in the damaged bowel.
- Immunological disturbances that may lead to autoimmune response against glial-neural components.
- Opportunistic infections secondary to the impairment of the immune system or because of the treatment for IBD.

These mechanisms can lead to neurological damage acting individually or in combination. The identification of the leading mechanism is essential to prevent greater neurological damage. Unfortunately, in many cases, it is not possible to identify the main pathological factor.

Nevertheless, disease-related mechanisms are not the only ones that need to be considered to understand the origin of neurological manifestations. The pharmacological agents usually used in IBD may also lead to the development of such manifestations. The appropriate selection of a therapeutic agent depends on the subtype of disease (CD or UC), location and phenotype of the disease [8].

Some of these treatments try to prevent new relapses of the disease, whereas others try to control the symptoms during a relapse. The vast majority of these therapeutic agents can produce neurological manifestations as an adverse effect (**Table 1**), thus clinicians always have to consider the possibility that neurological manifestations in IBD patients may have a pharmacological rather than a primary IBD-related origin.

Drug category		**High frequency (>1 case per 100 patients)**	**Low frequency (>1 case per 1000 patients)**	**Rare (>1 case per 10,000 patients)**	**Unknown frequency**
Steroids				Seizures. Development or worsening of psychiatric disorders (euphoria, mood and personality changes, depression and psychosis)	Dizziness, headache, insomnia
5-Aminosalicilates				Headache, dizziness and peripheral neuropathy	
Antibiotics	Metronidazole	Seizures, peripheral neuropathy. Others: dizziness, ataxia, incoordination, confusion, irritability depression, weakness, insomnia and encephalopathy			
	Ciprofloxacin		Headache, dizziness, sleep disorders, taste disorders, motor hyperactivity	Sensitive disturbances, tremor, seizures, migraine, incoordination, olfactory disorders, confusion, anxiety, depression, psychotic reactions	Peripheral neuropathy
Ciclosporin A		Tremor, headache, seizures, paresthesia	Encephalopathy, confusion, disorientation, decrease level consciousness, anxiety, insomnia, visual disturbances, cortical blindness, comma, paresia and ataxia	Motor polyneuropathy, optic nerve edema	Migraine

Methotrexate		Paresthesia	Motor weakness, encephalopathy, seizures and headache	Mood disorders and cognitive disturbances. Motor weakness, aphasia, cranial nerve disturbances	Intracranial hypertension, neurotoxicity, arachnoiditis, paraplegia, astonishment, ataxia, dementia, dizziness
Thiopurines	Azathioprine			Myasthenic crisis, paresia, polyneuritis	Progressive multifocal leucoencephalopathy when other immunosuppressors are combined
	6-Mercaptopurine	Not reported			
Anti-TNF	Infliximab	Headache, dizziness	Depression, confusion, amnesia, anxiety apathy, drowsiness. Demyelinating disease exacerbation		
	Adalimumab	Mood changes (depression), anxiety, insomnia. Headache, paresthesias, migraine, radicular compression	Cerebrovascular accident, tremor, neuropathy	Multiple sclerosis and other myelinating disorders (optic neuritis and Guillain-Barré syndrome)	
	Certolizumab pegol			Demyelinating disease, including multiple sclerosis (onset or exacerbation). Seizures, peripheral neuropathy	
	Golimumab	Dizziness, headache, paresthesias. Depression, insomnia	Instability	Multiple sclerosis and other demyelinating diseases, dysgeusia	
Vedolizumab		Headache, paresthesia			
Ustekinumab		Dizziness, headache	Depression. Facial palsy		

Table 1. IBD treatment-related neurological complications with categorization of their frequency.

3. Venous and arterial thrombotic and thromboembolic manifestations

Thromboembolic events are common in the context of IBD, secondary to the hypercoagulability state that exists in this disease. This hypercoagulability is associated with an increase of coagulation-associated factors and thrombin levels, as well as fibrin formation; a decrease of natural anticoagulant factors; a decrease in fibrinolytic activity; the presence of endothelial anomalies; and an increase in the count and activity of platelets [9].

Overall, the incidence of thrombotic complications is 1.2–7.5% in clinical studies, but this can rise to 39% when post-mortem studies are considered [10, 11]. Both arterial and venous system may be affected, but deep venous thrombosis and pulmonary thromboembolism are the most common thromboembolic complications in IBD [10–13].

Intracranial thromboembolic events are much less frequent. Cerebral venous thrombosis is more common in CU than in CD, and this may involve superficial or deep cerebral venous systems or even some of the brain venous sinus [11, 14]. The risk of thrombotic or thromboembolic complications in the brain is clearly associated with the activity of the disease. During these periods, IBD patients have a higher risk of cerebral thromboembolic complications than the normal population [9, 10]. These events are rarely reported during periods of non-activity of the disease [9, 10], although some authors have described a higher incidence of thromboembolic events in IBD patients than in healthy controls not only during a relapse of the disease but also during remission periods [15]. Larger cohort and case-control studies are needed to confirm this finding, because if IBD patients suffer more thromboembolic events even during remission periods, anticoagulant therapies might be routinely indicated.

In any case, the increase of thromboembolic events during relapses is clearly related to the inflammatory response whose effect in the coagulation and platelet system has been described above. Nevertheless, the use of steroids, dehydration, the increase of homocysteine and infections (all of which are associated with relapsing periods) may also contribute to the development of thrombotic complications [10–13, 16]. Furthermore, the presence of mutations in Leiden factor V in IBD patients leads to a higher incidence of thrombotic events [17].

Therefore, bearing in mind the high risk of thromboembolic events in IBD patients, mostly during relapses [18, 19], it is essential to rapidly initiate a primary prophylaxis, with an early mobilization, a correct rehydration and vitamin reposition, as well as the use of prophylactic anticoagulants (mainly low molecular weight heparins). All of these measures are proven to be useful in the prevention of venous thromboembolic events [20].

On the other hand, IBD patients also seem to present a higher incidence of arterial thromboembolic events. Indeed, many studies have reported an association between cardiovascular events and other chronic inflammatory diseases, like rheumatoid arthritis, lupus or psoriasis [21–23]. Active IBD is also associated with a higher risk of cardiovascular events (spontaneous or after surgical/invasive procedures), especially in young female patients [9].

When arterial thromboembolic events occur in the brain, they can be classified as ischemic stroke. Although the literature agrees about the high risk of thromboembolic events in IBD patients, the increase in the incidence of ischemic stroke in IBD patients is a matter of debate [9]. In this regard, Huang et al. [24], in a large retrospective cohort study, analyzed the risk of ischemic stroke in IBD patients of a Taiwanese population. Although the studied groups were not completely comparable in demographical and comorbidity features, the authors reported a higher prevalence of ischemic stroke in IBD patients (mainly in CD patients) than the general population (hazard ratios for UC and CD were 1.01 [95% confidence interval = 0.84–1.21] and 1.15 [95% confidence interval = 1.04–1.28], respectively) [24]. Similar results were reported in a Danish population-based setting (also with a mismatch in comorbidity distribution), showing a relative risk (RR) of 1.15 of suffering ischemic stroke in an IBD population (95% confidence interval 1.04–1.27) of suffering ischemic stroke in an IBD population [25]. Therefore, there is weak evidence of the higher incidence of ischemic stroke in IBD populations. In any case, it seems to be of the utmost importance to manage cardiovascular risk factors in IBD patients [9]. Their combination with the pro-thrombotic situation that may be present in any phase of IBD can play a major role in the development of brain ischemic complications, which are associated with a high level of dependence and an important worsening of quality of life.

However, vascular events may not be only associated with pro-thrombotic conditions. Vasculitis may also contribute to the presence of neurological manifestations. Bearing this in mind, systemic vasculitis is also considered an extra-intestinal manifestation of IBD. Wegener's granulomatosis, Takayasu arteritis, medial temporal arteritis and Cogan's syndrome (among others) have been reported in combination with IBD [4, 26]. For example, Takayasu arteritis is associated with IBD in 9.6% of cases [27], and this frequency seems to be higher in CD patients (9%) [28] than in UC (6.4%) [29]. The pathogenesis of vasculitis associated with IBD is mediated by immune complex deposits and cytotoxic lymphocytes [30]. The vasculitis of IBD patients involves medium and large caliber vessels and may lead to brain ischemic events [4], and some of them can directly affect the central nervous system (CNS) [31]. The global frequency of vasculitis associated with IBD is unknown, but it has been reported that such cases of vasculitis involving the CNS are rare [31]. Furthermore, this manifestation seems to be independent of the activity of the disease in the gastrointestinal tract [30, 32]. A correct diagnosis of CNS vasculitis is essential, because it allows the initiation of the appropriate treatment and the prevention of significant neurological impairment. Thus, when IBD patients present any CNS vascular event, vasculitis must be considered as a possible diagnosis and it has to be appropriately ruled out.

4. Demyelinating diseases

The association of demyelinating diseases has been proposed since the early 1980s. Rang et al. described a higher prevalence of multiple sclerosis (MS) than expected in UC patients [33]. Subsequently, this finding has been confirmed by many reports, but not only for UC but also for CD [34–36]. For instance, Gupta et al. described an increased risk of optic neuritis and other forms of MS in CD (odds ratio = 1.54) and UC (odds ratio = 1.75) [35]. In the same line, a recent meta-analysis concluded that IBD patients present a higher risk of suffering from concomitant MS and vice versa (i.e. MS patients have a higher risk of suffering from associated IBD) [36]. These authors found an increased risk of 50% [36].

However, some authors have proposed that the development of demyelinating diseases in IBD patients is more related to the use of anti-TNFα drugs [37]. In this regard, the Spanish registry of autoimmune adverse events of biological agents (BIOGEAS Project) reported 12 cases of MS and 25 cases of optic neuritis in IBD patients treated with anti-TNFα [38]. Furthermore, this phenomenon is not exclusive to IBD patients. Arthritis patients treated with anti-TNFα agents may develop MS or demyelinating lesions, with a partial or complete resolution of neurological symptoms after discontinuing the medication [39]. An increased number of new white matter lesions and new relapses have also been reported in MS patients treated with infliximab [40]. On the other hand, the use of Natalizumab, a monoclonal antibody against alfa4-integrin used in some cases of IBD, is associated with progressive multifocal leukoencephalopathy (PML). This disease appears after a reactivation of the JC virus infection, and the use of Natalizumab is clearly associated with this reactivation. PML is associated with a bad prognosis with a mortality rate at 6 months above 60% [37].

Apart from demyelinating diseases associated with IBD, there is strong evidence of a higher prevalence of white matter lesions in neurologically asymptomatic IBD patients than in healthy subjects [5, 41]. Although these lesions are usually asymptomatic, their number and volume tend to increase with age (mostly in CU patients) [41]. In any case, whenever these lesions become symptomatic, their association with other CNS complications (e.g. cerebrovascular complications) has to be identified.

Therefore, in spite of the plausible relationship between MS and IBD, the presence of white matter lesions is not evidence of the coexistence of both diseases. In fact, most of these lesions have no clinical relevance and their presence in IBD patients should not be used to infer active CNS disease [42]. Further research is needed about the origin of these lesions and their neurological and cognitive consequences in IBD patients.

5. Epilepsy

The relationship between epilepsy and IBD is uncertain. Lossos et al. reported a prevalence of 1.9% in a cohort of 638 IBD patients, although the majority of these patients had a structural and/or metabolic cause that may lead to epileptic seizures [32]. Other authors have reported an improvement of seizures in CD patients after treatment initiation, suggesting that immunological mechanisms may be associated with the development of this disorder [43]. This finding might also be supported by some case reports [44].

However, the most plausible explanation for the development of epileptic seizures in IBD patients is that other CNS complications (e.g. thromboembolic events or unspecific white matter lesions) or other systemic complications (e.g. dehydration, low levels of magnesium, etc.) may facilitate its development [45, 46]. Because of the above, a correct therapeutic management may help to resolve and/or prevent this condition.

6. Peripheral neuropathy

Peripheral neuropathy (PN) is one of the most common neurological complications in IBD patients [32, 43, 47]. Many factors have been associated with the development of PN, such as extraintestinal inflammation, immunological phenomena, nutritional disturbances (e.g. malabsorption-related vitamin deficit) and adverse effects of IBD therapeutic agents (e.g. metronidazole or anti-TNF agents) [48–50]. Whenever these causes are ruled out, the frequency of PN in IBD patients varies from 0 to 39% [51].

IBD-associated PN may be associated with axonal damage or demyelination and it may have an acute or chronic presentation [47, 51]. Cases of mononeuropathy, plexopathies, multiple mononeuritis, compressive neuropathies and cranial neuropathies have also been reported [50]. Bearing this in mind, IBD-related PNs present great clinical variability, although there is a certain dominance of non-demyelinating vs. myelinating forms [48].

Demyelinating forms have a better prognosis than non-demyelinating forms, because they have a more favorable response to immunotherapy. This situation may be related to the role that T lymphocytes seem to play in demyelinating IBD-associated PNs. On the other hand, the relationship between axonal PNs and immunological disturbances is less clear [47, 48].

7. Psychiatric disorders

IBD patients show a high prevalence of psychiatric disorders, with depression and anxiety as the main diagnosis [1, 52, 53]. The prevalence of depression in IBD patients varies from 15 to 30%, but the frequency of anxiety rises to 80%, mainly associated with the relapses of the disease [54, 55]. There is no overall difference in the frequency of psychiatric disorders between UC and CD [52].

Several factors have been associated with IBD-related depression: female gender, active intestinal disease, the presence of fistulas or perianal disease, use of biological treatments and the necessity of surgery because of IBD [55]. On the other hand, IBD patients with IBD seem to present more aggressive phenotypes of the disease, with more relapses and shorter periods of remission [52]. In any case, the prevalence of depression or anxiety is even higher when other psychiatric conditions coexist [1, 52, 53].

Anyway, depression and anxiety are not the only IBD- associated psychiatric disorders. The Manitoba IBD Cohort Study reported a higher prevalence in IBD patients than in general population of panic and obsessive-compulsive disorders [56]. Controversy exists around bipolar disorder. On the one hand, the Manitoba IBD Cohort Study reported a lower prevalence of bipolar disorder in IBD than in the general population. On the other hand, Eaton et al. (2010) reported a higher frequency of this psychiatric condition in IBD patients, more specifically in CD patients [57].

However, it is widely accepted that there is an infra-diagnosis and infra-treatment of psychiatric disorders, with no systematic screening established in clinical guidelines. There is a strong evidence of the presence of a bidirectional relationship between the degree of inflammation in the gastrointestinal tract and the development of depression. This can be explained by the brain-gut axis hypothesis. The brain and the gut are communicated by the autonomic nervous system (sympathetic and parasympathetic systems). The vagus nerve (the main parasympathetic afferent) transmits information to the CNS about luminal osmolarity, carbohydrate levels, mechanical distortion of the mucosa and the presence of bacterial or cytostatic drugs. On the other hand, sympathetic afferents transmit visceral pain [58].

Information sent by the gastrointestinal system reaches the medulla (nucleus tractus solitarius) and travels upstream until it reaches the paraventricular nucleus where it finally modulates the hypothalamic–pituitary–adrenal (HPA) axis [59].

Some authors proposed that an impairment in the gut-brain axis can be induced by stress. In this regard, stressful situations lead to a vagal inhibition and an overactivation of the sympathetic system. These conditions associated with other CNS-mediated responses involving the modulation of the immune system and the HPA axis may be associated with the appearance of a gastrointestinal immunoinflammatory response [58, 60]. For instance, during depression, an elevation of alpha-TNF, IL-1, reactive C protein and haptoglobin and a decrease of IL-10, TGF-B, albumin and transferrin are observed [61].

Therefore, there is a notable association between IBD and psychiatric disorders. New studies are necessary to elucidate in which cases the psychiatric condition is the cause or the consequence of IBD. This may help to understand pathophysiological aspects of IBD that are still unknown and ultimately may allow better management of the disease.

8. Conclusion

IBD patients may suffer from different neurological manifestations during their disease. The pathophysiological mechanisms involved in these complications are variable and, in many cases, they are still unrecognized. Anyway, clinicians must stay focused on the early identification of IBD neurological complications and to rapidly establish the appropriate management to prevent further impairment.

Author details

Julio Plata-Bello[1]* and Silvia Acosta-López[2]

*Address all correspondence to: jplata5@hotmail.com

1 Department of Neurosurgery, Hospital Universitario de Canarias, S/C de Tenerife, Spain

2 Department of Gastroenterology and Hepatology, Hospital Universitario Nuestra Señora de La Candelaria, S/C de Tenerife, Spain

References

[1] Abautret-Daly Á, Dempsey E, Parra-Blanco A, Medina C, Harkin A. Gut–brain actions underlying comorbid anxiety and depression associated with inflammatory bowel disease. Acta Neuropsychiatrica. 2017;**8**:1-22

[2] Burisch J, Jess T, Martinato M, Lakatos PL. The burden of inflammatory bowel disease in Europe. Journal of Crohn's and Colitis. 2013;**7**(4):322-337

[3] Montoro MA, García Pagán JC. Enfermedad inflamatoria intestinal. Enfermedad de Crohn. In: Gastroenterología y Hepatología Problemas comunes en la práctica clínica. 2nd ed. Madrid: Jarpyo Editores; 2012. pp. 443-458

[4] Bermejo PE, Burgos A. Complicaciones neurológicas de la enfermedad inflamatoria intestinal. Medicina Clínica (Barcelona). 2008;**130**(17):666-675

[5] Geissler A, Andus T, Roth M, Kullmann F, Caesar I, Held P, et al. Focal white-matter lesions in brain of patients with inflammatory bowel disease. Lancet (London, England). 1995 Apr;**345**(8954):897-898

[6] Lindgren S, Lilja B, Rosén I, Sundkvist G. Disturbed autonomic nerve function in patients with Crohn's disease. Scandinavian Journal of Gastroenterology. 1991 Apr;**26**(4): 361-366

[7] Mariño Suárez JE, Monedero Recuero I, Peláez Laguno C. Deficiencia de vitamina B12 y tratamiento por vía oral. Una opción tan eficaz como (todavía) poco utilizada. Atención Primaria. 2003;**32**(6):382-387

[8] Bernstein CN, Eliakim A, Fedail S, Fried M, Gearry R, Goh K-L, et al. Update. Journal of Clinical Gastroenterology. August 2015;**50**(10):803-818

[9] Zezos P, Kouklakis G, Saibil F. Inflammatory bowel disease and thromboembolism. World Journal of Gastroenterology. 2014;**20**(38):13863-13878

[10] Benarroch HS, Acosta AV. Complicaciones vasculares asociadas a la enfermedad inflamatoria intestinal. Anales de Medicina Interna. 2003;**20**:81-84

[11] Ashrafi MR, Hosseini F, Alizadeh H. Case report pseudotumor cerebri in a case of ulcerative colitis with sagittal sinus thrombosis case presentation. Iranian Journal of Pediatrics. 2013;**23**(1):109-112

[12] Lloyd-Still JD, Tomasi L. Neurovascular and thromboembolic complications of inflammatory bowel disease in childhood. Journal of Pediatric Gastroenterology and Nutrition. 1989 Nov;**9**(4):461-466

[13] Papa A, Gerardi V, Marzo M, Felice C, Rapaccini GL, Gasbarrini A. Venous thromboembolism in patients with inflammatory bowel disease: Focus on prevention and treatment. World Journal of Gastroenterology. 2014;**20**(12):3173-3179

[14] Cho Y, Chae MK, Cha JM, Il LJ, Joo KR, Shin HP, et al. Cerebral venous thrombosis in a patient with Crohn's disease. Intestinal Research. 2016;**14**(1):96-101

[15] Grainge MJ, West J, Card TR. Venous thromboembolism during active disease and remission in inflammatory bowel disease: A cohort study. Lancet. 2010;**375**(9715):657-663

[16] Twig G, Zandman-Goddard G, Szyper-Kravitz M, Shoenfeld Y. Systemic thromboembolism in inflammatory bowel disease: Mechanisms and clinical applications. Annals of the New York Academy of Sciences. 2005 Jun;**1051**:166-173

[17] Liebman HA, Kashani N, Sutherland D, McGehee W, Kam AL. The factor V Leiden mutation increases the risk of venous thrombosis in patients with inflammatory bowel disease. Gastroenterology. 1998 Oct;**115**(4):830-834

[18] Van Assche G, Dignass A, Reinisch W, van der Woude CJ, Sturm A, De Vos M, et al. The second European evidence-based consensus on the diagnosis and management of Crohn's disease: Special situations. Journal of Crohn's & Colitis. 2010 Feb;**4**(1):63-101

[19] Van Assche G, Dignass A, Bokemeyer B, Danese S, Gionchetti P, Moser G, et al. Second European evidence-based consensus on the diagnosis and management of ulcerative colitis part 3: Special situations. Journal of Crohn's & Colitis. 2013 Feb;**7**(1):1-33

[20] Dentali F, Douketis JD, Gianni M, Lim W, Crowther MA. Meta-analysis: Anticoagulant prophylaxis to prevent symptomatic venous thromboembolism in hospitalized medical patients. Annals of Internal Medicine. 2007 Feb;**146**(4):278-288

[21] Ahlehoff O, Gislason GH, Charlot M, Jørgensen CH, Lindhardsen J, Olesen JB, et al. Psoriasis is associated with clinically significant cardiovascular risk: A Danish nationwide cohort study. Journal of Internal Medicine. 2011 Aug;**270**(2):147-157

[22] Meune C, Touzé E, Trinquart L, Allanore Y. Trends in cardiovascular mortality in patients with rheumatoid arthritis over 50 years: A systematic review and meta-analysis of cohort studies. Rheumatology (Oxford, England). 2009 Oct;**48**(10):1309-1313

[23] Svenungsson E, Jensen-Urstad K, Heimbürger M, Silveira A, Hamsten A, de Faire U, et al. Risk factors for cardiovascular disease in systemic lupus erythematosus. Circulation. 2001 Oct;**104**(16):1887-1893

[24] Huang WS, Tseng CH, Chen PC, Tsai CH, Lin CL, Sung FC, et al. Inflammatory bowel diseases increase future ischemic stroke risk: A Taiwanese population-based retrospective cohort study. European Journal of Internal Medicine. 2014;**25**(6):561-565

[25] Kristensen SL, Ahlehoff O, Lindhardsen J, Erichsen R, Jensen GV, Torp-Pedersen C, et al. Disease activity in inflammatory bowel disease is associated with increased risk of myocardial infarction, stroke and cardiovascular death—A Danish nationwide cohort study. PLoS One. 2013;**8**(2):e56944

[26] Sy A, Khalidi N, Dehghan N, Barra L, Carette S, Cuthbertson D, et al. Vasculitis in patients with inflammatory bowel diseases: A study of 32 patients and systematic review of the literature. Seminars in Arthritis and Rheumatism. 2016 Feb;**45**(4):475-482

[27] Akiyama S, Fujii T, Matsuoka K, Yusuke E, Negi M, Takenaka K, et al. Endoscopic features and genetic background of inflammatory bowel disease complicated with Takayasu arteritis. Journal of Gastroenterology and Hepatology. 2017 May;**32**(5):1011-1017

[28] Reny J-L, Paul J-F, Lefèbvre C, Champion K, Emmerich J, Blétry O, et al. Association of Takayasu's arteritis and Crohn's disease. Results of a study on 44 Takayasu patients and review of the literature. Annales de Medecine Interne. 2003 Mar;**154**(2):85-90

[29] Terao C, Matsumura T, Yoshifuji H, Kirino Y, Maejima Y, Nakaoka Y, et al. Takayasu arteritis and ulcerative colitis: high rate of co-occurrence and genetic overlap. Arthritis & Rheumatology (Hoboken, NJ). 2015 May;**67**(8):2226-2232

[30] Scheid R, Teich N. Neurologic manifestations of ulcerative colitis. European Journal of Neurology. 2007 May;**14**(5):483-493

[31] Raj N, Arkebauer M, Waters B, Dickinson B. A case of cerebral vasculitis associated with ulcerative colitis. Case Reports in Rheumatology. 2015;**2015**:598273

[32] Lossos A, River Y, Eliakim A, Steiner I. Neurologic aspects of inflammatory bowel disease. Neurology. 1995 Mar;**45**(3 Pt 1):416-421

[33] Rang EH, Brooke BN, Hermon-Taylor J. Association of ulcerative colitis with multiple sclerosis. Lancet (London, England). 1982 Sep;**2**(8297):555

[34] Marrie RA, Reider N, Cohen J, Stuve O, Sorensen PS, Cutter G, et al. A systematic review of the incidence and prevalence of autoimmune disease in multiple sclerosis. Multiple Sclerosis. 2015 Mar;**21**(3):282-293

[35] Gupta G, Gelfand JM, Lewis JD. Increased risk for demyelinating diseases in patients with inflammatory bowel disease. Gastroenterology. 2005 Sep;**129**(3):819-826

[36] Kosmidou M, Katsanos AH, Katsanos KH, Kyritsis AP, Tsivgoulis G, Christodoulou D, et al. Multiple sclerosis and inflammatory bowel diseases: A systematic review and meta-analysis. Journal of Neurology. 2017 Feb;**264**(2):254-259

[37] Singh S, Kumar N, Loftus EV, Kane SV. Neurologic complications in patients with inflammatory bowel disease: increasing relevance in the era of biologics. Inflammatory Bowel Disease. 2013;**19**(4):864-872

[38] Ramos-Casals M, Roberto-Perez-Alvarez, Diaz-Lagares C, Cuadrado M-J, Khamashta MA, BIOGEAS Study Group. Autoimmune diseases induced by biological agents: A double-edged sword? Autoimmunity Reviews. 2010 Jan;**9**(3):188-93

[39] Mohan N, Edwards ET, Cupps TR, Oliverio PJ, Sandberg G, Crayton H, et al. Demyelination occurring during anti-tumor necrosis factor alpha therapy for inflammatory arthritides. Arthritis and Rheumatism. 2001 Dec;**44**(12):2862-2869

[40] van Oosten BW, Barkhof F, Truyen L, Boringa JB, Bertelsmann FW, von Blomberg BM, et al. Increased MRI activity and immune activation in two multiple sclerosis patients treated with the monoclonal anti-tumor necrosis factor antibody cA2. Neurology. 1996 Dec;**47**(6):1531-1534

[41] Dolapcioglu C, Guleryuzlu Y, Uygur-Bayramicli O, Ahishali E, Dabak R. Asymptomatic brain lesions on cranial magnetic resonance imaging in inflammatory bowel disease. Gut Liver. 2013 Mar;**7**(2):169-174

[42] Hart PE, Gould SR, MacSweeney JE, Clifton A, Schon F. Brain white-matter lesions in inflammatory bowel disease. Lancet (London, England). 1998 May;**351**(9115):1558

[43] Elsehety A, Bertorini TE. Neurologic and neuropsychiatric complications of Crohn's disease. Southern Medical Journal. 1997 Jun;**90**(6):606-610

[44] Masaki T, Muto T, Shinozaki M, Kuroda T. Unusual cerebral complication associated with ulcerative colitis. Journal of Gastroenterology. 1997 Apr;**32**(2):251-254

[45] Fagan C, Phelan D. Severe convulsant hypomagnesaemia and short bowel syndrome. Anaesthesia and Intensive Care. 2001 Jun;**29**(3):281-283

[46] Shorvon S, Andermann F, Guerrini R. The causes of epilepsy. In 2011. pp. 590-1

[47] Benavente L, Morís G. Neurologic disorders associated with inflammatory bowel disease. European Journal of Neurology. 2011;**18**(1):138-143

[48] Gondim FAA, Grannagan TH, Sander HW, Chin RL, Latov N. Peripheral neuropathy in patients with inflammatory bowel disease. Brain. 2005;**128**(4):867-879

[49] Deepak P, Stobaugh DJ, Sherid M, Sifuentes H, Ehrenpreis ED. Neurological events with tumour necrosis factor alpha inhibitors reported to the Food and Drug Administration adverse event reporting system. Alimentary Pharmacology & Therapeutics. 2013 Aug; **38**(4):388-396

[50] Pfeiffer RF. Gastroenterology and neurology. Continuum (Minneap Minn). 2017;**23**(3, Neurology of Systemic Disease):744-61

[51] Morís G. Inflammatory bowel disease: An increased risk factor for neurologic complications. World Journal of Gastroenterology. 2014;**20**(5):1228-1237

[52] Graff LA, Walker JR, Bernstein CN. Depression and anxiety in inflammatory bowel disease: A review of comorbidity and management. Inflammatory Bowel Diseases. 2009 Jul;**15**(7):1105-1118

[53] Nowakowski J, Chrobak AA, Dudek D. Psychiatric illnesses in inflammatory bowel diseases—Psychiatric comorbidity and biological underpinnings. Psychiatria Polska. 2016;**50**(6):1157-1166

[54] Bannaga AS, Selinger CP. Inflammatory bowel disease and anxiety: Links, risks, and challenges faced. Clinical and Experimental Gastroenterology. 2015;**8**:111-117

[55] Panara AJ, Yarur AJ, Rieders B, Proksell S, Deshpande AR, Abreu MT, et al. The incidence and risk factors for developing depression after being diagnosed with inflammatory bowel disease: A cohort study. Alimentary Pharmacology & Therapeutics. 2014 Apr;**39**(8):802-810

[56] Walker JR, Ediger JP, Graff LA, Greenfeld JM, Clara I, Lix L, et al. The Manitoba IBD cohort study: A population-based study of the prevalence of lifetime and 12-month anxiety and mood disorders. The American Journal of Gastroenterology. 2008 Aug;**103**(8): 1989-1997

[57] Eaton WW, Pedersen MG, Nielsen PR, Mortensen PB. Autoimmune diseases, bipolar disorder, and non-affective psychosis. Bipolar Disorders. 2010 Sep;**12**(6):638-646

[58] Bonaz BL, Bernstein CN. Brain-gut interactions in inflammatory bowel disease. Gastroenterology. 2013 Jan;**144**(1):36-49

[59] Benarroch EE. The central autonomic network: Functional organization, dysfunction, and perspective. Mayo Clinic Proceedings. 1993 Oct;**68**(10):988-1001

[60] Ghia J-E, Blennerhassett P, Deng Y, Verdu EF, Khan WI, Collins SM. Reactivation of inflammatory bowel disease in a mouse model of depression. Gastroenterology. 2009 Jun;**136**(7):2280-8.e1-4

[61] Martin-Subero M, Anderson G, Kanchanatawan B, Berk M, Maes M. Comorbidity between depression and inflammatory bowel disease explained by immune-inflammatory, oxidative, and nitrosative stress; tryptophan catabolite; and gut-brain pathways. CNS Spectrums. 2016 Apr;**21**(2):184-198

2

Psychiatric Comorbidities in Irritable Bowel Syndrome (IBS)

Mihaela Fadgyas Stanculete

Abstract

FA lot of research has pointed out that irritable bowel syndrome (IBS) is a multifactorial illness involving visceral hypersensitivity, alteration of communication between the enteric nervous system (ENS) and central nervous system (CNS), increased intestinal permeability, minimal intestinal inflammation, and altered intestinal microflora. Psychological, social, and genetic factors appear to be important in the development of IBS symptomatology through several mechanisms. This chapter addresses the relationships between irritable bowel syndrome (IBS) and psychiatric comorbidities. The aim of this chapter is to provide an overview of explanatory hypothesis and to describe a variety of approaches which integrate the vast research data about IBS and psychiatric comorbidities, including genetic, brain imaging, and neuropsychological findings. The section of this chapter which overlooks the psychotropic treatment reviews the comparative efficacy of various drugs.

Keywords: irritable bowel syndrome, neuroimaging, psychiatric comorbidities, psychosocial factors

1. Introduction

Irritable bowel syndrome (IBS) is a chronic functional gastrointestinal (GI) disorder that has been reported to be associated with increased use of health-care resources and impaired quality of life.

Over the last two decades, it is becoming increasingly clear that many factors are involved in IBS, and they interact in very complex ways, which have not been yet elucidated.

The biopsychosocial model has been developed to explain the IBS pathogenesis better. According to this model, the gastrointestinal function is modulated via brain-gut axis by psychosocial factors. Particular attention is given to stress, emotion, and psychological factors in the IBS pathogenesis.

Emerging data reveals the interaction between psychiatric disorders and IBS, which suggests that this association should not be ignored when developing strategies for screening and treatment. The simultaneous presence of a mental disorder and IBS worsen the prognosis of both diseases involved to a significantly greater extent.

It is very important to understand better how social and psychological factors influence biological processes both in IBS and psychiatric conditions. Several mechanisms have been proposed to explain this association. In this chapter, we highlight data from a wide range of research including genetic, neurotransmitter, and brain imaging studies.

Stressful life events can lead to the activation of hypothalamic-pituitary-adrenal (HPA) axis. Neurotransmitters including serotonin, norepinephrine, and corticotropin-releasing factor change the motility and the perception in the gut. Brain regions necessary for pain processing and pain and emotional regulation may be involved. The psychological burden of a chronic relapsing illness can increase the maladaptive behaviors and negative emotions and decrease the coping abilities. A better understanding of these processes will be crucial for developing more useful treatments.

Although pharmacological treatments have proven efficacy in IBS, the illness remains chronic with the symptomatic and functional problems only partially influenced for most patients.

A lot of papers have documented improved clinical prognosis in IBS through psychological and pharmacologic interventions. Despite these promising data, the evidence is still limited by underpowered sample sizes.

With this growing awareness of the importance of psychosocial factors in IBS care, medical professionals experience an increased need for accessible background information and practical guidelines for diagnosis and management of psychiatric comorbidities.

Over the last two decades, it is becoming increasingly clear that many factors are involved in IBS and they interact in very complex ways, which have not been yet elucidated.

2. Psychosocial factors linked to IBS

The biopsychosocial model aims to integrate the multidimensional mechanisms to understand how IBS can be developed under such multiple interactions. The most important characteristic of this model is the bidirectional causality: the psychosocial factors influence the brain and the gut, and the gut interacts with the brain via the autonomic nervous system and the hypothalamic-pituitary-adrenal (HPA) axis [1]. The principal psychological and social factors that have been reported to contribute to the onset, the severity, and the evolution of IBS are presented in **Table 1**.

Sociological factors	– Parental beliefs and behaviors – Illness behavior – Learning through positive reinforcement or reward and modeling – Adverse life events (sexual, emotional, physical abuse) – Chronic life stress – Social support – Culture (cultural beliefs, norms)
Psychological factors	– Anxiety, depression – Anger – Cognitive-affective processes: gastrointestinal anxiety, hypervigilance, and attentional bias, catastrophizing, alexithymia – Coping mechanisms

Table 1. Psychological and sociological factors involved in IBS.

- Parental beliefs and behaviors. It is accepted that there is a familial aggregation of IBS. Studies demonstrated that not only the genetic factors could explain why IBS tends to cluster in families, but the development of gastrointestinal symptoms could also be explained by reinforcement and modeling of gastrointestinal illness behavior by parents [2].

- Positive reinforcement of illness behavior. Children whose parents reinforce sickness behavior (through parental protective behaviors) report more severe pain and more school absences than other children. Studies of childhood learning have also suggested that social learning through modeling processes (children observing and learning to exhibit the behaviors they witness) may also contribute to the intergenerational transmission of GI illness behavior and play a significant role in development and maintenance of IBS symptoms [3–5].

- Various types of early adverse life events (EALs) are associated with the development of IBS, in particular sexual, emotional, and physical abuse [6]. The relationship between abuse and severity of gastrointestinal symptoms and poorer health-related quality of life (HRQOL) seems to be partially mediated by concomitant mood disturbances [7]. Studies have shown that other types of EALs have been associated with an increased vulnerability toward developing IBS (parental death, divorce, or separation) [8]. A substantial body of evidence suggests that epigenetic mechanisms play a major role in the causal link between EALs and IBS. Findings from animal models and human studies highlighted the long-term effects of exposure to stress in early life through changes in gene expression [9]. Furthermore, prospective studies have demonstrated that chronic life stress is the most significant predictor of IBS symptom severity over 16 months. Stress has a marked impact on mucosal immune activation, intestinal sensitivity, permeability, secretion, and motility and through various mechanisms can affect the IBS treatment outcomes [10–12].

- Social support is related to many aspects of IBS. It was shown that social support is reduced in chronic illnesses. The association between the quality of social support and the severity of IBS symptoms was mostly investigated. Perceived adequacy of social support appears to have a positive influence on pain possibly through a reduction in stress levels [13]. In contrast, negative social relationship correlates with increased symptom severity.
- Culture. The impact of culture on the perception and description of IBS symptoms is already known. It was emphasized that cultural beliefs, norms, and behaviors should be taken into account when evaluating the IBS presentation and management of the symptoms. Cultural norms could shape the acceptability of expressing symptomatology and the willingness to seek health-care assistance.
- Gastrointestinal-specific anxiety (GSA) represents "the cognitive, affective, and behavioral response stemming from fear of gastrointestinal symptoms, and the context in which these visceral symptoms occur" indicating awareness of and concern about gastrointestinal sensations. It has been suggested that GSA may be more relevant than general anxiety for symptom severity and health outcome and represents a key predictor of IBS diagnosis. Moreover, GSA was found to be associated with the mental component of quality of life, suggesting that GSA is an important endpoint for different interventions [14].
- Hypervigilance. IBS patients selectively attend to gastrointestinal sensations compared to healthy individuals. Some researchers indicated that visceral hypersensitivity is linked with the hypervigilance toward visceral sensations and a tendency to label them negatively [15]. Hypervigilance may reflect poor coping with gastrointestinal-specific anxiety.
- Attentional bias. Studies indicate that attentional bias toward gastrointestinal sensations is exaggerated and could represent a potential factor in IBS development and maintenance. Researchers reported that focusing attention on bodily sensations leads to increased physical symptom complaints and illness behavior.
- Catastrophizing has been defined as a psychological construct characterized by the tendency to have a distorted negative view of health problems and amplify the threat of symptoms. Cross-sectional studies have found that catastrophizing in IBS is associated with increased

- Alexithymia is a multidimensional construct defined as an inability in experiencing, expressing, and describing emotions in a verbal manner. Alexithymia can be conceptualized as a deficit in cognitive processing and emotional regulations. IBS patients present higher levels of alexithymia than general population. Also, studies suggest that alexithymia, a stable trait, could be a stronger predictor of IBS severity than GSA, thus implying that impaired affective awareness may weigh in the clinical presentation of IBS [17].
- Anger represents a negative emotional state that has several dimensions: anger experience, anger expression, and anger control. Inhibited anger expression is associated with depression, pain interference, and the frequency of pain behaviors. There are results that higher

levels of trait anger characterize IBS patients when compared to healthy population, and this may be associated with clinical manifestations [18]. Other studies demonstrated that IBS patients appear to have higher levels of anger than a group of patients with organic bowel diseases.

- Coping mechanisms. Studies have begun to focus on the coping mechanisms because these factors influence treatment options, patients' expectations, and treatment outcome. Coping represents the cognitive and behavioral efforts to deal (reduce or tolerate) with a perceived stressful situation. As mentioned above, the coping can influence the outcome of the illness. Therefore the quality of a coping strategy should be evaluated according to with its effect on the outcome. Lazarus has defined two categories of coping from the cognitive perspective: problem focused and emotion focused [19].

Problem-focused strategies strive for resolving the stressful situation or event or altering the source of the stress. It includes strategies such as:

– Problem solving (managing external aspects of the stressor)

– Seeking information or support in handling the situation (instrumental support)

– Accepting responsibility

– Removing oneself from a stressful situation

Emotion-focused coping represents the efforts to regulate the emotions associated with the situation. It involves strategies as:

– Positive reappraisal

– Distancing

– Escape-avoidance

– Seeking social support

Studies showed that in cases of chronic illnesses, the effects of coping are not influenced by the type of problem, or emotion-focus strategies are used but rather if active or avoidant methods are employed. Moreover, in IBS patients, it seems that the presence or absence of depression and/or anxiety influences how they cope with illness. Maladaptive coping and visceral sensitivity appear to be significantly associated with psychological distress, illness perception directly affecting the maladaptive coping.

Phillips et al. evaluated the role of psychosocial factors in predicting the belonging to IBS group and severity of IBS symptoms [20]. They found that four coping strategies (active coping, instrumental support, self-blame, and positive reframing) were best predictors of IBS.

Coping seems to be a relevant factor in mediating the adverse impact of IBS symptomatology on daily activities. Patients' quality of life could be impaired by the lack of adequate social support and by lower coping abilities acquired through social learning during childhood. Also, the impact of IBS symptoms on HRQOL impairment is mediated by dysfunctional attitudes and avoidant-oriented coping. Inefficient coping strategies represent important treatment targets for cognitive-behavioral therapy (CBT) because coping styles are modulated by the use of cognitive abilities [21].

3. Genes and IBS

As discussed before, IBS is a chronic disease characterized by familial clustering. In the recent years, the hypothesis of a genetic contribution to the development of IBS has gained some support [22].

It was postulated that IBS is a multifactorial, polygenic complex disorder. A candidate gene study evaluates a specific polymorphism or set of polymorphisms. Until now, approximately 60 candidate genes were investigated to determine whether specific genetic variants may be associated with IBS. Until now the data sustaining the genetic hypothesis are scarce, and some results have not been replicated.

Many epidemiological studies reported psychiatric comorbidities, and also reported higher rates of these comorbidities than in the general population. Different pathways could be affected in the subgroup of IBS patients with psychiatric comorbidities. Recent studies tried to evaluate if the IBS and mental disorders share common genetic pathways (primary corticotropin-releasing system and serotoninergic pathway).

Data are sustaining that HPA axis and serotoninergic system are likely to be involved in the genetic susceptibility to major depressive disorder, but currently, there is no clinical evidence for a common gene in IBS and major depression.

Eight genes involved in psychiatric disorders were investigated with mixed results:

1. FKBP5 gene (the gene encoding FK506-binding protein 51) is located on the short arm of chromosome 5; some variants were associated with stress reactivity and post-traumatic stress disorder (PTSD) risk.

2. Catechol-O-methyltransferase (COMT) gene: COMT Val158Met was related to IBS with constipation. The same variant was associated with obsessive-compulsive disorder (OCD), panic disorder (PD), and cognitive performance.

3. Opioid receptor Mu 1 (OPRM1) gene: diseases related to this gene include opioid dependence, pain sensitivity, and social sensitivity. OPRM1 118AG variant was associated with IBS-mixed and IBS-diarrhea (IBS-D).

4. Brain-derived neurotrophic factor (BDNF) gene: psychiatric diseases related to this gene include schizophrenia, anorexia and bulimia nervosa, PTSD, and mood disorders. BDNF Val166Met was associated with IBS with psychiatric comorbidities.

5. Neuropeptide Y (NPY) gene is implicated in stress response

6. Ankyrin repeat and kinase domain containing 1 (ANKK1) gene: it was associated with impulse control disorders and alexithymia.

7. Dopamine receptor D2 (DRD2) gene: it seems to have a role in cocaine dependence.
8. Fatty acid amide hydrolase (FAAH) gene also has a role in substance dependence.

A recent study found preliminary evidence that IBS patients with comorbid anxiety or depression are more likely to present functional variant alleles of serotonin transporters than IBS patients without psychiatric comorbidities.

Maybe the new technological advances in genomic studies will make it possible to identify common and rare variants on genomic deoxyribonucleic acid (DNA) [23]. Until now, based on candidate gene studies, it appears that there may be a different molecular basis for IBS with comorbid anxiety versus IBS without comorbid anxiety. Thus the role of environmental factor contributors to IBS development should not be underestimated.

4. Psychiatric comorbidity in IBS

Many studies reported an increased frequency of psychiatric comorbidities (diagnosis and symptoms) among patients with IBS. It has been estimated that IBS patients have high rates of psychiatric comorbidities (50 %–90 %). There are multiple factors involved in the determination of this comorbidity. The latest disease models of IBS encompass the overlap of brain circuits involved in emotion regulation, autonomic responses, and pain modulation as the most important features.

Clinical reports indicate that the relationship between IBS and psychiatric illnesses is bidirectional between the gastrointestinal tract and the brain, through various pathways (neural, neuroimmune, and neuroendocrine). Among mental disorders, mood disorders, anxiety disorders, and somatoform disorders have been the most frequently diagnosed conditions [24]. The complexity of the underlying pathophysiological processes is not completely understood. The hypothesis linking cognitive and emotional areas in the central nervous system (CNS) with the autonomic nervous system (ANS) and the enteric system (ENS) had a significant contribution to the understanding of the pathogenesis of IBS.

The increased comorbidity among IBS and psychiatric disorders is well established. Even though data refers to patients seen in tertiary gastroenterology centers, recent data pointed out that psychiatric comorbidity is also present in primary care.

Another important aspect that should be emphasized is that the majority of the study results are based on the administration of self-report screening instruments rather than a psychiatric interview. The screening tools only assess the probability of a psychiatric diagnosis, but further investigations are necessary. Moreover, studies of a causal relationship between IBS and psychiatric comorbidities are still limited in number and provide contradictory data.

Some authors argued that the data are applying only to those patients who have sought treatment and are not applicable to the non-consulters. Others suggested that could be a subset of patients with IBS characterized by high psychiatric comorbidity. Nevertheless, there is some evidence supporting the biological association between IBS and mental disorders.

Approximately 50 % of patients with a psychiatric disorder develop the disease before the GI symptoms became manifest, and psychiatric symptoms appear to develop at the same time in a majority of the remaining 50 %.

Many studies pointed out that worry-rumination can influence the brain-gut axis. Moreover, it has been identified as one fundamental factor that mediates the high co-occurrence of the two most frequent psychiatric comorbidities in IBS patients (anxiety and depression) [25].

It is noteworthy that the patients with severe IBS and comorbid psychiatric disorders have been found to have a higher impairment in HRQOL, elevated symptom burden, increased functional disability, and increased health-care costs.

4.1. Mood disorders and IBS

Many studies have investigated the prevalence of depression among IBS patients, but the results are vastly variable, ranging from high to much lower rates. There are also studies showing that patients with major depressive disorders present gastrointestinal symptoms.

Relevant findings from a large-scale population-based study suggest that depression and stress are independent risk factors for IBS. In this study, the incidence rate of IBS was higher in the patients with mild depression than in those with severe depression.

Several authors reported that IBS is associated with suicidality. The findings of one study indicate that 4 % of IBS patients who sought help from primary care, 16 % from secondary care, and 38 % from tertiary care endorsed suicidal ideation determined primary by the gastrointestinal symptoms. A systematic review indicated that IBS patients were two to four times more likely to recognize a history of suicidal behavior, even in the absence of depression.

A study conducted by Guthrie et al. revealed three definite groups of IBS patients [26]:

- Distressed high utilizers: characterized by multiple psychosocial comorbidities, increase levels of health-care utilization, high frequency of sexual abuse, and low pain thresholds to rectal balloon distension; the patients from this group reported suicidal ideation and self-harm history.
- Distressed low utilizers: marked by high psychiatric comorbidity, low physician consultations, low frequency of sexual abuse, and low pain threshold.
- Tolerant low utilizers: characterized by low rates of psychiatric comorbidities, low levels of consultations, and high pain thresholds.

It should be taken into account that an increase in suicidal ideation is not entirely explained by the symptom intensity and the presence of anxiety or depressive comorbidity. Therefore, IBS patients, especially distressed high utilizers, should be assessed for suicidality [27].

4.2. Anxiety disorders and IBS

As mentioned earlier, there is a higher prevalence of anxiety disorders among IBS patients than in the general population (47 % versus 26 %). According to the available literature, the most prevalent anxiety disorders among patients with IBS are generalized anxiety disorder (GAD) and panic disorder (PD). Some studies suggest that mixed IBS (IBS-M) patients are more likely to present higher scores for anxiety, especially in comparison with IBS with constipation (IBS-C) [25].

It must be noted that recent studies suggest that the strong association between GAD morbidity and IBS observed in tertiary centers was not a consequence of increased help-seeking behavior.

PD and IBS share common characteristics such as gastrointestinal symptoms, anticipatory anxiety, and avoidant behavior because of fear of symptoms. Based on results of different studies, it appears that the presence of IBS is associated with greater severity of agoraphobia, anticipatory anxiety, and panic attacks in PD patients. Moreover, patients with IBS reported having high scores of anxiety sensitivity, as the PD patients. Further information on IBS and PD came from a review emphasizing that the experience of feeling uncontrollable somatic symptoms, very common in IBS, could be a stimulating component for PD in patients with subclinical PD symptoms [28].

4.3. Somatoform disorders and IBS

IBS is considered a functional disorder, and it is congruent with the definition of somatoform disorders. The Diagnostic and Statistical Manual for Mental Disorders (DSM-4-TR) and the International Classification of Diseases (ICD) classify physical symptoms that cannot be medically explained together with persistent requests for medical investigations in a separate somatoform category. In the DSM-5 this category was renamed as "somatic symptoms disorder" (SSD) and redefined; there is no longer a demand for lack of "medical" explanation of symptoms. It means that this diagnosis could be a primary diagnosis (somatic symptoms may be medically unexplained) or could be a secondary diagnosis in patients who have an organic illness. The documented prevalence rates of somatoform disorders among IBS patients vary from 15 % to 48 % [29].

5. Neuroimaging in IBS

Studies using structural and functional techniques in IBS patients showed abnormalities that were associated with:

- Visceral hypersensitivity
- Impairment of affective processes involved in visceral pain modulation
- Alteration of descending pain inhibitory pathways

Data obtained from brain imaging studies in IBS demonstrated physiological differences that distinguish patients with IBS from a healthy population. The results obtained have varied maybe because of different study designs or due to the heterogeneity of study populations [30, 31].

5.1. Structural neuroimaging

Nowadays, structural approaches are provided mainly by diffusion tensor imaging (DTI) and by structural magnetic resonance imaging (sMRI). The studies focus on structural connectivity.

IBS patients with chronic pain have regional cortical thickness (CT) alterations in comparison with healthy controls. CT represents the results of neural reorganization of pain circuits and regions associated with sensorial processing.

IBS patients present decreased gray matter density in prefrontal and parietal regions and in emotional circuits. Ellingson et al. demonstrated in a study using DTI that IBS patients have microstructural changes in areas involved in the cortical pain modulatory areas and cortico-thalamic modulation. The anterior insula and basal ganglia (BS) have a prominent role in the integration of sensory and non-sensory information.

Another study demonstrated that IBS patients showed lower cortical thickness (CT) in the interoceptive association cortex (aINS) in the right hemisphere than in healthy controls.

The anterior insular subregion has multiple roles:

- Integration of food-related (olfaction and taste), interoceptive, emotional, and cognitive functions
- Provides output to autonomic and pain modulation systems
- Plays a key role in prediction, error processing, and self-awareness of sensations

In the relationship with these roles, insular regions seem to be involved in psychopathology. As already highlighted, patients with IBS have an abnormal processing of visceral pain in this area as a result of the dysfunctional inhibition of the pain in cortical areas. Patients reporting higher levels of pain intensity associated with their IBS symptoms presented an important CT in the bilateral orbitofrontal cortex (OFC). Also, it was observed that disease duration and pain intensity were correlated with CT in the dorsolateral prefrontal cortex (DLPFC) and OFC, bilaterally.

Other studies reported CT in the anterior midcingulate cortex (aMCC), ventrolateral prefrontal cortex (vlPFC), and thalamus. The structural changes of gray matter density in the periaqueductal gray (PAG) region may be a reflection of the compromised descending modulation of pain.

Blankstein evidenced increased gray matter density in the hypothalamus of the IBS patients.

Depression and anxiety have a well-established role in the modulation of pain. It was suggested that the decreased gray matter density in the anterior/medial thalamus in patients with IBS could be related to the clinical levels of anxiety or depression.

Interestingly, some authors suggested that structural changes in the primary interoceptive cortex, as well as in the attentional and emotional network, could represent endophenotypes of IBS.

5.2. Functional neuroimaging

Functional approaches are provided by single-positron emission computerized tomography (SPECT), positron emission tomography (PET), resting-state magnetic resonance (MRI) and functional magnetic resonance (fMRI), magnetic resonance spectroscopy (MRS), near-infrared spectroscopic imaging (NIRSI), and magnetoencephalography (MEG).

A recent meta-analysis of research on cortical responses to rectal distension suggests the conclusion that brain responses to rectal distension are different in IBS patients and healthy controls. IBS patients showed greater activation in brain regions involved in emotional processing, cognitive modulation, and interoceptive analysis.

Using the functional neuroimaging techniques in IBS patients, it was identified the hyperactivity of the amygdala (an essential component in the emotional arousal network). The amygdala network is involved in processing visceral input in relation to emotional stimuli, modulation of sensorial information, and emotional regulation.

Another area that exhibited functional alteration during experimental pain in IBS patients is represented by the basal ganglia (BG). The data obtained are consistent with the reduction of the dendritic density in cortico-basal ganglia-thalamic-cortical circuits involved in modulation of pain. Moreover, hypersensitive IBS patients present more DLPFC activation than normosensitive patients.

The results obtained in studies using neuroimaging techniques sustain the hypothesis that IBS have a biological substrate, but the same changes could be noticed in other chronic disorders. Furthermore, psychosocial factors (early-life trauma, catastrophizing, anxiety, and depression) have had a substantial impact on the neuroimaging correlations of IBS. An association was noticed (either positive or negative) between the level of psychopathology and neuroimaging findings, thus emphasizing the relevance of psychological factors in IBS determinism [32–34].

6. Neuropsychological findings in IBS

Stress induces changes in HPA axis functioning with neurobiological and cognitive consequences. The brain-gut axis appears to have a major importance of cognitive performance. The psychiatric comorbidity has also impact in the neurocognitive functioning [15, 35].

In general, normal cognitive functioning was reported in IBS, but some researchers demonstrated subtle cognitive deficits that remained after the correction for psychiatric comorbidity.

6.1. Attention and IBS

Attention is a behavioral and cognitive process involving the selection of sensory information to optimize current behavioral responses to specific stimuli relevant for the organism.

Researchers suggest that IBS patients have specific abnormalities in attentional network functioning. IBS patients present attentional biases for pain words. Attentional alterations are associated with increased pain report and illness behavior.

6.2. Memory and IBS

Currently, there are data suggesting impairment in visuospatial memory in patients with IBS. The researchers found that IBS patients displayed poorer performance in hippocampal-mediated visuospatial tasks than non-IBS controls. They made twice to three times as many errors on the visuospatial test as the healthy control group. It was suggested that visuospatial memory dysfunction could represent a common component of IBS [36].

6.3. Executive function and IBS

Cognitive flexibility in IBS patients was evaluated with Wisconsin Card Sorting Test (WCST). Recent researches have shown that IBS patients present latent impairments in the cognitive flexibility. The biological substrate for those findings seems to be the modified activity of the DLPFC, hippocampus, and insula. Also, the altered connectivity between the DLPFC and pre-supplementary motor area appears to be involved [37].

7. Psychopharmacology of IBS

Treatment of IBS could be classified in pharmacologic and non-pharmacological strategies. The choice of therapy depends on types of symptoms and their severity and frequency. It is clear that many aspects of IBS may be linked to psychosocial stressors and psychiatric comorbidities. More recent research emphasized that the psychotropic drugs can play a major role in the treatment of IBS patients [38].

7.1. Antidepressants

IBS is characterized by abnormalities in visceral sensations and dysregulation of central pain perception. Thus, the antidepressants represent a treatment option in patients with moderate and severe symptoms. The antidepressants were found to be efficacious for abdominal pain but have no effect on bowel habit. Moreover, their tolerance may represent a problem. Currently, antidepressants are used as a second-line therapy. The beneficial effects of antidepressants could be the results of influence in central pain threshold (an increase of threshold). Other mechanisms of action are represented by the anticholinergic effects (influence on gastrointestinal motility and secretion) and by reducing the pain sensitivity of peripheral nerves [39].

7.1.1. Tricyclics antidepressants (TCA)

Most recent research supports the use of TCAs in IBS treatment. The effects of several TCAs including clomipramine, nortriptyline, and imipramine were investigated in IBS patients. The results showed that the required dose of TCAs is lower than that used to treat patients with depression. TCAs are effective in IBS-D due to the prolongment of whole-gut transit times. A systematic review of 11 randomized controlled trials RCTs comparing TCAs and placebo revealed that the benefit attributable to TCA therapy relative to placebo was 12.5 %. The numbers needed to treat (NNT) were four, equal or superior to other pharmacological agents (like motility agents and probiotics). The TCAs slow gut-transit time and could be used in diarrhea-predominant IBS.

7.1.2. Selective serotonin reuptake inhibitors (SSRIs)

Efficacy of SSRIs in the treatment of IBS was evaluated in seven randomized trials comparing SSRIs with placebo. The SSRIs studied were fluoxetine, paroxetine, and citalopram. One small open trial demonstrated the efficacy of paroxetine on abdominal pain. A common limitation of all the studies is represented by the short duration of the study (12 weeks) and the small sample size. The relative risks (RR) in the treatment of IBS symptoms were 0.62, but significant heterogeneity characterized the studies. The SSRIs decrease orocecal transit and would be of greater benefit in constipation-predominant IBS. According to Cochrane database of systematic reviews, SSRIs are prescribed at dosages standard for treating psychiatric disorders and should be used as a third-line treatment.

7.1.3. Serotonin-noradrenaline reuptake inhibitors (SNRIs)

Both serotonin and norepinephrine have a role in visceral motility and visceral sensation. It was noticed that low-dose SNRIs (duloxetine and venlafaxine) seem to be more efficacious than SSRIs. One study performed on healthy volunteers showed that venlafaxine reduced pain sensation ratings in response to grade distensions but did not have a significant impact on the colonic transit. SNRIs are promising, but more studies need to be done.

7.2. Atypical antipsychotics

Quetiapine may help patients with IBS by decreasing the anxiety and ameliorating sleep disturbances. It also augments the effect of antidepressants and provides an independent analgesic effect [40].

7.3. Anticonvulsants

Preliminary data from animal models provides evidence suggesting that the γ-aminobutyric acidergic (GABA) agents (gabapentin) and $\alpha 2\delta$ ligand (pregabalin) may also be efficient in reducing central sensitization in hyperalgesia [41]. Gabapentin has more recently been used in the treatment of chronic pain. Pregabalin has been shown to be more potent than gabapentin. In patients with IBS, both gabapentin and pregabalin have been shown to reduce rectal sensitivity to balloon distension, but currently, there are no results published from clinical trials examining the efficacy of $\alpha 2\delta$ ligands on symptoms in IBS patients.

7.4. Anxiolytic agents

The rationale for the use of anxiolytic drugs for the treatment of IBS likely came from the observation that the majority of patients also present of comorbid anxiety. Buspirone, an azapirone, is an anti-anxiolytic nonbenzodiazepine drug. It is a partial serotonin 1A (5-HT1A) receptor agonist used to augment the effects of antidepressants. The effects on gastrointestinal motility are represented by the reduction of funding tone and the delay of emptying. Also, a relaxation effect on the rectal tone was observed [42].

8. Conclusions

There is a general agreement that a global assessment of IBS patient should be done. The significant overlap between IBS and mental disorders should encourage the clinicians to evaluate for comorbid psychiatric disorders routinely. It is very important to recognize the linkage between psychiatric diagnoses and IBS because these comorbid conditions are characterized by increased symptom burden and additive functional impairment. Thus, successful management of patients with IBS requires careful attention to all psychosocial factors involved.

Author details

Mihaela Fadgyas Stanculete[1,2*]

Address all correspondence to: mihaelastanculete@yahoo.com

1 Department of Neurosciences, Discipline of Psychiatry and Pediatric Psychiatry, University of Medicine and Pharmacy "Iuliu Hațieganu", Cluj-Napoca, Romania

2 Second Psychiatric Clinic, Emergency County Hospital Cluj, Cluj-Napoca, Romania

References

[1] Tanaka Y, Kanazawa M, Fukudo S, Drossman DA. Biopsychosocial model of irritable bowel syndrome. J Neurogastroenterol Motil. 2011;2:131–9. DOI: 10.5056/jnm.2011.17.2.131

[2] Levy RL, Whitehead WE, Walker LS, Von Korff M, Feld AD, et al. Increased somatic complaints and health-care utilization in children: effects of parent IBS status and parent response to gastrointestinal symptoms. Am J Gastroenterol. 2004;99(12):2442–51. DOI: 10.1111/j.1572-0241.2004.40478.x

[3] Van Oudenhove L, Levy RL, Crowell MD, Drossman DA, Halpert AD, Keefer L, Lackner JM, Murphy TB, Naliboff BD. Biopsychosocial aspects of functional gastrointestinal disorders: how central and environmental processes contribute to the development and expression of functional gastrointestinal disorders. Gastroenterology. 2016;150(6):1355–67. DOI: http://dx.doi.org/10.1053/j.gastro.2016.02.027

[4] Vervoort T, Huguet A, Verhoeven K, Goubert L. Mothers' and fathers' responses to their child's pain moderate the relationship between the child's pain catastrophizing and disability. PAIN®. 2011;152(4):786–93. DOI: 10.1016/j.pain.2010.12.010

[5] Van Tilburg MA, Levy RL, Walker LS, Von Korff M, Feld LD, Garner M, Feld AD, Whitehead WE. Psychosocial mechanisms for the transmission of somatic symptoms from parents to children. WJG. 2015;21(18):5532. DOI: 10.3748/wjg.v21.i18.5532.

[6] Bradford K, Shih W, Videlock EJ, Presson AP, Naliboff BD, Mayer EA, Chang L. Association between early adverse life events and irritable bowel syndrome. Clin Gastroenterol Hepatol. 2012;10(4):385–90. DOI: 10.1016/j.cgh.2011.12.018

[7] Drossman DA. Abuse, trauma, and GI illness: is there a link?. Am J Gastroenterol. 2011;106(1):14–25. DOI: 10.1038/ajg.2010.453

[8] Chitkara DK, van Tilburg MA, Blois-Martin N, Whitehead WE. Early life risk factors that contribute to irritable bowel syndrome in adults: a systematic review. Am J Gastroenterol. 2008;103(3):765–74. DOI: 10.1111/j.1572-0241.2007.01722.x

[9] O'Mahony SM, Hyland NP, Dinan TG, Cryan JF. Maternal separation as a model of brain–gut axis dysfunction. Psychopharmacology. 2011;214(1):71–88. DOI: 10.1007/s00213-010-2010-9

[10] Moloney RD, Johnson AC, O'Mahony SM, Dinan TG, Meerveld GV, Cryan JF. Stress and the microbiota–gut–brain axis in visceral pain: relevance to irritable bowel syndrome. CNS Neurosci Ther. 2016;22(2):102–17. DOI: 10.1111/cns.12490

[11] Vanuytsel T, van Wanrooy S, Vanheel H, Vanormelingen C, Verschueren S, Houben E, Rasoel SS, Tóth J, Holvoet L, Farré R, Van Oudenhove L. Psychological stress and corticotropin-releasing hormone increase intestinal permeability in humans by a mast cell-dependent mechanism. Gut. 2014;63(8):1293–9. DOI: 10.1136/gutjnl-2013-305690

[12] Van Oudenhove L, Aziz Q. Recent insights on central processing and psychological processes in functional gastrointestinal disorders. Dig Liv Dis. 2009;41(11):781–7. DOI: 10.1016/j.dld.2009.07.004

[13] Lackner JM, Brasel AM, Quigley BM, Keefer L, Krasner SS, Powell C, Katz LA, Sitrin MD. The ties that bind: perceived social support, stress, and IBS in severely affected patients. Neurogastroenterol Motil. 2010;22(8):893–900. DOI: 10.1111/j.1365-2982.2010.01516.x

[14] Jerndal P, Ringström G, Agerforz P, Karpefors M, Akkermans LM, Bayati A, Simrén M. Gastrointestinal-specific anxiety: an important factor for severity of GI symptoms and

quality of life in IBS. Neurogastroenterol Motil. 2010;22(6):646-e179. DOI: 10.1111/j.1365-2982.2010.01493

[15] Kennedy PJ, Clarke G, Quigley EM, Groeger JA, Dinan TG, Cryan JF. Gut memories: towards a cognitive neurobiology of irritable bowel syndrome. Neurosci Biobehav Rev. 2012;36(1):310–40. DOI: 10.1016/j.neubiorev.2011.07.001

[16] Hunt MG, Milonova M, Moshier S. Catastrophizing the consequences of gastrointestinal symptoms in irritable bowel syndrome. J Cogn Psychother. 2009;23(2):160–73. DOI: 10.1891/0889-8391.23.2.160

[17] Porcelli P, De Carne M, Leandro G. Alexithymia and gastrointestinal-specific anxiety in moderate to severe irritable bowel syndrome. Compr Psych. 2014;55(7):1647–53. DOI: 10.1016/j.comppsych.2014.05.022

[18] Fadgyas Stănculete M, Pojoga C, Dumitrascu DL. Experience of anger in patients with irritable bowel syndrome in Romania. Clujul Medical. 2014;87(2):98. DOI: 10.15386/cjmed-290

[19] Lazarus RS. Coping theory and research: past, present, and future. Psychosom Med. 1993;55(3):234–47.

[20] Phillips K, Wright BJ, Kent S. Psychosocial predictors of irritable bowel syndrome diagnosis and symptom severity. J Psychosom Res. 2013;75(5):467–74. DOI: 10.1016/j.jpsychores.2013.08.002.

[21] Grodzinsky E, Walter S, Viktorsson L, Carlsson AK, Jones MP, Faresjö Å. More negative self-esteem and inferior coping strategies among patients diagnosed with IBS compared with patients without IBS-a case–control study in primary care. BMC Fam Pract. 2015;16(1):1. DOI: 10.1186/s12875-015-0225-x

[22] Saito YA. The role of genetics in IBS. Gastroenterol Clin North Am. 2011;40(1):45–67. DOI: 10.1016/j.gtc.2010.12.011

[23] Henström M, D'Amato M. Genetics of irritable bowel syndrome. Mol Cell Pediatr. 2016;3(1):1. DOI: 10.1186/s40348-016-0038-6

[24] Garakani A, Win T, Virk S, Gupta S, Kaplan D, Masand PS. Comorbidity of irritable bowel syndrome in psychiatric patients: a review. Am J Ther. 2003;10(1):61–7. DOI: 10.1097/00045391-200301000-00014

[25] Fond G, Loundou A, Hamdani N, Boukouaci W, Dargel A, Oliveira J, Roger M, Tamouza R, Leboyer M, Boyer L. Anxiety and depression comorbidities in irritable bowel syndrome (IBS): a systematic review and meta-analysis. Eur Arch Psychiatry Clin Neurosci. 2014;264(8):651–60. DOI: 10.1007/s00406-014-0502-z

[26] Guthrie E, Barlow J, Fernandes L, Ratcliffe J, Read N, Thompson DG, Tomenson B, Creed F, North of England IBS Research Group. Changes in tolerance to rectal distension correlate with changes in psychological state in patients with severe

irritable bowel syndrome. Psychosom Med. 2004;66(4):578–82. DOI: 10.1097/01.psy.0000128899.22514.c0

[27] Spiegel BM. The burden of IBS: looking at metrics. Curr Gastroenterol Rep. 2009;11(4):265–9. DOI: 10.1007/s11894-009-0039-x

[28] Hausteiner-Wiehle C, Henningsen P. Irritable bowel syndrome: relations with functional, mental, and somatoform disorders. World J Gastroenterol WJG. 2014;20(20):6024–30. DOI: 10.3748/wjg.v20.i20.60240.6024

[29] Wouters MM, Boeckxstaens GE. Is there a causal link between psychological disorders and functional gastrointestinal disorders?. Expert Rev Gastroenterol Hepatol. 2016;10(1):5–8. DOI: 10.1586/17474124.2016.1109446

[30] Weaver KR, Sherwin LB, Walitt B, Melkus GD, Henderson WA. Neuroimaging the brain-gut axis in patients with irritable bowel syndrome. WJGPT. 2016;7(2):320–33. DOI: 10.4292/WJGPT.v7.i2.320

[31] Beauregard M. Mind does really matter: evidence from neuroimaging studies of emotional self-regulation, psychotherapy, and placebo effect. Prog Neurobiol. 2007;81(4):218–36.DOI: 10.1016/j.pneurobio.2007.01.005

[32] Mayer EA, Labus JS, Tillisch K, Cole SW, Baldi P. Towards a systems view of IBS. Nat Rev Gastroenterol Hepatol. 2015;12(10):592–605. DOI: 10.1038/nrgastro.2015.121

[33] Ma X, Li S, Tian J, Jiang G, Wen H, Wang T, Fang J, Zhan W, Xu Y. Altered brain spontaneous activity and connectivity network in irritable bowel syndrome patients: a resting-state fMRI study. Clin Neurophysiol. 2015;126(6):1190–7. DOI: 10.1016/j.clinph.2014.10.004

[34] Blankstein U, Chen J, Diamant NE, Davis KD. Altered brain structure in irritable bowel syndrome: potential contributions of pre-existing and disease-driven factors. Gastroenterology. 2010;138(5):1783–9. DOI: 10.1053/j.gastro.2009.12.043

[35] Attree EA, Dancey CP, Keeling D, Wilson C. Cognitive function in people with chronic illness: inflammatory bowel disease and irritable bowel syndrome. Appl Neuropsychol. 2003;10(2):96–104. DOI: 10.1207/S15324826AN1002_05

[36] Kennedy PJ, Clarke G, O'Neill A, Groeger JA, Quigley EM, Shanahan F, Cryan JF, Dinan TG. Cognitive performance in irritable bowel syndrome: evidence of a stress-related impairment in visuospatial memory. Psychol Med. 2014;44(07):1553–66. DOI: 10.1017/S0033291713002171

[37] Aizawa E, Sato Y, Kochiyama T, Saito N, Izumiyama M, Morishita J, Kanazawa M, Shima K, Mushiake H, Hongo M, Fukudo S. Altered cognitive function of prefrontal cortex during error feedback in patients with irritable bowel syndrome, based on FMRI

and dynamic causal modeling. Gastroenterology. 2012;143(5):1188–98. DOI: 10.1053/j.gastro.2012.07.104

[38] Sinagra E, Romano C, Cottone M. Psychopharmacological treatment and psychological interventions in irritable bowel syndrome. Gastroenterol Res Pract. 2012;2012:486067. DOI: 10.1155/2012/486067

[39] Ruepert L, Quartero AO, de Wit NJ, van der Heijden GJ, Rubin G, Muris JW. Bulking agents, antispasmodics and antidepressants for the treatment of irritable bowel syndrome. Cochrane Datbase Syst Rev. 2011. DOI: 10.1002/14651858.CD003460.pub3

[40] Halland M, Talley NJ. New treatments for IBS. Nat Rev Gastroenterol Hepatol. 2013;10(1):13–23. DOI: 10.1038/nrgastro.2012.207

[41] Lee KJ, Kim JH, Cho SW. Gabapentin reduces rectal mechanosensitivity and increases rectal compliance in patients with diarrhoea-predominant irritable bowel syndrome. Aliment Pharmacol Ther. 2005;22(10):981–8. DOI: 10.1111/j.1365-2036.2005.02685.x

[42] O'Mahony S, Chua AS, Quigley EM, Clarke G, Shanahan F, Keeling PW, Dinan TG. Evidence of an enhanced central 5HT response in irritable bowel syndrome and in the rat maternal separation model. Neurogastroenterol Motil. 2008;20(6):680–8. DOI: 10.1111/j.1365-2982.2007.01065.x

3

Portal Hypertensive Gastropathy (PHG)

Samia Ali Gamie

Abstract

Reversal of erosive gastritis in patients with portal hypertension by surgical shunts evolves the term of portal hypertensive gastropathy. In 1984, Sarfeh et al. addressed the term PHG to describe the distinctive erosive gastritis in patients with portal hypertension. Since that time, the recorded incidence of PHG in the studies has varied widely from 20 to 75% in patients with portal hypertension, with or without liver cirrhosis. As the underlying pathophysiology of the disease is unclear, not all the patients with portal hypertension developed PHG. Thus, portal hypertension cannot be the only factor for the development of PHG. Patients with PHG presented with either acute or chronic bleedings. Acute presentation is an emergency case. Anemia from chronic bleeding is a frequent presentation in PHG patients. The diagnosis is confirmed by a characteristic endoscopic appearance of PHG. Capsule endoscopy and dynamic CT are also used for the diagnosis of PHG. The goal of the treatment of PHG is reducing the portal pressure in patients with acute or chronic bleeding. Pharmacological treatment, endoscopic therapy, trans-jugular intrahepatic portosystemic shunt (TIPS), and shunt surgery are different modalities for treatment of PHG. Yet, primary prophylaxis treatment is not recommended in the patients with PHG.

Keywords: portal hypertensive gastropathy, portal hypertension, gastropathy, GAVE, liver cirrhosis

1. Introduction

1.1. Definition

Portal hypertensive gastropathy (PHG) is a painless condition of gastric mucosal ectasia and impaired mucosal defense, typically seen in patients with portal hypertension [1].

Portal hypertension (PH) exists when the hydrostatic pressure in the portal vein or its branches has increased. Two important factors are implicated; vascular resistance and blood flow, thus if the pressure gradient anywhere along the portal venous system (between the portal vein, and hepatic veins or the inferior vena cava (IVC)) is increased, portal hypertension develops.

The normal portal venous pressure ranges from 5 to 10 mm Hg, therefore, if the hepatic venous pressure gradient (HVPG) is ≥10 mm Hg, significant portal hypertension is considered, but if the HVPG is ≥12 mm Hg, severe portal hypertension is diagnosed [2].

The causes of portal hypertension are classified into three categories related to anatomical consideration. First, are causes originating in the portal venous system before it reaches the liver (pre-hepatic), e.g. portal vein thrombosis, schistosomiasis, primary biliary cholangitis/primary sclerosing cholangitis, or congenital hepatic fibrosis. Second, are causes within the liver (intrahepatic) e.g. cirrhosis as a result of viral, non alcoholic fatty liver disease (NAFLD), or autoimmune. Finally, are causes between the liver and the heart (post-hepatic) e.g. Budd-Chiari syndrome, inferior vena cava obstruction, or hepatic veno-occlusive disease (**Table 1**). The most common cause of PH is cirrhosis [3].

1.2. Essentials to diagnose PHG

- Portal hypertension with or without cirrhosis.
- Characteristic endoscopic findings.

Prehepatic	Hepatic	Posthepatic
Portal vein thrombosis	Cirrhosis of any cause, e.g. chronic viral hepatitis, alcoholic, autoimmune, NAFLD, biliary atresia, etc.	Inferior vena cava obstruction
Arteriovenous fistula	Primary biliary cholangitis	Hepatic vein thrombosis
Splenomegaly	Primary sclerosing cholangitis	Budd-Chiari syndrome
	Schistosomiasis	Right sided heart failure, e.g. from constrictive pericarditis
	Congenital hepatic fibrosis	
	Nodular regeneration hyperplasia	
	Granulomatous or infiltrative diseases (Gaucher, sarcoidosis, amyloid deposition	
	Toxicity (from arsenic, copper, methotrexate, amiodarone, ...)	
	Veno-occlusive disease	

NAFLD, non alcoholic fatty liver disease.

Table 1. Condition associated with portal hypertension.

2. History

In 1984, Sarfeh et al. recognized a distinct form of gastric mucosal hemorrhage in patients who had portal hypertension, they called it "portal hypertensive gastritis". They reported that this mucosal lesion in patients with portal hypertension was reversed after the portacaval shunt, in contrary to the mucosal lesion of patients without portal hypertension. Therefore, they concluded that there is a unique mucosal change excited with portal hypertension. 1 year later, it was discovered that this mucosal change was not a form of gastritis as there is no evidence of inflammation in the mucosa. Specific histopathological findings described this change, and the term "portal hypertensive gastropathy" was introduced by McCormack et al. in 1985 as a separate entity. However, there was no grading system of the endoscopic findings to put an accurate score for this condition. Several grading systems like the three- category system, and the two-category system have been proposed in 1994. The clinical importance of grading classification system resides in the fact that patients with severe PHG have a higher chance to bleed than patients with mild PHG [4].

The overall mortality from gastrointestinal bleeding is up to 25% of the mortality in patients with cirrhosis. In recent years however, PHG has been recognized as a distinct entity of gastrointestinal bleeding in patients with cirrhosis and portal hypertension. While variceal hemorrhage and peptic ulcer disease are known as significant causes of GI bleeding in cirrhosis, PHG and gastric antral vascular ectasia (GAVE) should also be considered as important causes. However, PHG should be differentiated from GAVE, GAVE occurs in patients with cirrhosis and portal hypertension, in addition to other conditions, such as chronic renal failure, connective tissue disorders, and bone marrow transplantation. On the other hand, PHG occurs only in patients with portal hypertension, whether with or without cirrhosis. In patients with cirrhosis, PHG is more common than GAVE [5].

However, although the endoscopic, histological and hemodynamic features of PHG mucosa have been extensively studied, the pathogenesis of PHG is still poorly understood, its natural history is not clearly documented and its treatment needs to be improved [6].

3. Epidemiology

The incidence of PHG varies greatly, it ranges between 20 and 75% of patients with portal hypertension, of those, approximately 65–90% have mild PHG, whereas 10–25% have severe PHG. This wide discrepancy in results may be attributed to the fact that the study was carried out on different groups of patients; patients with cirrhosis, patients without cirrhosis, patients with different Child-Pugh score of liver failure, and lastly patients with history of previous esophageal eradication therapy [7]. It was noticed that higher prevalence of PHG is found in patients with severe portal hypertension, advanced liver disease, and post-eradication therapy of esophageal varices [8]. Conversely, the incidence of acute gastrointestinal bleeding (hematemesis and/or melena) in PHG patients with cirrhosis were low; reported incidences ranged from 2.5 to 30%, with the greatest occurrences being observed in patients with severe PHG [9].

On the other hand, PHG as a marker of portal hypertension has conflicting results among the studies. Its sensitivity, positive predictive value (PPV) and negative predictive value (NPV), vary considerably between the studies, but its specificity has been reported to be above 95%. Snake-skin pattern has higher specificity (93–100%) for the diagnosis of PHG [10].

PHG can present at any age, including pediatric or adult patients [7].

4. Pathophysiology

The pathogenesis of PHG is still poorly understood. Portal hypertension is essential in the presence of PHG, due to the mechanical effect of the increased pressure in the portal vein which leads to hyper-dynamic congestion with a net increase in the gastric blood flow, this increase occurs in the submucosal, muscle, and serosal layers, while decreasing in the mucosal layer due to congestion and stasis. These hemodynamic changes impair gastric mucosal defense mechanisms, which lead to release of pro-inflammatory mediators, and alter the growth factors which render gastric mucosa more susceptible to injury, and impair mucosal healing. This defenseless mucosa may explain the increase in the rate of bleeding from PHG, additionally this abnormal gastric microcirculation, may render gastric mucosa more vulnerable to hypoxia, and more susceptible to noxious gastric factors, such as aspirin and ethanol [4].

Many other factors have also been implicated in the pathogenesis of PHG such as increased production of nitric oxide (NO), oxygen free radicals, endothelin-1, tumor necrosis factor-α, and prostaglandins. The most important factor, NO, is a potent vasodilator secreted by endothelial cells which may underlie the gastric vascular dilation and hyper-dynamic circulation in PHG. Furthermore, the expression of transforming growth factor α (TGF-α) and the epidermal growth factor (EGF) receptors in the gastric mucosa were reported to be highly elevated in areas of spontaneous gastric injury. Recently, studies found other factors, like p53-upregulated modulator of apoptosis (PUMA), to be markedly induced in the gastric mucosa of PHG patients [11]. Increased gastric mucosal apoptosis and decreased mucosal proliferation, were also noted in rats with PGH.

5. Factors influencing the development of portal hypertensive gastropathy

Many factors related to portal hypertension affect the presence and the severity of PHG. As the commonest cause of portal hypertension is liver cirrhosis, the presence or absence of cirrhosis, and its severity, may also affect the PHG.

5.1. Factors related to portal hypertension

- **Severity of portal hypertension:** The frequency of PHG is strongly correlated with the severity of portal hypertension, as indicated by hepatic venous pressure gradient (HVPG), esophageal intra-variceal pressure, and/or presence of esophageal varices and its size [12]. It was also found that portal hypertension associates with severe PHG, but not mild PHG, this was evident in patients with severe PHG, which were discovered to have elevated HVPG, high hepatic sinusoidal resistance, and low hepatic blood flow, all markers of severe portal hypertension [12].

This leads us to the conclusion that not all patients with portal hypertension exhibit evidence of, or develop PHG. On the other hand, resolution of PHG, which occurs after intervention to decrease portal hypertension (by pharmacotherapy, trans-jugular intrahepatic portosystemic shunt (TIPS), or liver transplantation), may suggest an association between PHG and portal hypertension [13].

Thus, although PHG cannot be diagnosed without portal hypertension, it is however not the only factor that evokes PHG.

- **Correlation with varices**: Severe PHG is more common in patients with esophageal varices than patients without varices. It also, correlated positively with the size of varices; denoting, it was higher in those with large varices than in those with medium-sized or small varices [12].
- **Location of varices:** PHG was more commonly seen in patients with coexisting gastric and esophageal varices than in patients with only esophageal varices. Additionally, moderate or severe PHG was noted to be higher (not to a significant level) in patients with common collateral circulation *vs* uncommon collaterals. Portosystemic common collateral circulation includes esophageal varices, gastric varices, and vein dilatation (whether abdominal, umbilical, or hemorrhoid), while uncommon collaterals include splenorenal, gastric, renal, retroperitoneal, or cardiac angle venous shunts [14].
- **Portal vein diameter:** It was proposed that PHG is promoted by minimal collateral circulation since significant collaterals would otherwise reduce portal hypertension and gastric mucosal congestion. Later on, it was found that portal vein diameter in cirrhotic patients with PHG and no esophageal varices is greater than the portal vein diameter in patients with esophageal varices. This concept was further supported by the finding that patients with portal vein diameter < 12 mm have a significantly higher prevalence of esophageal varices than patients with larger portal vein diameter. It was then believed that the absence of reversed blood flow in the portal vein (due to the absence of hepatofugal flow), in patients without esophageal varices, meant that the pressure in the portal vein was not affected [15].
- **Esophageal variceal eradication:** PHG may appear for the first time in patients with portal hypertension, or increase in severity in patients with pre-exciting PHG after eradication of esophageal varices by either endoscopic variceal ligation or endoscopic variceal sclerotherapy [16], thus patients with well developed fundal varices are more liable to develop PHG after obliteration of the varices than patients with poorly developed fundal varices. Since fundal varices are usually formed by a gastro-renal shunt, this finding supports the view that the presence of a gastro-renal shunt may play a protective role in the development of PHG after variceal obliteration. Therefore; some patients may exhibit minimum or no change in PHG after esophageal eradication [17].

Other techniques are also used for obliteration of the esophageal varices including angiographic variceal obliteration (which increases the PHG frequency), and percutaneous transhepatic variceal embolization; after which 38% of the patients develop *De-novo* PHG. The development of PHG for the first time or its increase in frequency and/or its severity is attributed to increased gastric mucosal congestion due to a decrease in the blood flow in the esophageal varices, which leads to an increase in the portal blood flow.

This phenomenon can be explained by obliteration of the blood flow after eradication of esophageal varices, this can lead to increased portal pressure and redistribution of residual blood flow that had passed through the previously patent varices. This mechanism is supported by the finding that gastric mucosal blood flow increases after variceal ligation [4].

Some investigators believe that the higher rate of PHG in patients undergoing endoscopic variceal eradication (sclerotherapy or banding) merely reflects other factors rather than the procedures *per se,* factors like; increased duration of portal hypertension, advanced liver disease, or severe portal hypertension in patients selected to undergo variceal eradication, must be evaluated in patients who developed PHG or showed an increase in its severity [18]. Nevertheless, higher frequency of PHG in patients undergoing sclerotherapy, suggest that portal hypertension is still the main underlying cause of PHG

5.2. Factors related to liver cirrhosis

- **Cirrhotic vs non-cirrhotic portal hypertension:** Primary liver disease usually occurs in PHG, but is not essential for PHG, provided another cause of portal hypertension exists. Consequently, PHG can occur in patients with other causes of portal hypertension; non-cirrhotic portal fibrosis, pre-hepatic or post-hepatic portal hypertension [19].

  Portal pressure is not the only factor that is determinant of PHG, other factors, like cirrhosis, may be implicated in the development of the mucosal lesions, which are characteristic of PHG. PHG was found to occur more commonly in patients with cirrhotic liver than in non-cirrhotic portal hypertension patients, also the patients with cirrhosis have a more aggressive course of PHG with faster progression to more severe PHG as time advances [19].

Taking this in consideration, other factors may also be involved in the pathogenesis of PHG. For example, in patients with portal hypertension and cirrhosis, there is an increase in the level of many vasodilator substances in systemic circulation e.g. gastrin, secretin, and VIP, this increase in the level of vasodilator or the decrease in the sensitivity to vasoconstrictor substance may have a role in the underlying mechanism of PHG [10]. However, these changes were also found in cirrhotic patients not suffering from PHG, thus the exact picture of the pathogenesis is not yet fully understood.

- **Duration of liver disease:** The duration of liver disease positively correlates with development of PHG, with average cumulative incidence of 3% at 1 year, 10% at 2 years, and 24% at 3 years [7].

- **Liver disease severity:** PHG is correlated with liver disease severity, as measured by Child-Turcotte-Pugh score (CTP score) (**Table 2**), Child-Pugh stage C cirrhosis is associated with more frequent and faster progression of PHG. Also, it was found that cirrhotic patients with severe PHG (especially those without esophageal varices) had more frequent CTP stage C than patients with mild PHG [7].

Model for end-stage liver disease (MELD) is another important scoring system for assessing liver disease severity, which was found to significantly correlate with PHG severity [20].

On the other hand, the severity of PHG was correlated to markers of advanced liver disease (like hypoalbuminemia and hyperbilirubinemia) which are biochemical markers of advanced liver disease. Markers of portal hypertension (thrombocytopenia) and of insulin resistance (hyperglycemia), were also significant independent predictors of PHG [21].

5.3. Other factors

Many other factors may be involved in the pathogenesis of PHG, this includes thrombocytopenia or splenomegaly which are associated with the severity of PHG. Additional factors like an increase in the thickness of the lesser omentum and the presence of a splenorenal shunt were found to correlate with PHG in patients with chronic liver disease [22].

5.3.1. Factors that do not affect the risk of PHG

Although, portal hypertension is essential for PHG diagnosis, there is still no association between the etiology of portal hypertension and PHG. Similarly, as cirrhosis is the common cause of portal hypertension, there is no correlation between the underlying causes of cirrhosis and PHG. Moreover, in cirrhotic patients, the role of Helicobacter pylori (H. pylori) in the pathogenesis of PHG is not fully understood. Some contributed that Helicobacter has no role in the pathogenesis of PHG in these patients [23]. However, there is evidence of association between H. pylori infection and PHG in cirrhotic patients, in these patients, Helicobacter infection may be related to the severity of PHG. This was strengthened by the fact that there was mild improvement of PHG after H. pylori eradication. Therefore, we can conclude that there may be a minor role for H. pylori in the pathogenesis of PHG in cirrhotic patients [23]. Further studies on large number of patients are conducted to show the effect of H. pylori eradication in the treatment of PHG, especially severe portal gastropathy in cirrhosis.

Parameter	Point assigned		
	1	2	3
Albumin (g/dl)	>3.5	2.8–3.5	<2.8
Bilirubin (mg/dl)	<2	2–3	>3
INR	<1.7	1.7–2.3	>2.3
Ascites	None	Slight-moderate	Tense
Encephalopathy	0	1–2	3–4

A total Child-Turcotte-Pugh score of 5–6 considered class A, 7–9 is class B, and 10– 15 is class C. INR, international normalized ratio.

Table 2. Child-Turcotte-Pugh score.

Also, there is no evidence that there is any increase in the prevalence or severity of PHG with the use of either nonsteroidal anti-inflammatory drugs (NSAIDs), or COX-(cyclooxygenase)-2 inhibitor [24]. Another negative correlation was found between alcohol and smoking alongside PHG, thus there is no benefit from abstinence or quitting smoking [25]. Likewise, the presence of PHG was independent of patient's age, or sex.

6. Whom should go for screening for PHG

Patients with portal hypertension and chronic iron deficiency anemia who are suspected to have chronic bleeding should go for PHG screening. Chronic bleeding is diagnosed when there is either decrease in hemoglobin level below 2 g/dL within 6-month, or if there is presence of iron deficiency anemia with a positive fecal occult blood test. For those patients, upper endoscopy can confirm the diagnosis of PHG [26].

7. Natural history

PHG may change in an individual patient over time, about 30% of the patients with cirrhosis and mild PHG, progress to severe PHG during a 10 year follow up period, considering that these patients did not receive any prophylactic treatment. Most of the patients with worsening PHG, severe lesions, or *de novo* PHG develop bleeding. There are only a few improved cases in PHG without treatment [27]. Furthermore, Patients who have PHG associated with cirrhosis-related portal hypertension have more frequently persistent and progressive PHG, which is more likely to bleed than patients with PHG related to non-cirrhotic portal hypertension [9].

Although, as mentioned above, patients with previous endoscopic therapy (sclerotherapy or endoscopic variceal ligation) have a higher prevalence of PHG, the clinical course of PHG in this context, particularly in non cirrhotic portal hypertension, may be milder and transient [28].

PHG is a dynamic condition emphasized by the observation that 30% of patients who have endoscopic features of PHG remained unchanged throughout follow-up period, whereas 25% of patients show either worsening or improvement of the condition during the follow up period. Thus, not only can PHG appear for the first time or progress from mild to severe condition over time, but it can also revert from severe to mild, and even disappear completely with treatment [23].

8. Clinical picture

Most patients with PHG are asymptomatic, but a significant number of patients exhibit symptoms related to iron deficiency anemia from chronic GI bleeding. Bleeding from PHG may be either chronic occult blood in the stool, or overt which occurs in a smaller proportion of patients. Endoscopic diagnosis of acute hemorrhage from PHG is established when there is active bleeding from gastropathy lesions, if non-removable clots overlying these lesions is observed, or when there is PHG and no other cause of acute bleeding can be demonstrated after thorough evaluation of the gastrointestinal tract [9]. Recurrent bleeding is common in PHG after the initial episode.

Although all PHG patients with chronic bleeding develop severe chronic iron deficiency anemia, no study has evaluated the prevalence of PHG in cirrhotic patients with chronic iron deficiency anemia. In patients with portal hypertension, with or without cirrhosis and chronic iron deficiency anemia, chronic bleeding from PHG must be suspected, its diagnosis is confirmed by upper endoscopy. Comprehensive study of the whole gastrointestinal tract in these patients by capsule endoscopy is mandatory to exclude similar lesion elsewhere along gastrointestinal tract e.g. colonopathy [27].

8.1. Diagnosis

The diagnosis of PHG is done mainly by upper endoscopy. The endoscopic findings of PHG diagnosis was classified by the New Italian Endoscopic Club according to its severity based on the presence of four elementary lesions: mosaic like pattern, red point lesions, cherry red spots, and black brown spots (**Figure 1**) [29]. Early change in PHG is called scarletina, which appears as a fine pink speckling. On the other side, severe PHG appear as cherry red spots that may become confluent and is very friable, so it can actively bleed during endoscopy. These lesions are present predominantly in the fundus and/or the corpus of the stomach, yet PHG–like lesions have been described in other sites in the gastrointestinal tract e.g. the rectum, colon, and small bowel in asymptomatic patients and in patients with bleeding [29].

8.2. Endoscopic evaluation of PHG

The elementary lesions of PHG according to the New Italian Endoscopic Club for the Study and Therapy of Esophageal Varices [NIEC] classification are as follows [30]:

(1) Mosaic-like pattern (MLP); it is described as the presence of small, polygonal areas in the center (areola) surrounded by a whitish-yellow depressed border. The term mosaic is further subdivided according to the color of the areola into; mild, when the areola is uniformly pink, moderate, if the center is red, and severe, when the areola is uniformly red.

(2) Red-point lesions (RPLs) are defined as red, small, flat lesions, and <1 mm in size.

(3) Cherry-red spots (CRSs) are defined as red, round lesions, >2 mm in diameter, which slightly protrude into the lumen of the stomach.

(4) Black-brown spots (BBSs) are defined as irregularly flat spots, either black or brown in color, does not disappear after washing, and it is due to intra-mucosal hemorrhage.

PHG is classified by endoscopy, into mild, moderate and severe forms. PHG mucosa can be seen as snakeskin (MLP) in mild cases, while RPLs, CRSs or BBCs that is liable to bleeding, are found in severe cases, however, the presence of red or brown spots without bleeding is considered a moderate disease [35].

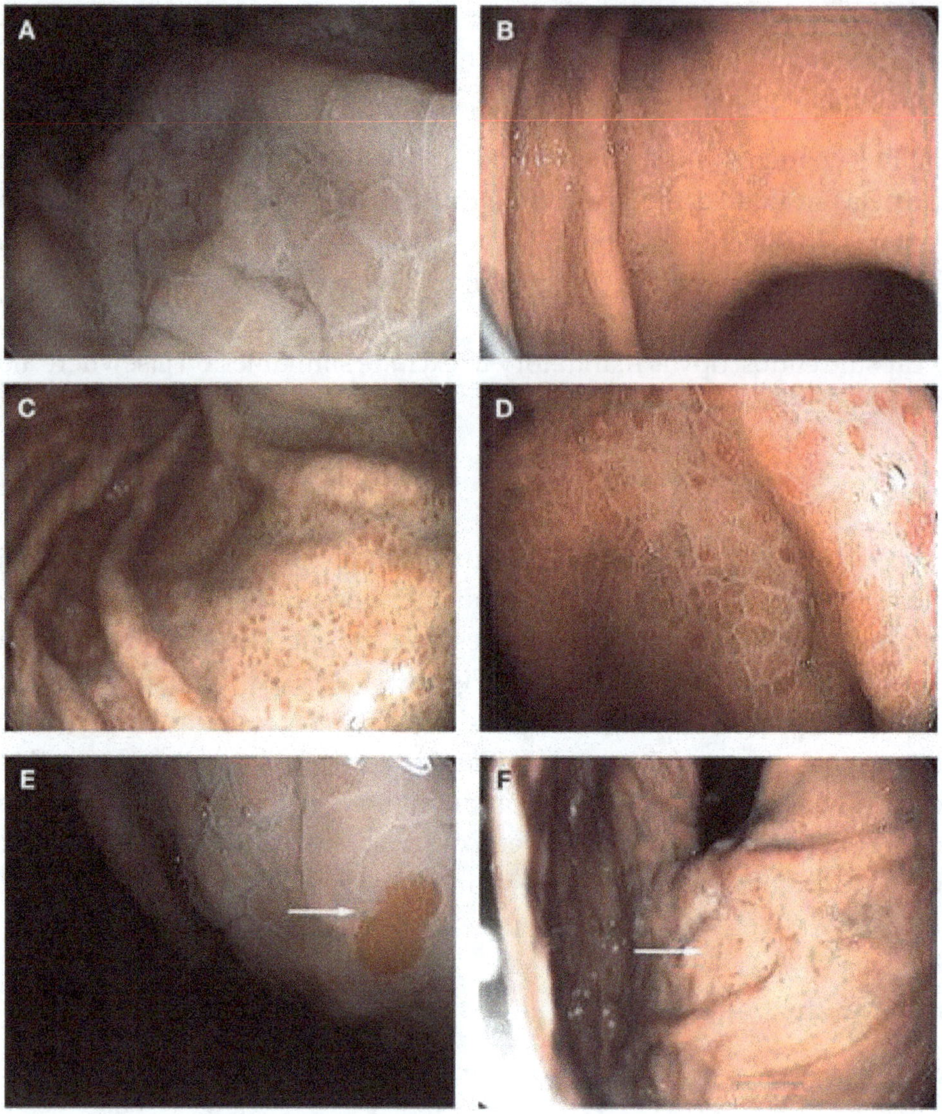

Figure 1. Endoscopic images of portal hypertensive gastropathy that show the four main findings of this condition. Mild (A) and moderate (B) mosaic-like gastric mucosal pattern, red point lesions (C), cherry-red spots (D), and black–brown spots, including an intramucosal hemorrhage (E) and a brown spot (F).

8.3. Classification of portal hypertensive gastropathy

PHG is classified on the basis of the condition's severity, therefore many classifications of the PHG mucosa have been proposed. McCormack's classification, NIEC's and Tanoue's classifications are the most popular used classifications (**Table 3**). McCormack classified the mucosal changes into two main categories, mild and severe, on the other hand, the NIEC classification has three categories; mild, moderate and severe, and further subdivided the mosaic-like pattern into three groups [28]. Finally, the McCormack classification, a two-category classification system, is the recommended one. The classification comprises of:

Mild portal hypertensive gastropathy: Only one change in the stomach mucosa is present, that of appearance of mosaic or snakeskin pattern on it.

	McCormack	NIEC	Tanoue
Mild	Scarlatina type rash		
	Snake skin	Pink in center mosaic	Mild redness
	Striped appearance		
Moderate	–	Flat red spots mosaic	Fine red speckling mosaic
Severe	Red spots	Diffusely red mosaic	Point bleeding
	Diffuse hemorrhagic lesions		

Table 3. Endoscopic finding and classification of PHG.

Severe portal hypertensive gastropathy: In addition to the mosaic or snakeskin pattern of the stomach mucosa; bulging, flat red or black-brown spots are seen. There also may be active bleeding.

In the rare instance where PHG cannot be clearly diagnosed on the basis of endoscopic appearance and location alone, biopsy for histology may prove useful [28].

8.4. Histologically

The unique histological features of PHG are marked dilatation of the capillaries and collecting venules in the gastric mucosa with markedly congested and tortuous submucosal venules (**Figure 2**) [31]. These vascular features are present in the absence of any inflammatory cell

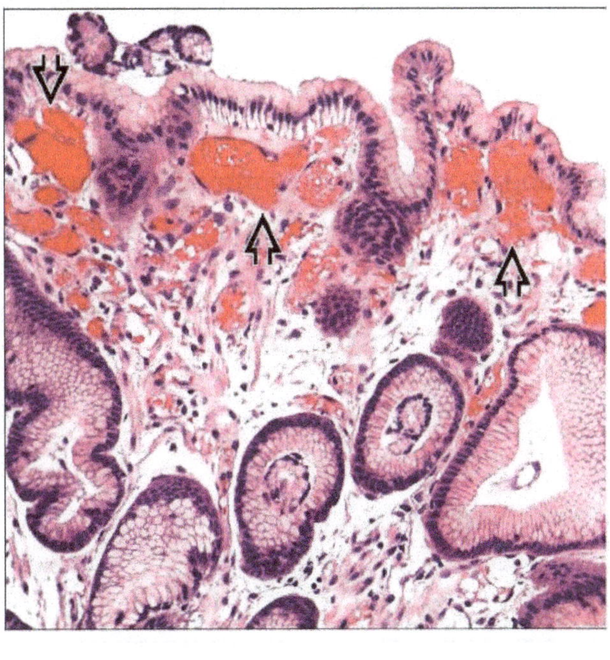

Figure 2. Hematoxylin and eosin shows numerous dilated capillaries in the superfacial gastric mucosa. These are not entirely specific for PHG.

infiltrate or erosion of the gastric mucosa. Stromal fibrosis and edema of the lamina propria can also be seen [31].

It may be difficult to differentiate between severe PHG and gastric antral vascular ectasia (GAVE) by endoscopic examination, so biopsy is beneficial in this case, as GAVE has distinct histological features that can set it apart from severe PHG. GAVE has many fibrin thrombi in the mucosal vessels with ectasia and spindle cell proliferation (smooth muscle and myofibroblast hyperplasia) in the superficial mucosa. Furthermore, fibrohyalinosis is more commonly present in GAVE. All of these findings provide additional features that help in differentiating between severe PHG and GAVE [32].

8.5. Portal gastropathy score calculation

Table 4 shows the scoring system to calculate the severity of PHG, the calculation depends on three categories: *Microscopic picture*; score 1 considered for mild findings, and score 2 for severe findings. *Red marks*; isolated lesion is considered score 1, whereas confluent red marks is scored 2. *GAVE*; if absent scored 0, while its presence is scored 2. If the total score was equal to 3 or less, the PHG is mild, on the other hand if the score is 4 or greater, PHG is severe [33].

8.6. Other diagnostic modalities

8.6.1. Non-endoscopic methods for diagnosis of HPG

Other non-endoscopic methods for the diagnosis of PHG such as MRI and CT are not yet considered as routine investigation for the diagnosis of PHG. Their results must be further evaluated to warrant their role in the diagnosis of PHG. Endoscopy still remains the main diagnostic method [34].

In CT scan, enhancement of the inner layer of the gastric walls due to gastric congestion, characterizes PHG lesion. Similarly, MRI is used to measure the diameter of collateral veins e.g. the left gastric, paraesophageal, and azygos veins to confirm the diagnosis of portal hypertension. In patients with PHG, the measurement of the diameters of these veins does not differ from those

Endoscopic findings	Parameter	Score
Mucosal mosaic pattern	Mild	1
	Severe	2
Red markings	Isolated	1
	Confluent	2
Gastric antral vascular ectasia (GAVE)	Absence	1
	Presence	2

Mild portal hypertensive gastropathy ≤ 3; severe portal hypertensive gastropathy ≥ 4.

Table 4. Portal hypertensive Gastropathy scoring system.

in patients without PHG, therefore it is not helpful in the diagnosis. These data suggest that these imaging techniques is still in its infancy period and best reserved for experimental purposes [35].

8.7. Differential diagnosis

The endoscopic findings of the gastric mucosa include many differential diagnoses of several disorders. When red spots are seen in the stomach by endoscopy, important diagnostic considerations are evoked. GAVE or watermelon stomach which is a common differential diagnosis of PHG, has characteristic endoscopic findings which are linear red stripes, separated by normal mucosa, these findings give the appearance of a watermelon, that is seen in the gastric antrum or proximal stomach. GAVE and PHG are distinct entities, however both are encountered in cirrhotic patients. While PHG routinely affects the gastric body and fundus, GAVE almost exclusively inhabits the antrum [32].

These findings have a diagnostic accuracy of 85% for GAVE and help distinguish it from PHG.

Table 5 further shows the differences between GAVE and PHG, however, there may be an overlap between GAVE and PHG in cirrhosis with portal hypertension [6].

Other conditions that increase the dilemma of PHG diagnosis include simple acute gastritis caused by non-steroidal anti–inflammatory drug (NSAIDS) or *H. pylori*, which may have a mosaic like pattern endoscopically but, the main histopathological feature in gastritis is inflammatory cell infiltration with minor vascular dilation, and it is also localized to the mucosa (superficial lesion). Lastly, endoscopic lesions similar to PHG may be also seen in some uncommon diseases e.g. polycythemia, gastric purpura, and Osler-Weber-Rendu disease [36].

	PHG	GAVE
Underlying etiology	Portal hypertension with or without cirrhosis	Can be present without portal hypertension, such as chronic renal failure, connective tissue disorders, and bone marrow transplantation
Predominant location	Fundus and corpus	Antrum
Endoscopic appearance	Mosaic like pattern or red marks	Linear red strips separated by normal mucosa
Pathological findings	Dilatation of the capillaries, and collecting venules in the gastric mucosa. Ectasia of submucosal veins, with intimal thickening	Fibrin microthrombi, myofibroplast hyperplasia, fibrinolysis
Management		
• **Response to beta blockers**	Yes	No
• **TIPS**	Yes	No
• **Endoscopic therapy ACP**	Used in refractory bleeding	Preferable as first line

ACP, argon plasma coagulation.

Table 5. Comparison between portal hypertensive gastropathy and gastric antral vascular ectasia.

9. Management of PHG

The goal of management of PHG is to reduce portal pressure.

9.1. Primary prophylaxis

PHG in asymptomatic patients who have no evidence of bleeding is discovered accidentally during screening for either chronic iron deficiency anemia or for esophageal varices in patients with cirrhosis. Till now, there is no recommendation to start any primary prophylaxis to prevent bleeding from PHG patients, except if there is an indication of beta-blocker for other reasons. However, in asymptomatic patients with both esophageal varices and PHG, if the patient undergoes esophageal eradication therapy, co-administration of a nonselective beta-blocker is beneficial. The dose of beta blocker should be titrated to a goal heart rate of 55–60 bpm or a 25% reduction from baseline. On the other hand, in patients with severe PHG and no varices, starting prophylaxis therapy with nonselective beta-blockers, should be considered. Yet, this approach is controversial, and more research is needed to clarify the prophylactic role of beta-blockers as primary prophylaxis for bleeding from PHG [34].

9.2. Secondary prophylaxis

Beta-blockers (like propranolol or nadolol) are used as secondary prophylaxis, and are the basis of therapy, to prevent recurrent bleeding from PHG. It is not only used to prevent the bleeding, but it also improves the severity score of PHG by endoscopy, changing it from severe to mild, or even completely curing it. On the other hand, about 50% of PHG patients especially cirrhotic during a 2-year follow up, show mild or even no response to beta blocker therapy. For those patients adding isosorbide 5-mononitrate may have a synergistic effect to reduce the portal pressure [37].

Addition of beta-blocker therapy to endoscopic management of varices is beneficial in reducing the progression of PHG after endoscopic therapy of varices. Propranolol, a non-selective beta-blocker (24–480 mg/day), has been commonly used in these cases. The dose of propranolol should be increased gradually to maximum dose (up to 160 mg twice daily) with targeted heart rate of 55–60 bpm, and should be continued as long as there is portal hypertension [37]. In patients with iron deficiency anemia, iron replacement therapy and beta blocker should be started simultaneously.

9.3. Treatment of chronic bleeding

Patients with PHG with or without cirrhosis, and chronic blood loss are commonly presented with iron deficiency anemia. Thorough investigation of these patients must be done to rule out other causes of iron deficiency anemia before attributing PHG as the cause. All patients with PHG and iron deficiency anemia should start iron-replacement therapy either; oral preparations, or intravenous (IV) iron.

To reduce chronic bleeding from PHG, with or without portal hypertension, portal pressure should be reduced, therefore non selective beta blocker is the first line of treatment. The use of beta blockers has proved efficient, based on both experimental and clinical investigations demonstrating that, propranolol reduces portal pressure and cause vasoconstriction in the overall splanchnic vascular bed.

Anti-oxidants have also been used to treat PHG. Experimentally, Vitamin E led to complete reversal of susceptibility of PHG mucosa to alcohol injury, in rats. Vitamin E also, led to the restoration of normal Extracellular signal-regulated kinase (ERK-2 signaling), which plays a pivotal role in healing after gastric mucosal injury. Thus, vitamin E may have a protective effect on the PHG mucosa [38].

Use of other pharmacological agents such as losartan, thalidomide and corticosteroids have been prescribed in the treatment of chronic bleeding from PHG. However, the evidence supporting their use in PHG bleeding is weak [39].

9.4. Treatment of acute bleeding

- For acute bleeding; initial stabilization with octreotide or terlipressin to stop the bleeding, followed by initiation of beta-blockers as secondary prevention is recommended. During acute bleeding from PHG, the patients may be hemodynamically unstable, therefore beta blocker therapy must be reserved, regarding its drawback, as it has a negative effect on heart and the circulation. Despite the drawbacks of beta-blocker therapy, it is considered immediately after the patient becomes hemodynamically stable, usually within 3 days. This highlights their important role in the management of acute as well as chronic GI bleeding.
- Octreotide, a somatostatin analogue (100 μg bolus followed by an infusion of 25 μg/h for 48 h), and Terlipressin, a vasopressin analogue, are both effective in the treatment of acute bleeding caused by PHG. Vasopressin and omeprazole when used together are more effective in controlling the acute bleeding than when vasopressin is used alone [40].

9.5. For refractory cases

When the patients do not respond to the previously mentioned treatments, invasive intervention must be done. Transjugular intrahepatic portosystemic shunt (TIPS) or surgical shunt are considered as salvage therapy only when they are performed in certain circumstances and in an expert center due to their significant morbidity and mortality results [41].

Surgical shunting has also proved beneficial in refractory bleeding from PHG however, this benefit is limited by an increase in the risk of deterioration of the hepatic function in patients with cirrhosis. Only cirrhotic patients with Child Pugh score A or B found improved outcomes from surgical shunting with reduced mortality. Comparing the results of TIPS with surgical shunt, it is reported that surgical shunt reduced re-bleeding, with fewer shunt complication e.g. shunt revisions, stent thrombosis, re-stenosis, and re-intervention of TIPS. However, long-term mortality was similar. On the other hand, similar results were found between TIPSS and distal splenorenal shunting with regards to re-bleeding, encephalopathy, and survival. Whatever the method of shunting in case of refractory bleeding from PHG, it should always be performed in expertise center. Surgical shunting may be an option only in CTP stage A cirrhosis with PHG or in patients with non-cirrhotic portal hypertension [42].

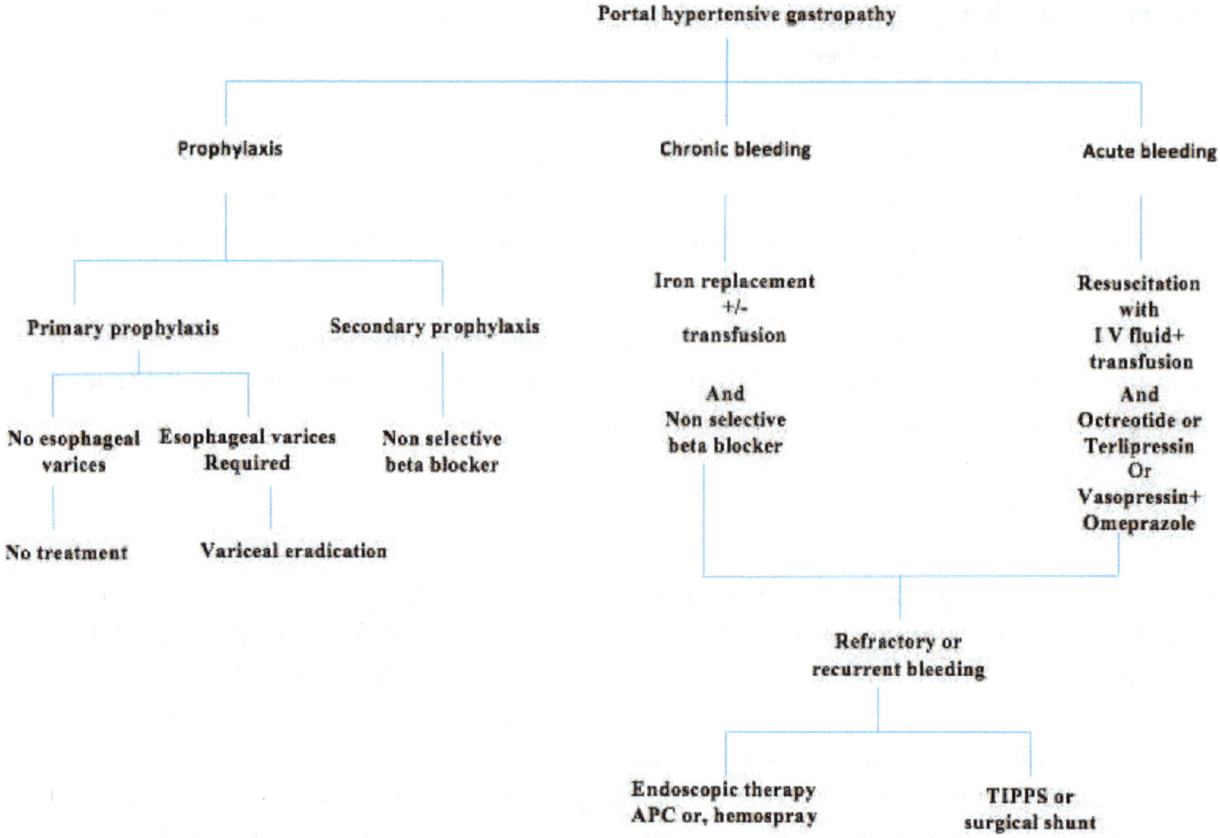

Figure 3. Treatment algorithm of portal hypertensive gastropathy.

Argon plasma coagulation (APC) is an electrosurgical technique used for treatment of bleeding of PHG. APC is a noncontact thermal coagulation, high frequency current, that is applied to the bleeding site through an argon plasma jet, this creates effective hemostasis and a homogenous surface coagulation with limited depth penetration. Treatment with APC decrease the need of transformation and improve the hemoglobin level in PHG patients, accordingly APC is an effective and rapid therapy to control bleeding from PHG, especially if there is a contraindication for beta blockers. If beta blocker can be used, co administration with APC has a synergistic effect in controlling PHG bleeding [5].

Hemospray: In patients with acute active bleeding due to PHG, it may be useful to use hemostatic powder that acts as a barrier to enhance the action of the clotting factors, giving time for the coagulation process to act and stop the bleeding [43]. A treatment algorithm for patients with PHG is described in **Figure 3**.

10. Mortality rates

Limited data on mortality due to bleeding from PHG is available, but the bleeding from PHG is rarely fatal. It represents a small percentage if compared with the mortality from other causes of gastrointestinal bleeding due to portal hypertension, and especially in comparison to variceal bleeding. Also, in cirrhotic patients it represents only <1% of the mortality, because the bleeding is typically mild [4]. As bleeding from PHG is an unusual direct cause of death, it does not affect the survival in cirrhotic patients. However, anemia from chronic bleeding or repeated acute bleeding may lead to deterioration of the liver function.

Acknowledgements

I would like to thank my family for their continuous support. Mohamed & Mennat Allah for the late nights they stayed up with me. To my husband Megahed and my daughter Reem, I'm grateful for them inspiring and pushing me to do this in the first place. I'm eternally grateful to all of you.

Author details

Samia Ali Gamie

Address all correspondence to: samia_ali5@hotmail.com

Faculty of Medicine, Helwan University, Cairo, Egypt

References

[1] Snyder P, Ali R, Poles M, Gross SA. Portal hypertensive gastropathy with a focus on management. Expert Review of Gastroenterology & Hepatology. 2015;**9**(9):1207-1216

[2] Bandali MF, Mirakhur A, Lee EW, Ferris MC, Sadler DJ, Gray RR, et al. Portal hypertension: Imaging of portosystemic collateral pathways and associated image-guided therapy. World Journal of Gastroenterology. 2017;**23**(10):1735-1746

[3] Bloom S, Kemp W. Portal hypertension: pathophysiology, diagnosis and management. Internal Medicine Journal. 2015;**45**(1):16-26

[4] Mihajlo GjeorgievskiAl, Cappell MS. Portal hypertensive gastropathy: A systematic review of the pathophysiology, clinical presentation, natural history and therapy. World Journal of Hepatology. 2016;**8**(4):231-262

[5] Amr Shaaban Hanafy, Amr Talaat El Hawary. Efficacy of argon plasma coagulation in the management of portal hypertensive gastropathy. Endoscopy International Open. 2016;**4**(10):E1057–E1062

[6] Patwardhan VR, Cardenas A. Review article: The management of portal hypertensive gastropathy and gastric antral vascular ectasia in cirrhosis. Alimentary Pharmacology & Therapeutics. 2014;**40**:354-362

[7] Merli M, Nicolini G, Angeloni S, Gentili F, Attili AF, Riggio O. The natural history of portal hypertensive gastropathy in patients with liver cirrhosis and mild portal hypertension The American Journal of Gastroenterology. 2004;**99**:1959-654

[8] Thuluvath PJ, Yoo HY. Portal hypertensive gastropathy. The American Journal of Gastroenterology. 2002;**97**:2973-2978

[9] Cristina Ripoll, Guadalupe Garcia-Tsao. Management of gastropathy and gastric vascular ectasia in portal hypertension. Clinical Liver Disease. 2010;**14**(2):281-295

[10] Eleftheriadis E. Portal hypertensive gastropathy a clinically significant puzzle. Annals of Gastroenterology. 2001;**14**(3):196-204

[11] Wang J, Han W, Zborowska E, Liang J, Wang X, Willson JK, Sun L, Brattain MG. Reduced expression of transforming growth factor beta type I receptor contributes to the malignancy of human colon carcinoma cells. The Journal of Biological Chemistry. 1996;**271**(29):17366-17371

[12] Abbasi A, Bhutto AR, Butt N, Munir SM, Dhillo AK. Frequency of portal hypertensive gastropathy and its relationship with biochemical, haematological and endoscopic features in cirrhosis. Journal of the College of Physicians and Surgeons Pakistan. 2011;**21**:723-726

[13] Kamath PS, Shah VH. Portal hypertension and bleeding esophageal varices. In: Boyer TD, Manns MP, Sanyal AJ, editors. In: Zakim and Boyer's Hepatology: A Textbook of Liver Disease. 6th ed. Philadelphia: Elsevier Saunders. 2012: pp. 296-326

[14] Wu Q, Shen L, Chu J, Ma X, Jin B, Meng F, Chen J, Wang Y, Wu L, Han J, et al. Characterization of uncommon portosystemic collateral circulations in patients with hepatic cirrhosis. Oncology Letters. 2015;**9**:347-350

[15] Zardi EM, Uwechie V, Gentilucci UV, Dobrina A, Petitti T, Laghi V, Picardi A, Afeltra A. Portal diameter in the diagnosis of esophageal varices in 266 cirrhotic patients: Which role? Ultrasound in Medicine & Biology. 2007;**33**:506-511

[16] Elnaser MS, Elebiary S, Bastawi MB, El Shafei A, Elmagd IM, Hamza MM. The prevalence of portal hypertensive gastropathy and duodenopathy in some Egyptian cirrhotic patients. Ultrasound in Medicine & Biology. 2004;**34**:915-923

[17] Iwao T, Toyonaga A, Oho K, et al. Portal-hypertensive gastropathy develops less in patients with cirrhosis and fundal varices. Journal of Hepatology. 1997;**26**:1235-1241

[18] Feldman M, Lee EL. Gastritis. In: Feldman M, Friedman LS, Brandt LJ, editors. Sleisenger and Fordtran's Gastrointestinal and Liver Disease: Pathophysiology, Diagnosis, Management. 10th ed. Philadelphia: Elsevier Saunders; 2010. pp. 868-883

[19] Sogaard KK, Astrup LB, Vilstrup H, Gronbaek H. Portal vein thrombosis; risk factors, clinical presentation and treatment. BMC Gastroenterology. 2007;**7**:34

[20] MY, Choi H, Baik SK, Yea CJ, Won CS, Byun JW, Park SY, Kwon YH, Kim JW, Kim HS, et al. Portal hypertensive gastropathy: Correlation with portal hypertension and prognosis in cirrhosis. Digestive Diseases and Sciences. 2010;**55**:3561-3567

[21] Zardi EM, Ghittoni G, Margiotta D, Viera FT, Di Matteo F, Rossi S. Portal hypertensive gastropathy in cirrhotics without varices: A case-control study. European Journal of Gastroenterology & Hepatology. 2015;**27**:91-96

[22] Kim MY, Choi H, Baik SK, Yea CJ, Won CS, Byun JW, Park SY, Kwon YH, Kim JW, Kim HS, et al. Portal hypertensive gastropathy: Correlation with portal hypertension and prognosis in cirrhosis. Digestive Diseases and Sciences. 2010;**55**:3561-3567

[23] Khaled Abd-Alazeim Eid, Muhammad Abd El-Gawad Shawky MD, Amro Metwaly Hassan, Ahmed Qasem Mohammed, Mostafa Ismail Mohammed. Prevalence of *Helicobacter pylori* infection in patients with portal hypertensive gastropathy owing to liver cirrhosis Al-Azhar Assiut Medical Journal. 2016;**14**(3):109-114

[24] Fontana RJ, Sanyal AJ, Mehta S, Doherty MC, Neuschwander-Tetri BA, Everson GT, Kahn JA, Malet PF, Sheikh MY, Chung RT, et al. Portal hypertensive gastropathy in chronic hepatitis C patients with bridging fibrosis and compensated cirrhosis: results from the HALT-C trial. The American Journal of Gastroenterology. 2006;**101**:983-992

[25] Herbst DA, Reddy KR. Risk factors for hepatocellular carcinoma. Clinical Liver Disease. 2012;**1**(6):180-182. DOI: 10.1002/cld.111

[26] Sanyal AJG, Grace ND, Carey W. Prevention and management of gastroesophageal varices and variceal hemorrhage in cirrhosis. Hepatology. 2007;**46**:922-938

[27] Misra SP, Dwivedi M, Misra V. Prevalence and factors influencing hemorrhoids, anorectal varices, and colopathy in patients with portal hypertension. Endoscopy. 1996;**28**(4): 340-345

[28] D'Amico G, Garcia-Tsao G, Pagliaro L. Natural history and prognostic indicators of survival in cirrhosis: A systematic review of 118 studies. Journal of Hepatology. 2006;**44**: 217-231

[29] Rafael F Perini, Paula RS Camara and Jose GP Ferraz. Nature clinical practice, pathogenesis of portal hypertensive gastropathy: Translating basic research into clinical practice. Gastroenterology & Hepatology. 2009;**6**:150-158. DOI: 10.1038/ncpgasthep1356

[30] Spina GP, Arcidiacono R, Bosch J. et al. Gastric endoscopic features in portal hypertension: Final report of a consensus conference, Milan, Italy. 19 September 1992. 1994. pp. 461-467

[31] Amitabh Srivastava MD. Pathology & laboratory medicine, basicmedical insight engine. http://basicmedicalkey.com/portal-hypertensive-gastropathy [Accessed: July 6, 2016]

[32] Burak KW, Lee SS, Beck PL. Portal hypertensive gastropathy and gastric antral vascular ectasia (GAVE). Journal of Hepatology. 2001;**49**:866-872

[33] Charmaine Stewart A, Arun Sanyal J. Grading portal gastropathy: Validation of a gastropathy scoring system. The American Journal of Gastroenterology. 2003;**98**:1758-1765. DOI: 10.1111/j.1572-0241.2003.07595

[34] Urrunaga NH, Don Rockey C. Portal hypertensive gastropathy and colopathy. Clinical Liver Disease. 2014;**18**(2):389-406

[35] Erden A, Idilman R, Erden I, et al. Veins around the esophagus and the stomach: Do their calibrations provide a diagnostic clue for portal hypertensive gastropathy? Clinical Imaging. 2009;**33**:22-24

[36] Raul Cubillas, Don Rockey C. Portal hypertensive gastropathy: A review article. Liver International . 2010;**30**(8):1094-1102. DOI: 10.1111/j.1478-3231.2010.02286

[37] Lo GH, Lai KH, Cheng JS, Hsu PI, Chen TA, Wang EM, Lin CK, Chiang HT. The effects of endoscopic variceal ligation and propranolol on portal hypertensive gastropathy: A prospective, controlled trial. Gastrointestinal Endoscopy. 2001;**53**:579-584

[38] Thuluvath PJ, Yoo HY. Portal hypertensive gastropathy. The American Journal of Gastroenterology. 2002;**97**:2973-2978

[39] Wagatsuma Y, Naritaka Y, Shimakawa T. et al. Clinical usefulness of the angiotensin II receptor antagonist losartan in patients with portal hypertensive gastropathy. Hepatogastroenterology. 2006;**53**(68):171-174

[40] Zhou Y, Qiao L, Wu J. et al. Comparison of the efficacy of octreotide, vasopressin, and omeprazole in the control of acute bleeding in patients with portal hypertensive gastropathy: A controlled study. Journal of Gastroenterology and Hepatology. 2002;**17**:973-979

[41] Kamath PS, Lacerda M, Ahlquist DA, McKusick MA, Andrews JC, Nagorney DA. Gastric mucosal responses to intrahepatic portosystemic shunting in patients with cirrhosis. Gastroenterology. 2000;**118**:905-911

[42] De Franchis R, Faculty BV. Revising consensus in portal hypertension: report of the Baveno V consensus workshop on methodology of diagnosis and therapy in portal hypertension. Journal of Hepatology. 2010;**53**:762-768

[43] Smith LA, Morris AJ, Stanley AJ. The use of hemospray in portal hypertensive bleeding; A case series. European association for the study of the liver. Journal of Hepatology. 2014;**60**:457-460

4

Diagnostic Scores in Acute Appendicitis

Alfredo Alvarado

Abstract

Diagnostic scores should be part of the initial evaluation of patients suspected of acute appendicitis. This approach could be very helpful in order to make an early diagnosis and to stratify the cases for observation, further investigation, or surgical intervention.

Keywords: diagnostic scores in acute appendicitis, Alvarado score, clinical approach

1. Introduction

Several scoring systems have been developed to help clinicians in the diagnosis of acute appendicitis. The best-known scores are the Alvarado score, the modified Alvarado score, the Pediatric Appendicitis Score, the Appendicitis Inflammatory Response score, and the RIPASA score. These tools not only can be used for diagnostic purposes but also for stratification, separating those patients who require observation and workup from those who can be assigned for certain specific treatment. The aim of these scores is to reduce the number of negative appendectomies without increasing the number of perforations.

The Alvarado score was described in 1986 [1] and since then has been evaluated and validated in many studies. It consists of three symptoms, three clinical signs, and two laboratory tests. This system uses a simple mnemonics (**MANTRELS**) that is easy to remember and can be applied in many settings without the need of a computer. The symptoms are migration (one point), anorexia-acetonuria (one point), and nausea/vomiting (one point). The clinical signs are tenderness in the right lower quadrant (two points), rebound pain (one point), and elevation of oral temperature (37.3°C or more) (one Point).

The basic laboratory tests are a complete blood count (CBC) to look for leukocytosis (>10,000 cells/mm^3) and a differential white blood count (WBC) looking for left **shift** (increased stabs >5% or segmented neutrophils >75%). A urinalysis is useful to determine if there is acetone, which indicates the presence of a fasting state related to anorexia, and also, it may show many red cells due to an inflammatory process around the appendix. If the urine shows too many red cells, it may point to a ureteral calculus, and further investigation should be done. The C-reactive protein (CRP) test is not included in the score because it is a nonspecific test that detects an inflammatory process only and is not diagnostic for any particular condition. Besides this, it would be a redundancy since the shift to the left and leukocytosis are doing the same thing. Furthermore, it will not help in the initial stages of acute appendicitis because it will defeat the purpose of the score, that is to say, to make an early diagnosis of acute appendicitis.

Direct tenderness on the right lower quadrant can be replaced by direct percussion with the fist, as a mallet, on the right lumbar area in cases of retrocecal appendicitis which occurs in 75–85% of cases.

Rebound pain can be replaced by other indirect signs such as the Rovsing sign, Dunphy sign (cough test) or the Markle's test (heel-drop jarring test), pain on walking, pain with jolts or bumps in the road, and the inspiration test. Uncommon tests of peritoneal irritation such as the psoas and the obturator tests can replace the rebound pain test also. In children who are unable to communicate well, cutaneous hyperesthesia can be added to replace the migration symptom.

In order of decreasing importance, the best predictive factors proved to be localized tenderness on the right lower quadrant, leukocytosis, migration of pain, shift to the left, temperature elevation, nausea or vomiting, anorexia or acetone in the urine, and direct rebound pain. Two points are assigned to the more important factors (tenderness and leukocytosis) and a value of 1 for each one of the others, for a possible total score of 10. A score of 4–5 is compatible with the diagnosis of acute appendicitis, a score of 7 or 8 indicates a probable appendicitis, and a score of 9 or 10 indicates a very probable appendicitis. To this score the clinician could subtract two points if the patient complains of headache because this symptom is very rare in cases of acute appendicitis. In this particular situation, the patient may need further investigation to rule out a different disorder.

Scores of 5 or 6 are in a gray area, and in this case, the clinician may want to observe the patient for a short time (reevaluate every 4–6 hours) for 12–24 hours, and if the score remains, the same consider other tests such as ultrasound or diagnostic laparoscopy. When the score is 3 or 4, the clinician has two options: the patient could be kept under observation and repeat the tests or, even more, order additional tests such as an US or a CT scan if they are available in that particular setting. Another option is to rely on the clinical impression of the examiner because, as I already mentioned in my original article, "there is always an intangible ingredient in the diagnosis of acute appendicitis."

The modified Alvarado score (MAS) [2] is a simplification of the Alvarado score by eliminating the neutrophil count because a differential WBC count is not available in certain facilities. The results are similar to the original score but with less capacity to detect the early stages of acute appendicitis.

The Pediatric Appendicitis Score (PAS), developed by Samuel in 2002 [3], is a modification of the Alvarado score in which the rebound sign has been replaced by cough/percussion/hopping tenderness in the right lower quadrant, and the elevation of temperature has been increased to 38°C. In this score the sign of tenderness in the right lower quadrant, the most relevant feature of the score, was given one point only.

The Appendicitis Inflammatory Response (AIR) score [4] is based along the same principles of the Alvarado score assigning patients to low, medium, or high probability of acute appendicitis. It was developed by Andersson and Andersson in 2008 and was constructed from eight independent variables (right lower quadrant pain, rebound tenderness, muscular defense, WBC count, proportion of neutrophils, CRP, body temperature, and vomiting). The AIR score contains rebound tenderness or muscular defense that is divided in three groups—light, medium, and strong—which makes these signs subjective and very difficult to evaluate, and this may deviate the final score one way or another. Besides this, the AIR score omits the symptom of migration of pain which is a very important and specific symptom in the diagnosis of acute appendicitis.

The Raja Isteri Pengiran Anak Saleha Appendicitis (RIPASA) score [5] was developed for the diagnosis of acute appendicitis in Brunei, Darussalam, in 2008. It contains 14 patient characteristics: gender, age, and symptoms, right iliac fossa (RIF) pain, migration to the RIF, anorexia, nausea and vomiting, duration of symptoms, and clinical signs RIF tenderness, guarding, rebound tenderness, Rovsing sign, and fever. It also contains two laboratory tests (WBC and urinalysis) and an additional parameter related to a foreign national card record. Some authors found that the Alvarado score was disappointing in the diagnosis of acute appendicitis in Asian and Mid-Eastern populations, so they decided to have a different score more suitable to them. Chong [6] found that the RIPASA score of >7.5 correctly classified 98% patients confirmed with histological findings of acute appendicitis in comparison with 68.3% patients with an Alvarado score of >7. However, RIPASA and Alvarado scores correctly classified 81.3% and 87.9% patients without acute appendicitis into the true negative groups with scores of >7.5 and <7, respectively. The negative appendectomy rate was 14.66% for the RIPASA score and 13.75% for the Alvarado score.

Khadda et al. [7] found that the RIPASA score has a sensitivity of 97.7% and a specificity of 77.4% and a negative appendectomy rate of 13.7% which is higher than many reports that had used the Alvarado score such as Menon et al. [8], in Pakistan, who reported a negative appendectomy rate of 1.9%. In other study, Pouget-Baudry et al. [9], in France, reported 3 out of 174 patients with a normal appendix on histological examination which equals to 1.72%. The good thing is that Khadda recognized that the Alvarado score is the simplest of all the scores used in current practice. Furthermore, Gaikwad et al. [10], in India, found that the false-positive rate is reduced to zero when ultrasonography is added to the Alvarado score.

Goel et al. [11], in India, evaluated the efficacy of the Alvarado score and the RIPASA score finding that the Alvarado score has a better specificity than the RIPASA score (100 vs. 50%) and also a better negative appendectomy rate (0 vs. 5%). Similar results were reported by Karami et al. [12], in Iran, who found that the Alvarado score was 100% specific as compared with the RIPASA and the AIR scores (91.6% for both).

Malik et al. [13], in Ireland, found that the RIPASA score has a PPV of 84.06% and a NPV of 72.86% with a negative appendectomy rate of 15.94% and an accuracy of 80%. This is the first study evaluating the utility of the RIPASA score predicting acute appendicitis in a Western population. However, Rodrigues and Sindhu [14], in India, found that the Alvarado score had a greater specificity, PPV, and positive likelihood than the RIPASA score. The negative appendectomy in this study was quite high (18.09%) as compared to different negative appendectomy rates reported with the Alvarado score that range between 0 and 10%. Similar results were reported by Rathod et al. [15] with a negative appendectomy rate of 20.69% and a perforated appendicitis of 8.05%. This indicates that the RIPASA score can reduce the number of complicated appendectomies at the expense of a high negative appendectomy rate.

In a recent study in India, Regar et al. [16] found that the Alvarado score is more specific (80%) than the RIPASA score (60%). The PPV of the Alvarado score was 98.46% as compared to 97.83% of the RIPASA score. The negative appendectomy rate for the Alvarado score was lower that the RIPASA score (1.54 vs. 2.17%).

In another recent study, Sinnet et al. [17], in India, found that the RIPASA score has more sensitivity than the Alvarado score (95.5 vs. 65%) but has less specificity (65 vs. 90%). The PPV was 92.89% for the RIPASA score and 96.6% for the Alvarado score which indicates that the negative appendectomy rate is higher for the RIPASA score than the Alvarado score (7.61 vs. 3.33%).

In a study to assess the reliability and practical application of the Alvarado, Eskelinen, Ohmann, and RIPASA scoring systems, Erdem et al. [18], in Turkey, found that the Alvarado score had the best negative appendectomy rate (12%) than the RIPASA score (25%). The negative appendectomy rate for the Ohmann and the Eskelinen scores was 22 and 21%, respectively.

Diaz-Barrientos et al. [19], in Mexico, found that the RIPASA score showed no advantage over the Modified Alvarado score taking into consideration that the ROC curve area was 0.59 for the RIPASA score vs. 0.71 for the modified Alvarado score.

In another study, in Mexico, Reyes-Garcia et al. [20] found 15.7% cases of necrotic appendicitis and 14.3% cases of perforated appendix when using the RIPASA score. The negative appendectomy rate was also high (18.6%).

Golden et al. [21] compared the physician-determined decision with the RIPASA, the Alvarado, and the modified Alvarado score systems in order to measure the physician gestalt in the diagnosis of acute appendicitis. They found that at the higher "rule-in" cutoff threshold, the RIPASA score had a high sensitivity (78%) but a low specificity (36%). Conversely, the modified Alvarado score had a low sensitivity (47%) and a high specificity (81%). The original Alvarado score had test characteristics between these two values. They also calculated the test characteristics for the clinical scoring systems at lower "rule-out" threshold. The NPV for each score varied from 75% for the modified Alvarado score to 89% for the RIPASA score. The NPV for the physician-determined decision was 83%. The area under the curve (AUC) was greatest for the Alvarado score and the physician-determined decision (72% for both), 70% for the MAS score, and 67% for the RIPASA score. These authors concluded that the physician-determined probability estimates were accurate as these scoring systems, which proves that the physician gestalt works well in the diagnosis of acute appendicitis.

All of these findings on the RIPASA score indicate that we need more studies to find out why the differences among the Western and South Asian and Middle Eastern populations. It is possible that these differences have to do with the anatomical position of the appendix and not precisely with the physiopathological process of acute appendicitis or the cultural differences of these populations.

2. Other scores

There are other less-known scores similar to the Alvarado score such as the Adult Appendicitis score of Sammalkorpi et al. [22] that was constructed by logistic regression analysis using multiple imputations for missing values. This score contains four symptoms and clinical signs including the sign of guarding divided into three graduations (mild, moderate, and severe) which is in reality a very subjective sign. It also contains two laboratory tests (WBC and CRP) divided at different levels that are very difficult to memorize. They reported sensitivities and specificities similar to the Alvarado score and areas under the ROC curve of 0.882 for the new score and 0.790 for the Alvarado score. The negative appendectomy rate for this new score is 18.2% which is much higher than the usual reported rates with the Alvarado score.

The Tzanakis scoring system [23] is a very simplified score that contains two clinical signs only: right abdominal tenderness (four points) and rebound tenderness (three points). The only laboratory test is a white blood cell count (WBC) greater than 12.000 cells/mm^3 (two points). The score relies on positive ultrasound scan findings (six points).

Sigdel et al. [24] carried out a prospective study of the Tzanakis score to compare this score with the Alvarado score and reported a sensitivity of 91.4% for the Tzanakis score and 81% for the Alvarado score. The specificity for both scores was the same (66.6%). The ROC curve gave an AUC of 0.867 for the Tzanakis score and 0.81 for the Alvarado score. The negative appendectomy rate was reported as 6% which is certainly low and is due to the addition of the ultrasound studies that are not available in many health facilities. The overall diagnostic accuracy for the Tzanakis score was 91.48% vs. 81.91% for the Alvarado score.

In a study to compare the sensitivity, specificity, and diagnostic accuracy of the Tzanakis score (TS) and the modified Alvarado score (MAS), Sharma et al. [25], in India, found that the sensitivity for the MAS was higher than the TS score (97.7 vs. 82.0%), but the specificity for the TS was higher (36.38 vs. 18%). The PPV for both scores was the same (19%), and the accuracy for the MAS was better than the TS (89 vs. 79%). They concluded that the MAS was better than the TS since in the TS there are chances of observer bias. Besides this, they could not wait till a leukocyte count goes up to 12,000 cells/cm^3 if clinical suspicion is present.

Kumar et al. [26], in India, found that the Tzanakis score is an effective modality in the establishment of accuracy in the diagnosis of acute appendicitis, but the limitation is observer bias which may vary the scoring results.

The Lintula score [27] was developed from 35 symptoms and clinical signs recorded for 131 Finnish children with abdominal pain and was modeled using logistic regression. This complicated score uses gender, intensity of pain, relocation of pain, vomiting, pain in the right lower quadrant, fever, guarding, bowel sounds, and rebound tenderness with different grades. Some of these signs are very difficult to evaluate which may alter the final scoring.

Konan et al. [28], in a study to compare the Alvarado and the Lintula scores in patients older than 65 years of age, found that the Alvarado score was better predictor than the Lintula score. Both scores have a high sensitivity and specificity in the diagnosis of acute appendicitis.

Ojuka and Sangoro [29], in a prospective study, carried out at Kenyatta National Hospital, found that the ROC curves for Lintula and Alvarado scores are almost identical (0.6824 and 0.6966), respectively. However, the sensitivity for the Lintula score is lower than the Alvarado score (60.8 vs. 83.3%), and the overall accuracy for the Lintula score was also lower (69.6 vs. 70.4%).

The Ohmann score [30] was developed in Germany using a computer-aided diagnosis. The variables of the score are tenderness, no micturition difficulties, steady pain, leukocytosis count >10,000 cells/mm^3, age >50 years, relocation of pain to the right lower quadrant, and rigidity. In spite of this computerized system, there was no improvement in the number of perforations or complications.

In an analysis of scores in the diagnosis of acute appendicitis in women, Horzic et al. [31] compared the modified Alvarado score, Ohmann score, and Eskelinen score finding that all patients with the modified Alvarado score of 7 or more had acute appendicitis (100% specificity) which can be used to determine the need for immediate appendectomy.

Recently, Wilasrusmee et al. [32] developed a new appendicitis score for patients with suspected appendicitis and compared it with the Alvarado score. This score, also known as RAMA-AS, includes seven variables (migration of pain, progression of pain, pain aggravation by cough or movement, temperature of 37.8°C or more, and rebound tenderness). Also, it includes two laboratory tests (WBC >10,000 cells/mm^3 and neutrophils <75%). In the evaluation of the variables of the score, there are serious questions. For example, they gave great importance to rebound tenderness (the only sign of the score) which contradicts the literature that always mentions direct tenderness in the right lower quadrant as the main variable. Besides this, their own statistic shows that rebound tenderness is present in 23.9%, whereas tenderness in the right lower quadrant is present in 88.4% of their cases. Another significant discrepancy is that they gave more importance to pain aggravation than anorexia (56.3 vs. 76.1%). Another objectionable symptom is progression of pain since this is a very subjective symptom that is difficult to evaluate. The C-statistics reported by Wilasrusmee et al. are better than the Alvarado score, but the RAMA-AS score did not perform well in the external data when compared to the derived data. Using the score in practice is not as easy as claimed by this group since it requires the use of the Fagan nomogram. In addition, the calculation of the score is difficult to obtain because the evaluation of the parameters is given in fractional numbers. For all of these reasons, the new score will need external evaluations to establish its usefulness in the real practice.

Khanafer et al. [33] made some modifications to the Alvarado score (AS) and the Pediatric Appendicitis score (PAS) to screen children at low risk for appendicitis who could be carefully observed at home without the need for laboratory investigation. In this study, a total of 180 children were enrolled with an average age of 11.2 years of which 56.7% were female. According to their findings, children with a score of >7 for the modified PAS and AS may be safely sent home with close follow-up, while those above this cut-off would benefit from a referral for further evaluation in the ED. They found similar sensitivities for all the scores but reduced specificities and predictive values for the modified PAS and AS scores. As expected, the ROC curves showed a reduced AUC using the modified scores. The negative appendectomy rate was 5.2% only.

3. Conclusion

A good diagnostic score for acute appendicitis should be simple, easy to memorize, repeatable, economical, and easy to apply in an emergency setting. It should contain elements with a good statistical significance. Also, a good diagnostic score for acute appendicitis could be useful for statistical purposes by providing a more precise indexing of the disease. For example, it could be used, as a clinical indicator, in the International Classification of Diseases at a fifth digit level.

Author details

Alfredo Alvarado[1,2,3,4,5*]

*Address all correspondence to: alfredoalvara@hotmail.com

1 Alma Mater Universidad Nacional de Colombia, Bogotá, Colombia

2 Certified by the American Board of Surgeons and the American Board of Emergency Medicine, Miami, FL, USA

3 International College of Surgeons, Chicago, IL, USA

4 Society of Laparoscopic Surgeons, Chicago, USA

5 American College of Emergency Physicians, Irving TX, USA

References

[1] Alvarado A. A practical score for the early diagnostic of acute appendicitis. Annals of Emergency Medicine. 1986;**15**(5):557-564

[2] Kalan M, Talbot D, Cunliffe WJ, Rich AJ. Evaluation of the modified Alvarado score in the diagnosis of acute appendicitis: A prospective study. Annals of the Royal College of Surgeons of England. 1994;**76**:418-419

[3] Samuel M. Pediatric appendicitis score. Journal of Pediatric Surgery. 2002;**37**:877-881

[4] Andersson M, Andersson R. The appendicitis inflammatory response score: A tool for the diagnosis of acute appendicitis that outperforms the Alvarado score. World Journal of Surgery. 2008;**32**:1843-1849

[5] Chong CF, Adi MI, Thien A, et al. Development of the RIPASA score: A new appendicitis scoring system for the diagnosis of acute appendicitis. Singapore Medical Journal. 2018;**51**:220-225

[6] Chong CF, Thien A, Mackie AJA, et al. Comparison of RIPASA and Alvarado scores for the diagnosis of acute appendicitis. Singapore Medical Journal. 2011;**52**(5):340-345

[7] Khadda S, Yadav AK, Anwar A, et al. Clinical study to evaluate the RIPASA scoring system in the diagnosis of acute appendicitis. American Journal of Advanced Medical and Surgical Research. 2015;**1**(29):67-73

[8] Menon AA, Vohra LM, Khalik T, Lehri AA. Diagnostic accuracy of Alvarado score in the diagnosis of acute appendicitis. Pakistan Journal of Medical Sciences. Jan 2009;**25**(1): 118-121

[9] Pouget-Baudry Y, Mucci S, Eyssartier E. Le score clinicobiologique d'Alvarado dans la prise en charge d'une douleur de fosse iliaque droite chez l'adulte. Journal de Chirurgie Viscerale. Apr 2010;**147**(2):128-132

[10] Gaikwad V, Murchite S, Chandra S, Modi P. To evaluate the efficacy of Alvarado score and ultrasonography in acute appendicitis. Journal of Dental and Medical Sciences. Sep 2016;**15**(9):14-18

[11] Goel P, Mishra K, Sharma, et al. The study to evaluate the efficacy of Alvarado score and RIPASA score in diagnosis of acute appendicitis and correlation with intraoperative and pathological findings. Annals of Medical and Dental Research. Oct 2017;**3**(6):33-39

[12] Karami MY, Niakan H, Zabedagheri N, et al. Which one is better? Comparison of acute inflammatory response, Raja Isteri Pengiran Anak Saleha appendicitis and alvarado scoring systems. Annals of Coloproctology. Dec 2017;**33**(6):227-231

[13] Malik MU, Connelly TM, Awan F, et al. The RIPASA score is sensitive and specific for the diagnosis of acute appendicitis in a western population. International Journal of Colorectal Disease. Apr 2017;**32**(4):491-494

[14] Rodrigues W, Sindhu S. Diagnostic importance of Alvarado score in acute appendicitis. International Journal of Scientific Study. Feb 2017;**4**(11):57-60

[15] Rathod S, Ali I, Bawa A, et al. Evaluation of Raja Isteri Pengiran Anak Saleha appendicitis scoring system. Medical Journal of D.Y. Patil University. 2015;**8**:744-749

[16] Regar MK, Choudhary GS, Nogia C, et al. Comparison of Alvarado and RIPASA scoring systems in diagnosis of acute appendicitis and correlation with intraoperative and histopathological findings. International Journal of Surgery. May 2017;**4**(5):1755-1761

[17] Sinnet P, Chellappa KS, et al. Comparative study on the diagnostic accuracy of the RIPASA score over Alvarado score in the diagnosis of acute appendicitis. Journal of Evidence Based Medicine Healthcare. 2016;**3**(80):4318-4321

[18] Erdem F, Cetincünar S, Dag K, et al. Alvarado, Esleinem, Ohmann and Raja Isteri Pengiran Anak Saleha appendicitis scores for diasgnosis of acute appendicitis. World Journal of Gastroenterology. Dec 2013;**1947**(47):9057-9062

[19] Diaz-Barrientos CZ, Aquino-Gonzalez A, Heredia-Montaño M, et al. Escala RIPASA para el diagnóstico de apendicitis aguda: Comparación con la escala de Alvarado. Revista de Gastroenterología de México. Feb 2018. Article in press (5 pages)

[20] Reyes-Garcia N, Zaldivar-Ramirez FR, Cruz-Martinez R, et al. Precisión diagnóstica de la escala de RIPASA para el diagnóstico de apendicitis aguda: análisis comparativo con la escala de Alvarado modificada. Cirujano General. Apr-Jun 2012;**34**(2):101-106

[21] Golden SK, Harringa JB, Pickhard PJ, et al. Prospective evaluation of the ability of clinical scoring systems and physician-determined likelihood of appendicitis to obviate the need for CT. Emergency Medicine Journal. 2016;**0**:1-7

[22] Sammalkorpi MP, Leppaniemi P. A new adult appendicitis score improves diagnostic accuracy of acute appendicitis: A prospective study. BMC Gastroenterology. 2014;**14**:114

[23] Tzanakis NE, Stamatis P, Danulidis K, et al. New approach to accurate diagnosis of acute appendicitis. World Journal of Surgery. 2005;**29**(9):1151-1155

[24] Sigdel GS, Lakhey PJ, Mishra PR. Tzanakis score vs Alvarado score in acute appendicitis. Journal of the Nepal Medical Association. Apr-Jun 2010;**49**(178):96-99

[25] Sharma A, Gharde P, Gharbe PM, et al. European Journal of Biomedical and Pharmaceutical Sciences. 2017;**4**(4):588-559

[26] Kumar SLA, Nagaraja AL, Srinivasaiah M. Evaluation of Tzanakis scoring system in acute appendicitis. International Journal of Surgery. Oct 2017;**4**(10):3338-3343

[27] Lintula H, Kokki H, Ketunnen R, Eskelinen M. Appendicitis score for children with suspected appendicitis. A randomized clinical trial. Langenbeck's Archives of Surgery. Nov 2009;**294**(6):999-1004

[28] Konan A, Hayran M, Kilic YA. Scoring systems in the diagnosis of acute appendicitis in the elderly. Ulusal Travma ve Acil Cerrahi Dergisi. Oct 2011;**17**(5):396-400

[29] Ojuka D, Sangoro M. Alvarado vs Lintula scoring system in acute appendicitis. The Annals of African Surgery. Jan 2017;**14**(1):21-25

[30] Ohmann C, Franke C, Yang Q. Clinical benefit of a diagnostic score for appendicitis: Results of a prospective interventional study. Archives of Surgery. 1999;**134**(9):993-996

[31] Horzic M, Salamon A, Kopljar M, et al. Analysis of scores in diagnosis of acute appendicitis in women. Collegium Antropologicum. 2005;**29**(1):133-138

[32] Wilasrusmee C, Sirimbumrungwong P, et al. Developing and validating of Ramathibodi appendicitis score (RAMA-AS) for diagnosis of appendicitis in suspected appendicitis patients. World Journal of Emergency Surgery. 2017;**12**:49

[33] Khanafer et al. Test characteristics of common appendicitis scores with and without laboratory investigations: A prospective observational study. BMC Pediatrics. Aug 30, 2016; **16**(1):147

5

Molecular Pathogenesis of Gastric Adenocarcinoma

Wei Kang, Jinglin Zhang and Ka Fai To

Abstract

The incidence and mortality of gastric cancer (GC) rank top five and top three, respectively, among cancers around the world. It is an intricate malignancy caused by the reciprocity of intrinsically genetic, environmental, and host-related elements. The silent property, advanced clinical characterization, and potential heterogeneity have made GC a thorny disease with a high death rate. The increasing knowledge of the abundant genetic abnormalities regarding GC will definitely elongate the patients' survival. Scientists have been working hard to discover the myths beneath gastric tumorigenesis: novel biomarkers have been established, and cell transduction cascades have been well described. The study grouping GC into four molecular subtypes by The Cancer Genome Atlas (TCGA) broadens our horizon of GC etiologies. Knowledge regarding to the sophisticated networks in tumor microenvironment also bring new insights into the mechanisms assist GC development. In the future, people will strive for translating more research achievements into clinical utility. Successful translational medicine will lead to new methods for early GC diagnosis and precise medical strategies for individuals.

Keywords: gastric adenocarcinoma, molecular classification, pathogenesis

1. Introduction

Gastric cancer (GC) is the fifth most common malignancy worldwide and third leading cancer-related death. Because of poor diagnosis, 5-year survival rate of GC is rather low, ranging from 15 to 52% [1, 2]. The incident rates are higher in men than in women. GC contributes over 20% of morbidity and mortality to cancer all over the world annually, following lung and liver cancer, which account for 23 and 28%, respectively. In 2012, approximate 723,000 deaths and more than 950,000 new GC cases were reported worldwide. Despite the incidence of GC has been declining in the North American and most of the west European countries, GC remains a type of prevailing cancer with increasing risk in regions including

Asia, Eastern Europe, and certain areas of Latin America [3]. Particularly, adenocarcinomas, which developed from the glands of the most superficial layer or the mucosa, take up 90% of GC. The rest types of GC include mucosa-associated lymphoid tissue (MALT) lymphomas, which originate from the muscles surrounding mucosa areas of the stomach [4].

The risk factors include environmental factors, such as *Helicobacter pylori* infection, cigarettes smoking and high-salt diet, and host genetic alterations. Although the incidence of GC has shown a dramatic decrease in recent years due to *H. pylori* eradication, the overall survival is still quite poor due to its silent nature, late clinical presentation, and genetic heterogeneity. Thus, comprehensive understanding of the detailed molecular mechanisms and accurate pathogenesis of GC will improve patient outcome. Recently, several kinds of molecular classification of GC have been provided to reveal the genomic landscape of GC and decipher the crucial molecular changes. Among them, The Cancer Genome Atlas (TCGA) classification is a milestone for the molecular characterization of GC. Clinical translation of these molecular findings will provide novel strategies for early GC detection and promote precision therapies for GC patients.

2. The risk factors of GC

GC is defined as a tumor with multifactorial etiologies. Environmental alteration and genetic factors play major roles in GC, particularly, virus infection, dietary habits, and lifestyles are recognized to be critical factors.

H. pylori is a common human pathogen, contributing to both malignant and benign diseases. Among all the risk factors of GC, *H. pylori* is considered to be the most predominant factor, up to 80% of GC cases are led by *H. pylori* infection. At least 660,000 new diagnoses are making annually [5, 6]. Data in western countries indicated that *H. pylori* is a major risk factor for only non-cardia GC instead of cardia GC [5]. It has been noted that the death number of GC is decreasing in many developed regions, partially related to eradication therapy and improved living condition in certain populations and regions [7]. Given the worldwide aging problem and the migration trend of people from high to low prevalence regions, the mortality is very likely to increase in the future [8]. *H. pylori* infection alone is not sufficient to trigger GC. Chiba et al. suggested *H. pylori* infection contributed to GC development via two potential mechanisms, either caused chronic inflammation or directly acted on epithelial cells [9]. In general, *H. pylori* colonizes the gastric mucosal epithelium and induces chronic inflammation at the beginning of infection, while persistent inflammation resulted in GC [10, 11]. Cytokines and chemokines produced by the tumor microenvironment facilitate cell proliferation and migration, and keep cells from apoptosis and immune detection [12]. Cytokines released by different cell sources have been described as suggestive indicators in the progression of GC. The serum level of Tumor necrosis factor-α (TNF--α) in GC was found greatly reduced, however, levels of TNF-α in stage III or IV GC patients showed a significant elevation when compared to levels in earlier stage patients [13]. Besides, the secretion of Interleukin-1 (IL-1) contributes to tumor cell proliferation and progression. In addition, IL-6, IL-10, and Transforming growth factor-β (TGF-β) improve survival of GC cells by promoting cell invasion and suppression of antitumor immunity. IL-11, IL-17, IL-18, IL-22, and chemokines secreted by a specific cell type also improve the progression of GC [14]. Major types of virulence factors of *H. pylori* include cytotoxin VacA, the type IV secretion system (T4SS), and the CagA effector protein. These factors are associated with multiple cellular responses, such as induction of oxidative stress and epithelial barrier disruption, in various model systems [15].

Epstein-Barr virus (EBV), also termed as human herpesvirus 4 (HHV-4), is one of the most prevalent viruses in humans. EBV was the first virus identified in human carcinoma in 1964 [16]. Approximately 95% of adults in the world are infected by EBV due to the positive detection of serological EBV markers. EBV infection may not cause severe symptoms and disease. After primary infection, EBV establishes a carrier state called latent stage. However, latent EBV infection could subsequently become high-risk oncogenic factors associated with human malignancies. EBV has been known as another significant pathogen exists in GC cells. According to worldwide data, EBV-associated GC (EBVaGC) accounts for 10%, in average, of total GC cases. Most of the EBVaGC cases were epithelial tumors, while lymphoepithelioma-like carcinomas take up 90% of the rest rare EBVaGC cases. EBVaGC presents distinct clinic properties, such as predominance among male and younger individuals and predominant proximal stomach location [17]. EBV infection can be achieved by two different entry mechanisms, either via B cell entry or fusion with epithelial cells directly [18, 19]. EBVaGC occurs in the upper and middle stomach in the majority. Fukayama et al. indicated the tumor distribution in the stomach, with the proportion that 58% in the cardia, 33% in the body, and 9% in the antrum [20, 21]. They also depicted the appearance of EBVaGC as ulcerated or saucer-like, with obvious thickened gastric wall. Moreover, the lymph node was less frequently involved during early stage within the submucosa. These characteristics are proposed to be favorable prognosis indicators. Histological studies provide evidence that immune cell infiltration was a feature of EBVaGC. For instance, infiltrating lymphocytes, containing EBV-specific cytotoxic T cells, communicate with carcinoma cells directly, in the opposite, cytokine IL-1β was upregulated to recruit noninfiltrating lymphocytes against this cell-cell contact [22, 23]. Therefore, in EBVaGC, immune responses in tumor microenvironment also accompany with the progression of EBVaGC [24].

Dietary factors: dietary risks, including salty and spicy food intake, cigarettes smoking, frequent coffee, and high-temperature drinking habits are positively associated with GC. Intriguingly, excess salt intake showed susceptibility to EBVaGC and *H. pylori*-induced GC. Habitual excess salt intake was suggested to progressively increase the risk across consumption levels of GC via a meta-analysis [25]. The association between salty food intake and *H. pylori* infection was also evaluated in a cross-sectional study of 634-middle age male cohort. The result supported habitual salt-rich Japanese food intake was prevalent in *H. pylori*-induced GC cases [26]. It is probably due to the increase of *H. pylori* colonization and persistent infection [27]. Besides salty food intake, Camargo et al. indicated that smoking was strongly associated with EBVaGC by a case-case comparison between EBV-positive tumors and EBV-negative tumors [28]. Although alcohol drinking was a suggestive risk factor of GC, heavy alcohol drinking, rather than moderate alcoholic drinks, was significantly correlated with GC development [29, 30].

3. Molecular classification and pathogenies of GC

Up to 90% of stomach malignancies are adenocarcinomas. Non-Hodgkin's lymphomas and gastrointestinal stromal tumor (GIST) make up most of the remaining 10% [31]. Even though infrequently, adenosquamous, squamous, and undifferentiated carcinomas also occur. In regard to clinical diagnosis, several pathological characterization varied from time to time. Several histological classification systems for gastric adenocarcinoma have been described, but the most frequently used are those of the World Health Organization (WHO) and Lauren [32]. In the World Health Organization (WHO) classification, there are 10 histological types [33]. The Lauren classification is commonly applied and it makes the distinction between intestinal and diffuse types. The intestinal GC consists of cohesive neoplastic cells forming gland-like structures while the diffuse type has lost cell cohesion and resulting in diffuse discohesive cellular infiltration [31]. Men and elderly are more likely to suffer intestinal type, whereas diffuse type carcinomas are relatively more common among the younger population with an equal male-to-female ratio [32]. Recently, a project named The Cancer Genome Atlas (TCGA) has proposed a brand new classification, in which GC is grouped by four subtypes: EBV-positive (EBV), microsatellite instability (MSI), genomically stable [34], and chromosomal instability [35, 36].

According to previous studies, about 9% of GC cases are infected by EBV [37]. All the EBV-positive GCs harbor the property of CpG island methylator phenotype (CIMP) [36, 38, 39]. EBV-positive tumors exhibited a higher incidence of whole-genomic DNA hypermethylation than any molecular subtypes. The genes with promoter hypermethylation showed most differentially silenced expression in EBV-associated GC [36]. Moreover, PI(3)-kinase inhibition was also strongly detected in EBV-positive GC, which offered a new method for the evaluation of this subtype [36]. The most highly transcribed EBV viral, message RNAs (mRNAs) and microRNAs (miRNAs), fell within the BamH1A region of the viral genome and showed similar expression patterns across tumors [36]. The mutation rate of PIK3CA is exclusively high in EBV-positive gastric cancer compared with other molecular subtypes. The mutation rate of PIK3CA in this subtype is about 80 and 68% of the mutations belongs to recurrent mutation in this dataset. In contrast, in other molecular subtypes, the mutation rates of PIK3CA are from 3 to 42%. So, this result provides a hint that using PI3K inhibitor might have the clinical therapeutic potential for this kind of molecular subtype.

The next subtypes of GC are abundant in MSI, which display increased mutation rates (in major histocompatibility complex class I genes, including B2M and HLA-B) and hypermethylation (containing hypermethylation at the *MLH1* promoter). The most obvious difference between EBV-CIMP (CpG island methylator phenotype) and MSI-associated gastric-CIMP methylation profiles is that all EBV-positive gastric tumors show promoter hypermethylation of *CDKN2A* ($p16^{INK4A}$), but the *MLH1* hypermethylation was only detected in MSI-associated CIMP [38].

In genomically stable subtype, *RHOA* mutation was detected [36]. When binding with Guanosine-5'-triphosphate (GTP), RHOA behaves through a great number of downstream effectors, such as ROCK1, mDIA, and protein kinase N. This will lead to actin-myosin-dependent cell contractility and cellular motility [40, 41] and activation of STAT3 to promote carcinogenesis [42, 43]. Except from activating mDia or ROCK1, the *RHOA* mutation Y42C has been confirmed to attenuate the activationof protein kinase N. Because RHOA is strongly associated with cell motility, the *RHOA* mutations might contribute to the invasive growth patterns. In diffuse type GC or genomically stable GC, the lack of cellular cohesion is a hallmark for this diffuse phenotype. Apart from RHOA mutation, an inter-chromosomal translocation called CLDN18-ARHGAP26 fusion gene was identified. ARHGAP26 is a GTPase-activating protein that converts GTP-RHO to GDP-RHO and it is been reported to facilitate cellular motility. CLDN18 is a tight junction component that involves in cell adhesion. This fusion gene thus was thought to correlate with cell metastasis in this kind of molecular subtype.

With the somatic copy-number aberrations (SCNAs), the last group of GC was clustered as CIN subtype. In this subtype, a bunch of genes shows dysregulated, such as *TP53* mutations (in 71% of tumors) as well as *CDH1* somatic mutations (enriched in the genomically stable subtype, about 37% of cases).

4. The dysregulated miRNAs involved in GC

MicroRNAs (miRNAs) are one predominant category of small (roughly 20–30 nucleotides) non-coding RNAs that participate in gene expression and control [44]. Their effects are mostly lead to the degradation of message RNAs (mRNAs) or inhibitory of the translations, and subsequently affect a series of biological behaviors of cells, such as inflammation, cell proliferation, apoptosis and differentiation. In the nucleus, together with its cofactor Pasha (DGCR8), the RNase III enzyme Drosha cut out primary miRNA transcripts into a fragment of approximately 60 nucleotides named precursor miRNAs (pre-miRNAs), and initiate the biogenesis of miRNAs [45]. A cytoplasmic RNase III called Dicer will be responsible for the further processing of the pre-miRNAs and makes them mature after they are transported to the cytoplasm [46, 47]. A mature miRNA, with the length of about 18–24 nucleotides, is single-stranded, which can sometimes aim at multiple targets. These mature miRNAs always bind to the complementary sequences of targeted mRNAs directly to make mRNAs degrade or bind directly to 3′-untranslated regions (3′-UTR) of mRNAs to decrease their translation, so that miRNAs can exert their effects on regulating certain gene expression [44, 48]. Accordingly, miRNAs regulate at least 30% of genes of human as it is estimated [49].

In other words, miRNAs are capable of acting as a switch to control genes related to cell proliferation and apoptosis under pathogenic circumstances, consequently, they may have a chance to be involved in both cancer initiation and progression. It seems that no matter how clear the mechanism of malignancy behaviors or an effective therapy that might prevent tumorigenesis from the beginning, an increasing knowledge of these miRNAs is crucial. During the physiological periods, miRNAs present or absent in proper time of different stage of lives. However, they are produced abnormally in tumors, that the levels of some miRNAs are highly detected while some are lower or even none. Hence, those which are upregulated called onco-miRs, whereas the downregulated ones called tumor-suppressive miRNAs. As the names suggested, genes controlled by onco-miRs are oncogenes whose products may promote tumor cells in many aspects, whereas the opposite site of genes is tumor suppressive, which plays a role of inhibitor among the initiation or development of tumors (e.g., miR-15a and miR-16-1, which target a member of Hippo pathway called YAP1, are downregulated in GC) [50]. Thus, identifying the target genes of these miRNAs is crucial and it may lead us to a better understanding of the miRNAs themselves.

For example, miR-21 was the first miRNA which was influenced by *H. pylori*. In tissues of both GC and *H. Pylori* infection, it was highly detected [51, 52]. Several data have reported that this miRNA can be used as a biomarker in GC diagnosis in the clinic [53–55]. And most recently, a research conducted in China suggested this miR-21 to be a GC biomarker in both diagnosis and prognosis, for the reason that, besides the high levels found in tumor tissues compared with the normal ones, miR-21 was revealed to be associated with poor survivals in clinical patients [56]. Behind the phenomena, the molecular mechanism is still unclear in GC. In other types of cancer, however, such as colorectal cancer, miR-21 decreased the tumor suppressor protein programmed cell death 4 (PDCD4) and exhibited an oncogenic function [57]. Additionally, in nonsmall cell lung carcinoma, miR-21 was found to deregulate PTEN, a tumor suppressor, to promote carcinogenesis [58].

5. The tumor microenvironment and gastric carcinogenesis

More and more evidence supported the idea that not only malignant GC cells, but also those nonmalignant cells involved in the tumor microenvironment play indispensable roles throughout GC pathogenesis. Generally, nonmalignant cells participate in various mechanisms related to GC development, such as stromal interactions, angiogenesis, and some immune responses.

Stromal components, including fibroblasts and extracellular matrix (ECM) adjacent to cancer cells, create a suitable environment for GC development. Stromal fibroblasts are known to play a central role in tumor microenvironment by interacting with cancer cells [59, 60]. However, other than ordinary fibroblasts, cancer-associated fibroblasts (CAFs) undergo a phenotypic change into myofibroblasts. Also, CAFs exhibit distinct gene expression patents that pertain to aberrant cell growth, focal adhesion, and ECM remodeling [61]. The remodeling ECM promotes the survival ability and distant colonization cancer cells by synthesizing components, such as type I and type III collagens, fibronectins, tenascin, and versican [62–64], as well as proteases like urokinase, plasminogen activator, fibroblast activation protein (FAP), and matrix metalloproteinases (MMPs) [65–67]. These characteristics are usually associated with poor prognostics. Moreover, tumor-related stromal fibroblasts secrete small molecules, such as IL-6 to stimulate cell growth, as well as factors associated with TGF-β signaling, triggering epithelial-mesenchymal transition (EMT) [68–70].

Angiogenesis is also a pivotal process contributes to tumor progression. Cell population in GC tumor microenvironment regulates the density and architecture of new blood vessels by stimulating the proliferation and differentiation of myofibroblasts and vascular endothelial cells [71, 72]. The growing number of new vessels was reported to facilitate GC metastasis [73, 74]. To promote angiogenesis, GC cells provide numerous angiogenic factors, including VEGF, FGF-2, CXCL1, and Ang-2, to microenvironment [75–78]. It has been noted that high level of VEGF-A contributed to endothelium-dependent angiogenesis. VEGF-A signaling increased both the new blood vessel number and permeability in GC [79]. VEGF-A strongly promotes the angiogenesis and aggressive phenotype of human intestinal-type GC [80]. Bevacizumab is a specific antibody against VEGF-A, and dominantly regulates normal and pathological angiogenesis. Clinical trials of bevacizumab in phase II advanced GC suggested a satisfied curative effect [81]. Unfortunately, in the randomized phase III Avastin in Gastric Cancer (AVAGAST) study, the combination of chemotherapy and bevacizumab did not show a better overall survival extension in the first-line treatment when compared to advanced GC patients, who only subjected chemotherapy [82]. Intriguingly, REGARD and RAINBOW trials using VEGFR2 targeting antibody ramucirumab have also shown a significant increase in the overall survival of patients with advanced GC [83]. It can be partially explained by the geographical differences of GC patients.

Immune reactivity in GC development is based on various types of immune cells in different stages [84]. First, in eliminating stage, macrophages and dendritic cells recruit to secrete chemokines and cytokines, such as IL-12 and IFN-γ, to phagocytize and remove apoptotic cancer cells [85]. Cancer cells survived from elimination subsequently under equilibrium stage and adapted to immune-suppression. The number of tumor-infiltrating lymphocytes (TILs) was noted as independent predictors to evaluate lymph node metastasis and GC patient survival in this stage. Interestingly, TILs exert either oncogenic or tumor-suppressive influence in GC cells, attributing to their unique functions. In a recent report, tumor-associated macrophages with high levels of CD163 expression exhibited aggressive characteristics and expression of cancer stem cell markers in recurrent GC cases. CD163$^+$ macrophages might, therefore, related to independent worse prognosis [86]. T-lymphocyte subsets are also significant cell types associated with both early onset of tumor and tumor progression. It has been reported that the high ratio of CD8$^+$ cytotoxic TILs/FOXP3$^+$ regulatory T cells (Treg) correlated with high overall survival rate and good prognosis, especially in MSI gastric cancer [87, 88]. Eventually, cancer cells escape from immune responses.

Immunogenicity could be blunted by releasing cytokines including TGF-β, TNF-α, and IL-10. Therefore, cancer cells can evade the detection by immune effectors in the tumor microenvironment [89]. PD-1 is one of the most important receptors expressed by T cells and monocytes. PD-1 negatively regulates the effectors by binding to its ligands PD-L1 and PD-L2. Blocking PD-1/PD-L1 has been suggested as a promising immune-therapeutic option [90, 91]. The relationship between PD-L1 level and prognosis remains under debate, however, a recent meta-analysis pooled all present data and suggested PD-L1 to be a valuable prognostic indicator of GC patients by dividing patients into different groups [92].

Collectively, tumor microenvironment composed of multiple subjects, such as tumor stromal fibroblasts, lymphocytes, and angiogenic factors. All these components cooperate together, configuring a context for GC development.

6. Conclusion

There is still a large realm of the unknown area about GC pathogenies even though the related research studies have been going deeper and our horizon has been broadened in the past few years. Epigenetically, we are seeking to unravel the mechanisms of gastric tumorigenesis affected by chromatin remodeling. Besides, there are miRNAs, lncRNAs, and some other classic molecules that are involved in GC development, which requires a more detailed investigation regarding these aspects. The most crucially and urgently, we are struggling to explore specific and precise therapies for patients who are suffering or likely to suffer from GC, especially genomically stable GC (a type of GC with a high mortality).

When it comes to the novel small entities, there are even more issues waiting to be addressed, such as how lncRNAs interact with chromatin alterations during gastric carcinogenesis. Moreover, in addition to *H. pylori* and EBV, scientists have identified a wild variety of bacteria in the stomach through DNA sequencing. These uncultivatable bacteria have formed a complicated community and there are few clues about how they interact with *H. pylori* and host immunity during GC initiation and progression. In the early detection field, molecular findings may facilitate new approaches for diagnosing GC early, by identifying high-risk potential sufferers via the molecular features of precancerous lesions. Finally, therapeutic strategies need to be designed precisely for each GC subtypes, according to their somatic driver change of genome or tumor-associated cell compartments, such as stromal cells and tumor-infiltrating immune cells.

Acknowledgements

This work is supported by the General Research Fund (RGC Reference No. CUHK14114414 and CUHK14110016) from the Research Grants Council of Hong Kong.

Author details

Wei Kang*, Jinglin Zhang and Ka Fai To

*Address all correspondence to: weikang@cuhk.edu.hk

Department of Anatomical and Cellular Pathology, State Key Laboratory of Oncology in South China, State Key Laboratory of Digestive Diseases, The Chinese University of Hong Kong, Hong Kong SAR, PR China

References

[1] Marchet A, Mocellin S, Ambrosi A, Morgagni P, Vittimberga G, Roviello F, Marrelli D, de Manzoni G, Minicozzi A, Coniglio A, Tiberio G, Pacelli F, Rosa F, Nitti D. Validation of the new AJCC TNM staging system for gastric cancer in a large cohort of patients (n = 2,155): Focus on the T category. European Journal of Surgical Oncology. 2011;**37**:779-785

[2] Nashimoto A, Akazawa K, Isobe Y, Miyashiro I, Katai H, Kodera Y, Tsujitani S, Seto Y, Furukawa H, Oda I, Ono H, Tanabe S, Kaminishi M. Gastric cancer treated in 2002 in Japan: 2009 annual report of the JGCA nationwide registry. Gastric Cancer. 2013;**16**:1-27

[3] International Agency for Research on Cancer. GLOBOCAN Database. IARC; 2008

[4] Karimi P, Islami F, Anandasabapathy S, Freedman ND, Kamangar F. Gastric cancer: Descriptive epidemiology, risk factors, screening, and prevention. Cancer Epidemiology Biomarkers & Prevention. 2014;**23**:700-713

[5] Helicobacter and Cancer Collaborative Group. Gastric cancer and Helicobacter pylori: a combined analysis of 12 case control studies nested within prospective cohorts. Gut. 2001;**49**:347-353

[6] de Martel C, Ferlay J, Franceschi S, Vignat J, Bray F, Forman D, Plummer M. Global burden of cancers attributable to infections in 2008: A review and synthetic analysis. Lancet Oncology. 2012;**13**:607-615

[7] O'Connor A, O'Morain CA, Ford AC. Population screening and treatment of Helicobacter pylori infection. Nature Reviews Gastroenterology & Hepatology. 2017;**14**:230-240

[8] Yeh JM, Goldie SJ, Kuntz KM, Ezzati M. Effects of Helicobacter pylori infection and smoking on gastric cancer incidence in China: A population-level analysis of trends and projections. Cancer Causes Control. 2009;**20**:2021-2029

[9] Chiba T, Marusawa H, Seno H, Watanabe N. Mechanism for gastric cancer development by Helicobacter pylori infection. Journal of Gastroenterology and Hepatology. 2008;**23**:1175-1181

[10] Correa P. Human gastric carcinogenesis: A multistep and multifactorial process—First American Cancer Society Award Lecture on Cancer Epidemiology and Prevention. Cancer Research. 1992;**52**:6735-6740

[11] Sheibani S, Mahmoudian RA, Abbaszadegan MR, Chamani J, Memar B, Gholamin M. Expression analysis of matrix metalloproteinase-13 in human gastric cancer in the presence of Helicobacter Pylori infection. Cancer Biomarkers. 2017;**18**(4):349-356

[12] Hanahan D, Weinberg RA. Hallmarks of cancer: The next generation. Cell. 2011;**144**: 646-674

[13] Wu CW, Chi CW, Hsieh MC, Chao MF, Lui WY, P'Eng FK. Serum tumor necrosis factor in patients with gastric cancer. Anticancer Research. 1998;**18**:1597-1599

[14] Bagheri V, Memar B, Momtazi AA, Sahebkar A, Gholamin M, Abbaszadegan MR. Cytokine networks and their association with Helicobacter pylori infection in gastric carcinoma. Journal of Cellular Physiology. 2017;**9999**:1-13

[15] Naumann M, Sokolova O, Tegtmeyer N, Backert S. Helicobacter pylori: A paradigm pathogen for subverting host cell signal transmission. Trends in Microbiology. 2017;**25**:316-328

[16] Epstein MA, Achong BG, Barr YM. Virus particles in cultured lymphoblasts from Burkitt's lymphoma. Lancet. 1964;**1**:702-703

[17] Fukayama M, Hino R, Uozaki H. Epstein–Barr virus and gastric carcinoma: Virus–host interactions leading to carcinoma. Cancer Science. 2008;**99**:1726-1733

[18] Tsang CM, Deng W, Yip YL, Zeng MS, Lo KW, Tsao SW. Epstein-Barr virus infection and persistence in nasopharyngeal epithelial cells. Chinese Journal of Cancer. 2014;**33**:549-555

[19] Tsai MH, Raykova A, Klinke O, Bernhardt K, Gartner K, Leung CS, Geletneky K, Sertel S, Munz C, Feederle R, Delecluse HJ. Spontaneous lytic replication and epitheliotropism define an Epstein-Barr virus strain found in carcinomas. Cell Reports. 2013;**5**:458-470

[20] Abe H, Maeda D, Hino R, Otake Y, Isogai M, Ushiku AS, Matsusaka K, Kunita A, Ushiku T, Uozaki H, Tateishi Y, Hishima T, Iwasaki Y, Ishikawa S, Fukayama M. ARID1A expression loss in gastric cancer: Pathway-dependent roles with and without Epstein-Barr virus infection and microsatellite instability. Virchows Archiv. 2012;**461**:367-377

[21] Abe H, Kaneda A, Fukayama M. Epstein-Barr Virus-Associated gastric carcinoma: Use of host cell machineries and somatic gene mutations. Pathobiology. 2015;**82**:212-223

[22] Chong JM, Sakuma K, Sudo M, Osawa T, Ohara E, Uozaki H, Shibahara J, Kuroiwa K, Tominaga S, Hippo Y, Aburatani H, Funata N, Fukayama M. Interleukin-1beta expression in human gastric carcinoma with Epstein-Barr virus infection. Journal of Virology. 2002;**76**:6825-6831

[23] Fukayama M. Epstein-Barr virus and gastric carcinoma. Pathology International. 2010; **60**:337-350

[24] Cho J, Kang MS, Kim KM. Epstein-Barr Virus-Associated gastric carcinoma and specific features of the accompanying immune response. Journal of Gastric Cancer. 2016;**16**:1-7

[25] D'Elia L, Rossi G, Ippolito R, Cappuccio FP, Strazzullo P. Habitual salt intake and risk of gastric cancer: A meta-analysis of prospective studies. Clinical Nutrition. 2012;**31**:489-498

[26] Tsugane S, Tei Y, Takahashi T, Watanabe S, Sugano K. Salty food intake and risk of Helicobacter pylori infection. Japanese Journal of Cancer Research. 1994;**85**:474-478

[27] Fox JG, Dangler CA, Taylor NS, King A, Koh TJ, Wang TC. High-salt diet induces gastric epithelial hyperplasia and parietal cell loss, and enhances *Helicobacter pylori* colonization in C57BL/6 mice. Cancer Research. 1999;**59**:4823-4828

[28] Camargo MC, Koriyama C, Matsuo K, Kim WH, Herrera-Goepfert R, Liao LM, Yu J, Carrasquilla G, Sung JJ, Alvarado-Cabrero I, Lissowska J, Meneses-Gonzalez F, Yatabe Y, Ding T, Hu N, Taylor PR, Morgan DR, Gulley ML, Torres J, Akiba S, Rabkin CS. Case-case comparison of smoking and alcohol risk associations with Epstein-Barr virus-positive gastric cancer. International Journal of Cancer. 2014;**134**:948-953

[29] Tramacere I, Negri E, Pelucchi C, Bagnardi V, Rota M, Scotti L, Islami F, Corrao G, La Vecchia C, Boffetta P. A meta-analysis on alcohol drinking and gastric cancer risk. Annals of Oncology. 2012;**23**:28-36

[30] Everatt R, Tamosiunas A, Kuzmickiene I, Virviciute D, Radisauskas R, Reklaitiene R, Milinaviciene E. Alcohol consumption and risk of gastric cancer: A cohort study of men in Kaunas, Lithuania, with up to 30 years follow-up. BMC Cancer. 2012;**12**:475

[31] Kelley JR, Duggan JM. Gastric cancer epidemiology and risk factors. Journal of Clinical Epidemiology. 2003;**56**:1-9

[32] Lauren P. The two histological main types of gastric carcinoma: Diffuse and So-Called Intestinal-Type carcinoma. An attempt at a Histo-Clinical classification. Acta Pathologica et Microbiologica Scandinavica. 1965;**64**:31-49

[33] Brunicardi FC, Schwartz SI. Schwartz's Principles of Surgery. 8th ed. New York: McGraw-Hill, Medical Pub. Division; 2005

[34] Nguyen LH, Robinton DA, Seligson MT, Wu L, Li L, Rakheja D, Comerford SA, Ramezani S, Sun X, Parikh MS, Yang EH, Powers JT, Shinoda G, Shah SP, Hammer RE, Daley GQ, Zhu H. Lin28b is sufficient to drive liver cancer and necessary for its maintenance in murine models. Cancer Cell. 2014;**26**:248-261

[35] Finkielstain GP, Forcinito P, Lui JC, Barnes KM, Marino R, Makaroun S, Nguyen V, Lazarus JE, Nilsson O, Baron J. An extensive genetic program occurring during postnatal growth in multiple tissues. Endocrinology. 2009;**150**:1791-1800

[36] The Cancer Genome Atlas Research Network. Comprehensive molecular characterization of gastric adenocarcinoma. Nature. 2014;**513**:202-209

[37] Murphy G, Pfeiffer R, Camargo MC, Rabkin CS. Meta-analysis shows that prevalence of Epstein-Barr virus-positive gastric cancer differs based on sex and anatomic location. Gastroenterology. 2009;**137**:824-833

[38] Matsusaka K, Kaneda A, Nagae G, Ushiku T, Kikuchi Y, Hino R, Uozaki H, Seto Y, Takada K, Aburatani H, Fukayama M. Classification of Epstein-Barr virus-positive gastric cancers by definition of DNA methylation epigenotypes. Cancer Research. 2011;**71**:7187-7197

[39] Toyota M, Ahuja N, Suzuki H, Itoh F, Ohe-Toyota M, Imai K, Baylin SB, Issa JP. Aberrant methylation in gastric cancer associated with the CpG island methylator phenotype. Cancer Research. 1999;**59**:5438-5442

[40] Ridley AJ, Schwartz MA, Burridge K, Firtel RA, Ginsberg MH, Borisy G, Parsons JT, Horwitz AR. Cell migration: Integrating signals from front to back. Science. 2003;**302**: 1704-1709

[41] Thumkeo D, Watanabe S, Narumiya S. Physiological roles of Rho and Rho effectors in mammals. European Journal of Cell Biology. 2013;**92**:303-315

[42] Aznar S, Valeron PF, del Rincon SV, Perez LF, Perona R, Lacal JC. Simultaneous tyrosine and serine phosphorylation of STAT3 transcription factor is involved in Rho A GTPase oncogenic transformation. Molecular Biology of the Cell. 2001;**12**:3282-3294

[43] Yu H, Jove R. The STATs of cancer—New molecular targets come of age. Nature Reviews Cancer. 2004;**4**:97-105

[44] Carthew RW, Sontheimer EJ. Origins and mechanisms of miRNAs and siRNAs. Cell. 2009;**136**:642-655

[45] Lee Y, Han J, Yeom KH, Jin H, Kim VN. Drosha in primary microRNA processing. Cold Spring Harbor Symposia on Quantitative Biology. 2006;**71**:51-57

[46] Han J, Lee Y, Yeom KH, Kim YK, Jin H, Kim VN. The Drosha-DGCR8 complex in primary microRNA processing. Genes & Development. 2004;**18**:3016-3027

[47] Lund E, Guttinger S, Calado A, Dahlberg JE, Kutay U. Nuclear export of microRNA precursors. Science. 2004;**303**:95-98

[48] Bartel DP. MicroRNAs: Genomics, biogenesis, mechanism, and function. Cell. 2004;**116**: 281-297

[49] Miranda KC, Huynh T, Tay Y, Ang YS, Tam WL, Thomson AM, Lim B, Rigoutsos I. A pattern-based method for the identification of MicroRNA binding sites and their corresponding heteroduplexes. Cell. 2006;**126**:1203-1217

[50] Kang W, Tong JH, Lung RW, Dong Y, Zhao J, Liang Q, Zhang L, Pan Y, Yang W, Pang JC, Cheng AS, Yu J, To KF. Targeting of YAP1 by microRNA-15a and microRNA-16-1 exerts tumor suppressor function in gastric adenocarcinoma. Molecular Cancer. 2015;**14**:52

[51] Volinia S, Calin GA, Liu CG, Ambs S, Cimmino A, Petrocca F, Visone R, Iorio M, Roldo C, Ferracin M, Prueitt RL, Yanaihara N, Lanza G, Scarpa A, Vecchione A, Negrini M, Harris CC, Croce CM. A microRNA expression signature of human solid tumors defines cancer gene targets. Proceedings of the National Academy of Sciences of the United States of America. 2006;**103**:2257-2261

[52] Zhang Z, Li Z, Gao C, Chen P, Chen J, Liu W, Xiao S, Lu H. miR-21 plays a pivotal role in gastric cancer pathogenesis and progression. Laboratory Investigation; A Journal of Technical Methods and Pathology. 2008;**88**:1358-1366

[53] Shiotani A, Murao T, Kimura Y, Matsumoto H, Kamada T, Kusunoki H, Inoue K, Uedo N, Iishi H, Haruma K. Identification of serum miRNAs as novel non-invasive biomarkers for detection of high risk for early gastric cancer. British Journal of Cancer. 2013;**109**:2323-2330

[54] Li BS, Zhao YL, Guo G, Li W, Zhu ED, Luo X, Mao XH, Zou QM, Yu PW, Zuo QF, Li N, Tang B, Liu KY, Xiao B. Plasma microRNAs, miR-223, miR-21 and miR-218, as novel potential biomarkers for gastric cancer detection. Plos One. 2012;**7**:e41629

[55] Cui L, Zhang X, Ye G, Zheng T, Song H, Deng H, Xiao B, Xia T, Yu X, Le Y, Guo J. Gastric juice MicroRNAs as potential biomarkers for the screening of gastric cancer. Cancer. 2013;**119**:1618-1626

[56] Wang D, Fan Z, Liu F, Zuo J. Hsa-miR-21 and Hsa-miR-29 in tissue as potential diagnostic and prognostic biomarkers for gastric cancer. Cellular Physiology and Biochemistry: International Journal of Experimental Cellular Physiology, Biochemistry, and Pharmacology. 2015;**37**:1454-1462

[57] Asangani IA, Rasheed SA, Nikolova DA, Leupold JH, Colburn NH, Post S, Allgayer H. MicroRNA-21 (miR-21) post-transcriptionally downregulates tumor suppressor Pdcd4 and stimulates invasion, intravasation and metastasis in colorectal cancer. Oncogene. 2008;**27**:2128-2136

[58] Zhang JG, Wang JJ, Zhao F, Liu Q, Jiang K, Yang GH. MicroRNA-21 (miR-21) represses tumor suppressor PTEN and promotes growth and invasion in non-small cell lung cancer (NSCLC). Clinica Chimica Acta; International Journal of Clinical Chemistry. 2010;**411**:846-852

[59] Orimo A, Gupta PB, Sgroi DC, Arenzana-Seisdedos F, Delaunay T, Naeem R, Carey VJ, Richardson AL, Weinberg RA. Stromal fibroblasts present in invasive human breast carcinomas promote tumor growth and angiogenesis through elevated SDF-1/CXCL12 secretion. Cell. 2005;**121**:335-348

[60] Pietras K, Ostman A. Hallmarks of cancer: Interactions with the tumor stroma. Experimental Cell Research. 2010;**316**:1324-1331

[61] Bhowmick NA, Neilson EG, Moses HL. Stromal fibroblasts in cancer initiation and progression. Nature. 2004;**432**:332-337

[62] Lagace R, Grimaud JA, Schurch W, Seemayer TA. Myofibroblastic stromal reaction in carcinoma of the breast: Variations of collagenous matrix and structural glycoproteins. Virchows Archiv A Pathological Anatomy and Histology. 1985;**408**:49-59

[63] Brown LF, Guidi AJ, Schnitt SJ, Van De Water L, Iruela-Arispe ML, Yeo TK, Tognazzi K, Dvorak HF. Vascular stroma formation in carcinoma in situ, invasive carcinoma, and metastatic carcinoma of the breast. Clinical Cancer Research. 1999;**5**:1041-1056

[64] Hanamura N, Yoshida T, Matsumoto E, Kawarada Y, Sakakura T. Expression of fibronectin and tenascin-C mRNA by myofibroblasts, vascular cells and epithelial cells in human colon adenomas and carcinomas. International Journal of Cancer. 1997;**73**:10-15

[65] Park JE, Lenter MC, Zimmermann RN, Garin-Chesa P, Old LJ, Rettig WJ. Fibroblast activation protein, a dual specificity serine protease expressed in reactive human tumor stromal fibroblasts. Journal of Biological Chemistry. 1999;**274**:36505-36512

[66] DeClerck YA. Interactions between tumour cells and stromal cells and proteolytic modification of the extracellular matrix by metalloproteinases in cancer. European Journal of Cancer. 2000;**36**:1258-1268

[67] Huang WB, Zhou XJ, Chen JY, Zhang LH, Meng K, Ma HH, Lu ZF. CD10-positive stromal cells in gastric carcinoma: Correlation with invasion and metastasis. Japanese Journal of Clinical Oncology. 2005;**35**:245-250

[68] Wu X, Tao P, Zhou Q, Li J, Yu Z, Wang X, Li C, Yan M, Zhu Z, Liu B, Su L. IL-6 secreted by cancer-associated fibroblasts promotes epithelial-mesenchymal transition and metastasis of gastric cancer via JAK2/STAT3 signaling pathway. Oncotarget. 2017;**8**:20741-20750

[69] Landskron G, De la Fuente M, Thuwajit P, Thuwajit C, Hermoso MA. Chronic inflammation and cytokines in the tumor microenvironment. Journal of Immunology Research. 2014;**2014**:149185

[70] Huang L, Wu RL, Xu AM. Epithelial-mesenchymal transition in gastric cancer. American Journal of Translational Research. 2015;**7**:2141-2158

[71] Direkze NC, Hodivala-Dilke K, Jeffery R, Hunt T, Poulsom R, Oukrif D, Alison MR, Wright NA. Bone marrow contribution to tumor-associated myofibroblasts and fibroblasts. Cancer Research. 2004;**64**:8492-8495

[72] Matsumoto T, Kuroda R, Mifune Y, Kawamoto A, Shoji T, Miwa M, Asahara T, Kurosaka M. Circulating endothelial/skeletal progenitor cells for bone regeneration and healing. Bone. 2008;**43**:434-439

[73] Takahashi Y, Cleary KR, Mai M, Kitadai Y, Bucana CD, Ellis LM. Significance of vessel count and vascular endothelial growth factor and its receptor (KDR) in intestinal-type gastric cancer. Clinical Cancer Research. 1996;**2**:1679-1684

[74] Chung HW, Lim JB. Role of the tumor microenvironment in the pathogenesis of gastric carcinoma. World Journal of Gastroenterology. 2014;**20**:1667-1680

[75] Maeda K, Chung YS, Ogawa Y, Takatsuka S, Kang SM, Ogawa M, Sawada T, Sowa M. Prognostic value of vascular endothelial growth factor expression in gastric carcinoma. Cancer. 1996;**77**:858-863

[76] Tanimoto H, Yoshida K, Yokozaki H, Yasui W, Nakayama H, Ito H, Ohama K, Tahara E. Expression of basic fibroblast growth factor in human gastric carcinomas. Virchows Archiv. B, Cell Pathology Including Molecular Pathology. 1991;**61**:263-267

[77] Kasashima H, Yashiro M, Nakamae H, Kitayama K, Masuda G, Kinoshita H, Fukuoka T, Hasegawa T, Nakane T, Hino M, Hirakawa K, Ohira M. CXCL1-Chemokine (C-X-C Motif) receptor 2 signaling stimulates the recruitment of bone Marrow-Derived mesenchymal cells into Diffuse-Type gastric cancer stroma. American Journal of Pathology. 2016;**186**:3028-3039

[78] Huang MM, Guo AB, Sun JF, Chen XL, Yin ZY. Angiotensin II promotes the progression of human gastric cancer. Molecular Medicine Reports. 2014;**9**:1056-1060

[79] Wang L, Zhou R, Zhao Y, Dong S, Zhang J, Luo Y, Huang N, Shi M, Bin J, Liao Y, Liao W. MACC-1 promotes Endothelium-Dependent angiogenesis in gastric cancer by activating TWIST1/VEGF-A signal pathway. PLoS One. 2016;**11**:e0157137

[80] Yancopoulos GD, Davis S, Gale NW, Rudge JS, Wiegand SJ, Holash J. Vascular-specific growth factors and blood vessel formation. Nature. 2000;**407**:242-248

[81] Shah MA, Ramanathan RK, Ilson DH, Levnor A, D'Adamo D, O'Reilly E, Tse A, Trocola R, Schwartz L, Capanu M, Schwartz GK, Kelsen DP. Multicenter phase II study of irinotecan, cisplatin, and bevacizumab in patients with metastatic gastric or gastroesophageal junction adenocarcinoma. Journal of Clinical Oncology. 2006;**24**:5201-5206

[82] Ohtsu A, Shah MA, Van Cutsem E, Rha SY, Sawaki A, Park SR, Lim HY, Yamada Y, Wu J, Langer B, Starnawski M, Kang YK. Bevacizumab in combination with chemotherapy as first-line therapy in advanced gastric cancer: A randomized, double-blind, placebo-controlled phase III study. Journal of Clinical Oncology. 2011;**29**:3968-3976

[83] Shan F, Miao R, Xue K, Li Z, Bu Z, Wu A, Zhang L, Wu X, Zong X, Wang X, Li S, Ji X, Jia Z, Ji J. Controlling angiogenesis in gastric cancer: A systematic review of anti-angiogenic trials. Cancer Letters. 2016;**380**;598-607

[84] Blankenstein T, Coulie PG, Gilboa E, Jaffee EM. The determinants of tumour immunogenicity. Nature Reviews Cancer. 2012;**12**:307-313

[85] Subhash VV, Yeo MS, Tan WL, Yong WP. Strategies and advancements in harnessing the immune system for gastric cancer immunotherapy. Journal of Immunology Research. 2015;**2015**:308574

[86] Zhang WJ, Zhou ZH, Guo M, Yang LQ, Xu YY, Pang TH, Gao ST, Xu XY, Sun Q, Feng M, Wang H, Lu CL, Wu GZ, Guan WX, Xu GF. High infiltration of polarized CD163+ tumor-associated macrophages correlates with aberrant expressions of CSCs markers, and predicts prognosis in patients with recurrent gastric cancer. Journal of Cancer. 2017;**8**:363-370

[87] Kim KJ, Lee KS, Cho HJ, Kim YH, Yang HK, Kim WH, Kang GH. Prognostic implications of tumor-infiltrating FoxP3+ regulatory T cells and CD8+ cytotoxic T cells in microsatellite-unstable gastric cancers. Human Pathology. 2014;**45**:285-293

[88] Liu K, Yang K, Wu B, Chen H, Chen X, Jiang L, Ye F, He D, Lu Z, Xue L, Zhang W, Li Q, Zhou Z, Mo X, Hu J. Tumor-Infiltrating immune cells are associated with prognosis of gastric cancer. Medicine (Baltimore). 2015;**94**:e1631

[89] Mittal D, Gubin MM, Schreiber RD, Smyth MJ. New insights into cancer immunoediting and its three component phases—Elimination, equilibrium and escape. Current Opinion in Immunology. 2014;**27**:16-25

[90] Tumeh PC, Harview CL, Yearley JH, Shintaku IP, Taylor EJ, Robert L, Chmielowski B, Spasic M, Henry G, Ciobanu V, West AN, Carmona M, Kivork C, Seja E, Cherry G, Gutierrez AJ, Grogan TR, Mateus C, Tomasic G, Glaspy JA, Emerson RO, Robins H, Pierce RH, Elashoff DA, Robert C, Ribas A. PD-1 blockade induces responses by inhibiting adaptive immune resistance. Nature. 2014;**515**:568-571

[91] Herbst RS, Soria JC, Kowanetz M, Fine GD, Hamid O, Gordon MS, Sosman JA, McDermott DF, Powderly JD, Gettinger SN, Kohrt HE, Horn L, Lawrence DP, Rost S, Leabman M, Xiao Y, Mokatrin A, Koeppen H, Hegde PS, Mellman I, Chen DS, Hodi FS. Predictive correlates of response to the anti-PD-L1 antibody MPDL3280A in cancer patients. Nature. 2014;**515**:563-567

[92] Zhang M, Dong Y, Liu H, Wang Y, Zhao S, Xuan Q, Zhang Q. The clinicopathological and prognostic significance of PD-L1 expression in gastric cancer: A meta-analysis of 10 studies with 1,901 patients. Scientific Reports. 2016;**6**:37933

6

Dietary Management in IBS Patients

Francesca Pasqui, Carolina Poli,

Caterina Magrino and Davide Festi

Abstract

Irritable bowel syndrome (IBS) is a chronic, relapsing functional disorder of the gastrointestinal tract characterized by abdominal pain, bloating, and changes in bowel habits lacking a known structural or anatomic explanation. According to the Rome IV criteria, IBS consists of a set of altered bowel habits over a period of time and includes abdominal pain and discomfort. The pathogenesis of IBS is not completely understood, although it has been noted that various mechanisms are involved determining the onset of symptoms. The risk factors include antibiotics, enteric infection, food intolerance, altered pain perception, altered brain-gut interaction, dysbiosis, increased intestinal permeability, visceral hypersensitivity, and increased activation of the gut mucosal immune system. There has been interest regarding the possible role of food in IBS. Diet is crucial for managing IBS; it plays an important role both in the genesis and in the improvement of symptoms. The aim of the study was to summarize the evidence from the literature, which explains those causes tending to promoting IBS symptoms, such as food content short-chain carbohydrates and the presence of food allergy or food intolerance.

Keywords: IBS, FODMAPs, microbiota, diet, food allergy

1. Introduction

Irritable bowel syndrome (IBS) is a chronic functional gastrointestinal disorder; it is not associated with organic causes which can be detected using current diagnostic tools [1–3]. It is characterized by abdominal pain, distension, bloating and stool irregularities and its prevalence is 10–20%. The prevalence of IBS differs among countries; this may be due to varying application of the diagnostic criteria, demographic differences and other factors, such as lifestyle including physical activity, dietary habits, distress, and pharmacological treatment [4].

The incidence of IBS in women is twofold that of men, the majority in the <50-year-old age group and having a lower socioeconomic status [5]. Symptom severity varies in different patients, from tolerable to severe, possibly interfering with daily activity [6]; in fact, patients with IBS have a reduction in the quality of life and work productivity, and they sometimes tend to isolate themselves socially [5, 7]. Many patients report avoiding social events due to embarrassment from postprandial symptoms and lack of access to toilet facilities [2, 8].

The pathogenesis of IBS is not completely understood, although it has been suggested that various mechanisms are involved [9], such as the use of antibiotics, enteric infection, food intolerance, altered pain perception, altered brain-gut interaction, dysbiosis, increased intestinal permeability, visceral hypersensitivity, and increased activation of the gut mucosal immune system [7].

Since the etiology of IBS is unknown, there is no specific therapeutic strategy; in fact, treatment is often symptomatic, namely the alleviation of symptoms. The diagnosis of IBS is clinical, based on symptoms according to the Rome IV Criteria [10], which have updated the previous criteria:

The term "discomfort" has been eliminated since it was ambiguous for the patients.

In the past, the relative frequency of abdominal pain as a diagnostic criterion had to be at least 3 days a month.

"Improvement of symptoms with defecation" is no longer quoted; instead "related to defecation" is used since a large number of patients did not have improvement in abdominal pain with defecation but, rather, a worsening [3].

Symptom onset should occur at least 6 months before diagnosis, and the symptoms should be present for three successive months [10, 11].

The following IBS subtypes can be identified according to the predominant change in bowel habit:

- (IBS-C) with predominant constipation
- (IBS-D) with diarrhea
- (IBS-M) mixed
- (IBS-U) unsubtyped [1]

Over time, patients may migrate between the different IBS subtypes, most commonly from IBS-C or IBS-D to IBS-M [7].

2. Diet and lifestyle in IBS

As has already been pointed out, IBS patients frequently report that symptom exacerbation occurs after the ingestion of some foods. In fact, it has been reported that approximately 90% of patients voluntarily restrict their diet in order to prevent or improve their symptoms [2, 7]. Over time, excessive limitation of the quality and/or quantity of foods assumed can lead to malnutrition [12, 13].

Furthermore, the occurrence of exaggerated symptoms after food ingestion, such as gastric hypersensitivity to distension, small intestinal hypersensitivity to fat, and hypersensitivity to the effect of gut hormones, acid, capsaicin, and the products of colonic fermentation, has been observed [1, 14, 15].

This exaggerated response to the ingestion of lipids probably reflects the complexity of digestion and absorption, which is also present in physiological conditions. Another aspect regards the short-chain carbohydrates, which are poorly absorbed in the small bowel; therefore, the increased osmotic load increases the intestinal water content.

Short-chain carbohydrate malabsorption leads to their rapid fermentation which, in turn, leads to the production of short-chain fatty acids and gas, mainly hydrogen, carbon dioxide and methane, which may induce the bloating responsible for the abdominal pain [16, 17].

Owing to the strict relationship between food and symptom development present in patients with IBS, therapeutic management includes dietary and lifestyle advice and, in case of necessity, psychotherapy and pharmacological therapy targeted toward the symptoms [18].

In clinical practice, the following items need to be evaluated in patients with IBS, in order to identify their possible pathogenetic role:

1. Fermentable Oligo-, Di-, Monosaccharide and Polyols (FODMAPs)
2. Food allergy
3. Non-celiac gluten sensitivity (NCGS)
4. Interaction between diet and gut microbiota

2.1. FODMAPs

The term FODMAP was first coined by researchers at Monash University in Melbourne, Australia, to describe a group of short-chain carbohydrates and polyols [16, 19].

In recent years, the intake of FODMAPs has increased in Western diets, in particular, that of fructose due to the greater availability and consumption of fruit and fruit juice, and the extensive use of high fructose corn syrup in a wide variety of processed food and beverages [20].

2.1.1. Fructose

Fructose is a monosaccharide which is dose-dependently and variably absorbed; when an excess of glucose is present, it is taken up by a low-capacity facultative transporter called GLUT 5 [16, 21].

When the concentration of fructose is greater in the lumen with respect to that in the epithelial cells, a gradient of concentration is created which permits the fructose, by means of transport proteins, to enter into the interior of the epithelial cells, thereby being absorbed.

The transport proteins, however, saturate at low fructose concentrations which, in turn, lead to malabsorption [22]. However, when fructose is present with glucose, the fructose is taken up more efficiently by means of the GLUT2 transporter. The fructose-glucose ratio is crucial for adequate fructose absorption, and a 1:1 ratio is considered optimal [16, 21]. It has been observed that 40% of the population has "fructose malabsorption" due to its scarce capacity of absorption at the intestinal level [22–24].

2.1.2. Fructans and galacto-oligosaccharides (GOS)

Fructans are oligo or polysaccharides made up of small chains of fructose units having a terminal molecule of glucose. Fructans with a 2–9 unit length are defined as oligofructose and those with >10 units as inulins [22, 25, 26]. Due to the lack of enzymes capable of completely hydrolyzing the glycosidic bonds of these polysaccharides, the human body absorbs only 5–15% of the fructans; the fructans which are not absorbed are released into the colon where they undergo fermentation [26]. Wheat represents the major source of fructans in the diet (1–4%) [22, 27]. Rye also contains fructans; its chain length is longer than that found in wheat, which could make it less osmotically active or less rapidly fermented. The principal sources of galacto-oligosaccharides (GOS) are raffinose, which is made up of one fructose, one glucose, and one galactose molecule, and stachyose, which has the same composition as raffinose with the exception of having an additional galactose molecule. The human body is not capable of digesting raffinose and stachyose due to the lack of enzymes able to hydrolyze the bonds. Galactooligosaccharides are present, above all, in vegetables [22, 28]. Fructans and galactooligosaccharides are defined as "prebiotics" due to their ability to selectively stimulate the growth of beneficial colonic bacteria, specifically *Bifidobacteria* and *Lactobacilli* [16, 29, 30].

2.1.3. Polyols

Sorbitol, mannitol, xylitol, maltitol, erythirol, polydextrose, and isomalt are sugar alcohols. Sorbitol and mannitol are the major types found in food, and they are found naturally in fruits and vegetables, or as added sweeteners in low-calorie food products [16]. They are identified on food packaging with the following numbers: E420 (sorbitol), E421 (mannitol), E965 (maltitol), E967 (xylitol), and E953 (isomalt) [22]. Their rates of absorption depend largely on molecular size; their absorption is passive and varies between individuals [22, 31].

2.1.4. *Lactose*

Lactose is a disaccharide consisting of galactose bound to glucose; intestinal absorption requires hydrolysis to its component monosaccharides by brush-border enzyme lactase. Lactase begins its activity at approximately the eighth week of gestation; activity increases until week 34 and the peak of activity is at birth [32].

After the first few months of life, lactase activity begins to decrease; this condition is defined as "lactase non-persistence." However, approximately 30% of the population retains its capacity to digest lactose (lactase persistence); in particular, this is observed in the populations of Northern Europe as a result of the introduction of dairy farming approximately 10,000 years ago [17, 33]. Only 50% of lactase activity is necessary for the efficient digestion of lactose without causing symptoms of intolerance [17]. Lactase deficiency determines lactose intolerance and is defined as markedly reduced brush-border lactase activity, whereas lactose malabsorption occurs when a substantial amount of lactose is not absorbed in the intestine. Three distinct forms of deficiency exist: congenital, primary and secondary. The congenital form is extremely rare; it can be observed in newborns and is characterized by diarrhea from the first exposure to breast milk and by growth defects [32]. "Primary lactase deficiency" refers to the condition of lactase non-persistence, already described above, whereas secondary or acquired lactase deficiency refers to the loss of lactase activity in individuals with lactase persistence. This could be secondary to a gastrointestinal disease, which damages the brush border and is usually reversible. The primary aim in treating lactose intolerance is the improvement of symptoms. Therefore, it is necessary to reduce the malabsorption, and limiting the intake of the lactose found in milk and its derivatives is recommended.

In order to avoid the onset of symptoms, patients with self-reported lactose intolerance, even those with IBS, can ingest at least 12 g of lactose per day [17, 34, 35]. However, it has also been observed that, in many individuals, the restriction of lactose alone was not sufficient for improving functional GI symptoms. This is because lactose intolerance is part of a wider intolerance to FODMAPs [17, 36]. Lactase enzyme replacement products can be found commercially, but they should be used only by those individuals who have isolated lactose intolerance and wish to enjoy dairy products [17]. It is important to remember that dairy products are the major source of calcium in many individuals; therefore, it is reasonable to recommend increasing calcium intake from other foods, water rich in calcium or supplements, especially in the presence of other risk factors for osteoporosis [17].

2.2. Food allergy

Food allergy is an adverse immune response toward food proteins or a form of food intolerance associated with a hypersensitive immune response. There are three types of food allergies: IgE mediated, mixed IgE/non-IgE, which involves eosinophilic and other cellular components, and non-IgE mediated [37].

Food allergy has rapidly increased in prevalence. It suggests the important role of environmental factors in disease susceptibility [37]. Of the 20–30% of the population reported to be allergic or to have allergic children, the presence of allergy can be ascertained in only 6–8% of children under 5 years of age and in 3–4% of adults [38, 39].

In the presence of food allergies, a small quantity of food can cause an immediate reaction. The symptoms involving the gastrointestinal tract can include nausea, vomiting, abdominal cramps and diarrhea, other signs can involve the oropharyngeal tract or the skin [38, 40]. There has been interest regarding the possible role of food allergies in IBS, but few data are available to support this association [38].

In order to exclude food allergies, it is necessary to proceed on the basis of the results of the following tests:

1. *Total serum IgE*: High values may indicate the presence of some food allergies [38, 41].

2. *Immunoglobulin G (IgG):* It often produces false positive, and it is not recommended, as a diagnostic test, by national and international guidelines [38, 42].

3. *The radioallergosorbent test (RAST) of food/serum food-specific IgE:* A direct correlation exists between increasing concentrations of food-specific serum IgE and the probability that an individual will react to an ingested food [38, 43–45].

4. *The skin prick or scratch test:* Positivity indicates the presence of IgE to specific foods [38, 42, 44–47].

Furthermore, it is necessary to make an interview and administer an accurate food questionnaire in order to identify the correlation between specific food and symptoms.

2.3. Non-celiac gluten sensitivity (NCGS)

Currently, the gluten-related disorders actually documented are celiac disease (CD), non-celiac gluten sensitivity (NCGS) and wheat allergy (WA) [48]. Celiac disease is an autoimmune condition, which is characterized by an immunological response to ingesting gluten, which results in small-intestine villous atrophy with increased permeability and malabsorption of nutrients [48, 49].

Wheat allergy is characterized by an IgE-mediated response against various wheat components, which cause gastrointestinal and respiratory symptoms [48–50].

A food allergy to wheat begins with different symptoms as vomiting, abdominal pain, asthma, allergic rhinitis, urticaria/angioedema, acute exacerbation of atopic dermatitis, and exercise-induced anaphylaxis. The prevalence of IgE-mediated food allergies to wheat, confirmed by a food induce, is unknown.

At the moment, the management of IgE-mediated wheat allergy is mainly based on the avoidance of both food and inhaled wheat allergens. Patients allergic to wheat must be trained to identify relevant food allergens on labels, and written instructions should be given to effectively eliminate wheat from their diet [51].

Non-celiac gluten sensitivity is an emerging clinical problem characterized by various manifestations, in particular by IBS-like gastrointestinal symptoms and extra-intestinal symptoms, such as malaise, fatigue, headache, mental confusion, anxiety, sleep abnormality, and skin rash related to the ingestion of gluten-containing foods in patients who are not affected by either celiac disease or wheat allergy [52].

The symptoms generally improve after the removal of wheat products from the diet. Due to the lack of biomarkers, the diagnosis of NCGS is mainly based on clinical criteria [52, 53] after having excluded the presence of CD, WA, gluten ataxia, and dermatitis herpetiformis [52].

Similar to IBS, NCGS affects more young women (in their third decade of life; female:male = 3:1) [52]. The consumption of wheat has increased and is correlated not only to its adaptability and potential for high yields but also to its viscoelasticity, which allows it to be processed into several food items, such as bread, baked products, and pastas [54].

There are two components of wheat which could evoke IBS symptoms: proteins (primarily gluten) and short-chain carbohydrates (primarily fructans and galactans) [52].

Various studies have been carried out to verify which of these two components is responsible for the onset of symptoms. A study was carried out on patients with IBS who autonomously started a gluten-free diet; it was observed that the gastrointestinal symptoms significantly and consistently improved with a low-FODMAP diet, and symptoms did not worsen with either a low- or a high-dose challenge with gluten [54, 55].

Another study involving adults who believed that they had NCGS concluded that it was not gluten to induce the clinical picture [54]. Trials carried out on patients with suspected NCGS support the data regarding a greater improvement of the symptoms with a low-FODMAP diet as compared to a gluten-free diet [56–58].

A recent systematic review regarding NCGS concluded that there is insufficient evidence to support the efficacy of a gluten-free diet for NCGS [59].

2.4. Interaction between diet and microbiota

From birth, the gut microbiota plays various roles in the gastrointestinal tract. Postnatal gut function and immune development are largely influenced by intestinal microbiota. In fact, it has a role in gastrointestinal motility and the immune system, it provides protection against infection, it contributes to the development of gut function and the regulation and maintenance of the intestinal barrier, and it promotes food tolerance. Microbial species promote symbiotic host-bacteria interactions, which are fundamental for human health [12, 60, 61].

The gastrointestinal microbiota is determined by host genetic and environmental factors [12, 60, 62]. The composition of the microbiota varies according to prenatal events, delivery methods, infant feeding, infant care environment, and antibiotic use. Emerging evidence has shown that early microbiota colonization may influence the occurrence of eventual diseases [61]. Gut microbiota interferes with the intestinal functions it can be the cause of irregularity of intestinal sensitivity, motility, neuroimmune signaling, such as the alterations of the mucosal barrier and pattern recognition receptor expression and dysfunctions of the hypothalamus-pituitary-adrenal axis [63].

It has an important role in the digestion of dietary components, resulting in metabolites which may directly or indirectly contribute to IBS symptoms [12]. The vast majority of microbial commensal species give rise to symbiotic host-bacterial interactions, which are fundamental for human health [64]. Disruption and/or imbalance of the establishment of stable normal gut microbiota, dysbiosis, may be associated with the pathogenesis of several gastrointestinal conditions, such as inflammatory bowel disease (IBD) and irritable bowel syndrome, and wider systemic manifestations of disease, such as obesity, type 2 diabetes and atopy [12, 64, 65]. In the healthy gut, intestinal microbiota can prevent the adherence of pathogenic bacteria to the wall of the gastrointestinal tract [66]. In addition, dysbiosis in the gut may facilitate the adhesion of enteric pathogens, which could be associated with IBS symptoms [67]. Alteration of the composition of the normal microbiota and disturbed colonic fermentation in IBS patients may play an important role in the development of IBS symptoms, with a significant increase in the ratio of Firmicutes to Bacteroidetes [65, 68]. Dysregulated intestinal immune function, chronic low-grade mucosal inflammation and increased mucosal permeability and barrier dysfunction have all been suggested to be pathogenic mechanisms in IBS in which the intestinal microbiota might have a role [12, 69, 70]. Part of the etiology of IBS may involve the use of antibiotics; in these cases, probiotics are effective in ameliorating symptoms, even if the consistency of benefits across clinical studies is difficult to discern due to variation in strains, product dosages and the duration of the trials [68, 71–73].

Manipulation of the gut microbiota represents a new strategy for the treatment of IBS. Modulating the gut bacterial composition, expanding the bacterial species considered to be beneficial (*Lactobacilli* and *Bifidobacteria*) and reducing the bacterial species considered to be harmful (*Clostridium, Escherichia coli, Salmonella, Shigella,* and *Pseudomonas*) should attenuate IBS symptoms [63].

Several studies using culture-based and culture-independent methods have shown that the microbiota differs between IBS patients and healthy controls [12, 74, 75].

However, the association between IBS symptoms and specific bacterial species is uncertain [12, 76]. Decreased levels of *Lactobacilli* and *Bifidobacteria,* increased levels of anaerobic bacteria, such as *Streptococci* and *Escherichia coli,* as well as increased ratios of Firmicutes, Bacteroidetes, and *Clostridium* species, have been confirmed in several studies [12, 77, 78]. Studies have indicated that the microbiota, its function and its metabolic output are influenced by dietary patterns [79].

Habitual long-term dietary patterns have been directly linked to intestinal microbial enterotypes. Protein and animal fat intake have been associated with the Bacteroides enterotype, whereas a high-carbohydrate intake has been associated with the Prevotella enterotype [12, 80].

Preliminary data suggest that a diet with a low content of FODMAPs can reduce the growth of important species, such as Bifidobatteri [81]. The effect of short-term dietary interventions on the microbiota composition appears to have only a modest effect [12, 80, 82]. Diet and composition of the microbiota are two major interrelated factors, which can modify susceptibility to food allergy [37].

The number of publications describing an altered microbiota in allergic disease has significantly increased in recent years. The increasing use of antibiotics, in both humans and agriculture, and the increasing consumption of a high-fat/low-fiber diet have had a major impact on the gut microbiota and have been associated with an increased allergic response to food in industrialized countries in recent decades [83–85].

The use of probiotics to stabilize microbial homeostasis seems to be promising, but, to better understand the potential beneficial impact from probiotics, prebiotics, and bacterial-produced metabolites in the treatment of allergic disease, additional studies are needed [85].

3. Role of diet

Therefore, diet is crucial for managing IBS despite the lack of solid evidence involving many dietary recommendations for IBS; this issue must be addressed in clinical practice. The British Dietetic Association and NICE guidelines (National Institute for Health and Clinical Excellence) recommend that dietary and lifestyle advice should be routinely provided to patients [2]:

- Patients with IBS should be educated about the importance of self-help in effectively managing their IBS through information regarding lifestyle, physical activity, diet, and symptom-targeted medication.
- Professionals should encourage people with IBS to use their available leisure time to make relax.
- People should be motivated to increase their activity levels.
- In people with IBS diet and nutrition have to be assessed and general advice should be given:
    - Have regular meals during the day and take time to eat with calm.
    - Avoid skip meals and stay for long time without eating.
    - Drink at least 1500 ml of liquid/day, preferring water or other non-caffeinated drinks.
    - No more than three cups per day of tea and coffee.
    - Reduce alcohol and fizzy drinks.
    - Limit the intake of high-fiber food; reduce the intake of "resistant starch" (RS) because they resist to digestion in the small intestine and reaches the colon intact.
    - No more than three portions of fresh fruit per day.
    - In case of diarrhea, it is advisable to avoid sorbitol, an artificial sweetener found in sugar-free sweets, light drinks, and in some diabetic and diet products.
    - In case of wind and bloating, it is advisable to eat oats and linseeds.
- Healthcare professionals should review the fiber intake of people with IBS, adjusting it while monitoring its effect on the symptoms. People with IBS should be discouraged from eating

insoluble fiber. If an increase in dietary fiber is advised, it should be soluble fiber. People with IBS could try probiotics, and they should take the product for at least 4 weeks while monitoring the effect. Probiotics should be taken at the dosage recommended by the manufacturer.

- Discourage the use of aloe vera in the treatment of IBS.
- If a person's IBS symptoms persist while following general lifestyle and dietary advice, offer advice on additional dietary management.
    - Include single food avoidance and exclusion diets such as a low-FODMAP diet.
    - Only be given by a healthcare professional with expertise in dietary management.

A low-FODMAP diet provides for the restriction of all short-chain carbohydrates by finding low-FODMAP alternatives in each food group. The aim is that of reducing the malabsorption induced by these nutrients and the consequences, such as luminal distension and fermentation caused by the bacteria of the colon, which give rise to the symptoms [52].

In healthy adults, FODMAPs do not cause gastrointestinal symptoms; conversely, in IBS patients, this probably is a consequence of the previously mentioned abnormalities in gut physiology and visceral sensation [7, 86, 87].

There is evidence of low-FODMAP diet efficacy; in fact, it has been observed that it reduces and controls the GI symptoms with respect to a high-FODMAP diet [2, 88, 89], and this has also been confirmed by clinical trials [5, 90].

The low-FODMAP diet was compared with the indications of the NICE guidelines in order to verify which of the two approaches was better in controlling the symptoms.

In particular, in one study, it emerged that there was significantly greater satisfaction with symptom response with the low-FODMAP diet (76%) as compared to the NICE guidelines (54%) [5, 89].

Instead, a recent single-blinded random controlled trial (RCT) compared the efficacy of a low-FODMAP diet to the NICE guidelines for a 4-week period at the end of which an improvement in the IBS Symptom Severity Score (IBS SSS) was observed in both groups but without significant differences. At the end of the study, 56% of the patients on the low FODMAP diet and 46% on the traditional IBS diet responded to the treatment, and the IBS SSS was reduced to ≥ 50 relative to baseline. Food diaries demonstrated good adherence to the dietary advice [16, 91].

A recent meta-analysis, which compared IBS patients who followed a Westernized diet with patient who followed a low FODMAPs diet, showed that adherence to a low-FODMAP diet help to ameliorate all the functional IBS's symptoms and their severity also improving the quality of life score [20].

The symptom with the least improvement was constipation; in fact, a typical FODMAP diet can often be lacking in fiber content. If one decides to follow a low-FODMAP diet, it should be followed for at least 2–6 weeks in order to be able to verify whether there is effectively an improvement in the symptomology [5].

If patients report improvement, dietary rechallenge with FODMAPs may be tried gradually, that is, one food at a time can be reinserted, starting with small quantities [5]. The risk of inserting more than one food at a time is that of not being able to verify which, effectively, is that responsible for the worsening of the symptoms [5].

Decisions related to the food allowed or to that which should be avoided should always be based on individual tolerance; one valid evaluation instrument is a food diary in which patients have to report what they eat qualitatively, thereby being able to identify potential trigger foods [5].

The effect of a long-term FODMAP diet is not clear; few data are available regarding its long-term efficacy and safety. Presumably, a long-term low-FODMAP diet could lead to nutritional inadequacy. In one study evaluating the effect of fermentable carbohydrate restriction as compared with a control diet, no difference was found in micronutrient intake, except for a lower calcium intake, presumably as a result of the lower intake of dairy products [16, 90].

This might pose a problem principally for children and postmenopausal women [16]. The psychosocial risks of imposing a dietary change and the various difficulties encountered by an IBS patient, difficulties in socialization and eating disorders, such as orthorexia nervosa, should not be underestimated [52, 92].

4. Conclusions

The symptoms of IBS can be similar to those of other pathological conditions; it is necessary to exclude them by means of diagnostic examinations. From a nutritional point of view, the symptoms of IBS patients linked to food as well as to their present food habits must be evaluated carefully in order to reach a nutritional diagnosis and the specific objectives to reach, verifying the relative changes by means of successive checkups. Furthermore, a careful evaluation of the nutritional state is recommended with the aim of identifying, if present, the eventual lack of macro/micronutrients. It is possible to consider a dietetic regimen, which has a behavioral checkup linked to the indications of the NICE guidelines; successively, or in association with the execution of the guidelines, a low-FODMAP diet can be proposed which foresees a reduction in the intake of foods containing high quantities of short-chain carbohydrates and polyols in favor of substitutes for each food group in order to avoid undesired weight losses and nutritional deficits. A low-FODMAP diet must be limited to a precise period of time, and the patient must be monitored by keeping a daily food diary where the food consumed over a 24-h period, the subdivision of the meals and the clinical picture present is reported. Use of a diary makes patients feel more understood, with a consequent perception of greater interest in their problems and needs. With the reduction or disappearance of the clinical picture, the foods previously excluded can be reinserted, one at a time, evaluating individual tolerance with the aim of restoring a complete and balanced diet, always with the help of a food diary.

Author details

Francesca Pasqui*, Carolina Poli, Caterina Magrino and Davide Festi

*Address all correspondence to: francesca.pasqui@unibo.it

Department of Medical and Surgical Sciences, University of Bologna, Bologna, Italy

References

[1] Enck P., Aziz Q., Barbara G., Farmer AD., Fukudo S., Mayer EA., et al. Irritable bowel syndrome. Nat Rev Dis Primer. 2016;2:16014. doi: 10.1038/nrdp.2016.14

[2] Hayes PA., Fraher MH., Quigley EMM. Irritable bowel syndrome: the role of food in pathogenesis and management. Gastroenterol Hepatol. 2014;10:164–74.

[3] Mearin F., Lacy BE., Chang L., Chey WD., Lembo AJ., Simren M., Spiller R. Bowel disorders. Gastroenterology. 2016;150:1393–407. doi: 10.1053/j.gastro.2016.02.031

[4] Nanayakkara WS., Skidmore PM., O'Brien L., Wilkinson TJ., Gearry RB. Efficacy of the low FODMAP diet for treating irritable bowel syndrome: the evidence to date. Clin Exp Gastroenterol. 2016;9:131–42. doi: 10.2147/CEG.S86798

[5] Khan MA., Nusrat S., Khan MI., Nawras A., Bielefeldt K. Low-FODMAP Diet for irritable bowel syndrome: is it ready for prime time? Dig Dis Sci. 2015;60:1169–77. doi: 10.1007/s10620-014-3436-4

[6] Mansueto P., D'Alcamo A., Seidita A., Carroccio A. Food allergy in irritable bowel syndrome: the case of non-celiac wheat sensitivity. World J Gastroenterol. 2015;21:7089–109. doi: 10.3748/wjg.v21.i23.7089

[7] Chey WD., Kurlander J., Eswaran S. Irritable bowel syndrome: a clinical review. JAMA. 2015;313:949. doi: 10.1001/jama.2015.0954

[8] Bertram S., Kurland M., Lydick E., Locke GR., Yawn BP. The patient's perspective of irritable bowel syndrome. J Fam Pract. 2001;50:521–5.

[9] Soares RL. Irritable bowel syndrome: a clinical review. World J Gastroenterol. 2014;20(34):12144–60. doi: 10.3748/wjg.v20.i34.12144

[10] Mearin F., Ciriza C., Mínguez M., Rey E., Mascort JJ., Peña E., Cañones P., Júdez J. Clinical practice guideline: irritable bowel syndrome with constipation and functional constipation in the adult. Rev Esp Enfermedades Dig. 2016;108:332–63. doi: 10.17235/reed.2016.4389/2016

[11] Drossman DA., Hasler WL. Rome IV—Functional GI disorders: disorders of Gut-Brain interaction. Gastroenterology. 2016;150:1257–61. doi: 10.1053/j.gastro.2016.03.035

[12] El-Salhy M. Recent developments in the pathophysiology of irritable bowel syndrome. World J Gastroenterol. 2015;21:7621–36. doi: 10.3748/wjg.v21.i25.7621

[13] El-Salhy M., Gundersen D. Diet in irritable bowel syndrome. Nutr J. 2015;14:36. doi: 10.1186/s12937-015-0022-3

[14] Kellow JE., Miller LJ., Phillips SF., Zinsmeister AR., Charboneau JW. Altered sensitivity of the gallbladder to cholecystokinin octapeptide in irritable bowel syndrome. Am J Physiol. 1987;253:G650–5.

[15] Barbara G., Feinle-Bisset C., Ghoshal UC., Quigley EM., Santos J., Vanner S., Vergnolle N., Zoetendal EG. The intestinal microenvironment and functional gastrointestinal disorders. Gastroenterology. 2016;150:1305–18. doi: 10.1053/j.gastro.2016.02.028

[16] Molina-Infante J., Serra J., Fernandez-Bañares F., Mearin F. The low-FODMAP diet for irritable bowel syndrome: lights and shadows. Gastroenterol Hepatol. 2016;39:55–65. doi: 10.1016/j.gastrohep.2015.07.009

[17] Deng Y., Misselwitz B., Dai N., Fox M. Lactose intolerance in adults: biological mechanism and dietary management. Nutrients. 2015;7:8020–35. doi: 10.3390/nu7095380

[18] Does a low FODMAP diet help IBS? Drug Ther Bull. 2015;53:93–6. doi: 10.1136/dtb.2015.8.0346. http://dtb.bmj.com/content/53/8/93.full.pdf+html.

[19] Gibson PR., Shepherd SJ. Personal view: food for thought - western lifestyle and susceptibility to Crohn's disease. The FODMAP hypothesis. Aliment Pharmacol Ther. 2005;21:1399–409. doi: 10.1111/j.1365-2036.2005.02506.x

[20] Marsh A., Eslick EM., Eslick GD. Does a diet low in FODMAPs reduce symptoms associated with functional gastrointestinal disorders? A comprehensive systematic review and meta-analysis. Eur J Nutr. 2016;55:897–906 doi: 10.1007/s00394-015-0922-1

[21] Fernández-Bañares F., Esteve M., Viver JM. Fructose-sorbitol malabsorption. Curr Gastroenterol Rep. 2009;11:368–74.

[22] Mansueto P., Seidita A., D'Alcamo A., Carroccio A. Role of FODMAPs in patients with irritable bowel syndrome. Nutr Clin Pract. 2015;30:665–82. doi: 10.1177/0884533615569886

[23] Latulippe ME., Skoog SM. Fructose malabsorption and intolerance: effects of fructose with and without simultaneous glucose ingestion. Crit Rev Food Sci Nutr. 2011;51:583–92. doi: 10.1080/10408398.2011.566646

[24] Douard V., Ferraris RP. The role of fructose transporters in diseases linked to excessive fructose intake. J Physiol. 2013;591:401–14. doi: 10.1113/jphysiol.2011.215731

[25] Roberfroid MB. Introducing inulin-type fructans. Br J Nutr. 2005;93(Suppl. 1):S13–25. doi: 10.1079/BJN20041350

[26] Fedewa A., Rao SS. Dietary fructose intolerance, fructan intolerance and FODMAPs. Curr Gastroenterol. 2014;16:370. doi: 10.1007/s11894-013-0370-0

[27] Roberfroid MB., Delzenne NM. Dietary fructans. Annu Rev Nutr. 1998;18:117–43. doi: 10.1146/annurev.nutr.18.1.117

[28] Sangwan V., Tomar SK., Singh RRB., Singh AK., Ali B. Galactooligosaccharides: novel components of designer foods. J Food Sci. 2011;76:R103–11. doi: 10.1111/j.1750-3841.2011.02131.x

[29] Roberfroid MB. Inulin-type fructans: functional food ingredients. J Nutr. 2007;137:2493S–2502S.

[30] Macfarlane GT., Steed H., Macfarlane S. Bacterial metabolism and health-related effects of galacto-oligosaccharides and other prebiotics. J Appl Microbiol. 2008;104:305–44. doi: 10.1111/j.1365-2672.2007.03520.x

[31] Yao CK., Tan H-L., van Langenberg DR., Barrett JS., Rose R., Liels K., et al. Dietary sorbitol and mannitol: food content and distinct absorption patterns between healthy individuals and patients with irritable bowel syndrome. J Hum Nutr Diet. 2014;27:263–75. doi: 10.1111/jhn.12144

[32] Lomer MCE., Parkes GC., Sanderson JD. Review article: lactose intolerance in clinical practice: myths and realities. Aliment Pharmacol Ther. 2008;27:93–103. doi: 10.1111/j.1365-2036.2007.03557.x

[33] Swallow DM. Genetics of lactase persistence and lactose intolerance. Annu Rev Genet. 2003;37:197–219. doi: 10.1146/annurev.genet.37.110801.143820

[34] Shaukat A., Levitt MD., Taylor BC., MacDonald R., Shamliyan TA., Kane RL., Wilt TJ. Systematic review: effective management strategies for lactose intolerance. Ann Intern Med. 2010;152:797–803. doi: 10.7326/0003-4819-152-12-201006150-00241

[35] Savaiano DA., Boushey CJ., McCabe GP. Lactose intolerance symptoms assessed by meta-analysis: a grain of truth that leads to exaggeration. J Nutr. 2006;136:1107–13.

[36] Parker TJ., Woolner JT., Prevost AT., Tuffnell Q., Shorthouse M., Hunter JO. Irritable bowel syndrome: is the search for lactose intolerance justified? Eur J Gastroenterol Hepatol. 2001;13:219–25.

[37] Benedé S., Blázquez AB., Chiang D., Tordesillas L., Berin MC. The rise of food allergy: environmental factors and emerging treatments. EBioMedicine. 2016;7:27–34. doi: 10.1016/j.ebiom.2016.04.012

[38] Pasqui F., Poli C., Colecchia A., Marasco G., Festi D. Adverse Food reaction and functional gastrointestinal disorders: role of the dietetic approach. J Gastrointestin Liver Dis. 2015;24:319–27. doi: 10.15403/jgld.2014.1121.243.paq

[39] Ho MH-K., Wong WH-S., Chang C. Clinical spectrum of food allergies: a comprehensive review. Clin Rev Allergy Immunol. 2014;46:225–40. doi: 10.1007/s12016-012-8339-6

[40] Burks AW., Tang M., Sicherer S., Muraro A., Eigenmann PA., Ebisawa M., Fiocchi A., Chiang W., Beyer K., Wood R., Hourihane J., Jones SM., Lack G., Sampson HA. ICON: food allergy. J Allergy Clin Immunol. 2012;129:906–20. doi: 10.1016/j.jaci.2012.02.001

[41] Sampson HA. Food allergy: accurately identifying clinical reactivity. Allergy. 2005;60:19–24. doi: 10.1111/j.1398-9995.2005.00853.x

[42] Caubet J-C., Sampson HA. Beyond skin testing: state of the art and new horizons in food allergy diagnostic testing. Immunol Allergy Clin North Am. 2012;32:97–109. doi: 10.1016/j.iac.2011.11.002

[43] Turnbull JL., Adams HN., Gorard DA. Review article: the diagnosis and management of food allergy and food intolerances. Aliment Pharmacol Ther. 2015;41:3–25. doi: 10.1111/apt.12984

[44] Lieberman JA., Sicherer SH. Diagnosis of food allergy: epicutaneous skin tests, in vitro tests, and oral food challenge. Curr Allergy Asthma Rep. 2011;11:58–64. doi: 10.1007/s11882-010-0149-4

[45] Stiefel G., Roberts G. How to use serum-specific IgE measurements in diagnosing and monitoring food allergy. Arch Dis Child Educ Pract Ed. 2012;97:29–36. doi: 10.1136/archdischild-2011-300569

[46] Siles RI., Hsieh FH. Allergy blood testing: a practical guide for clinicians. Cleve Clin J Med. 2011;78:585–92. doi: 10.3949/ccjm.78a.11023

[47] Bergmann MM., Caubet J-C., Boguniewicz M., Eigenmann PA. Evaluation of food allergy in patients with atopic dermatitis. J Allergy Clin Immunol Pract. 2013;1:22–8. doi: 10.1016/j.jaip.2012.11.005

[48] Makharia A., Catassi C., Makharia GK. The overlap between irritable bowel syndrome and non-celiac gluten sensitivity: a clinical dilemma. Nutrients. 2015;7:10417–26. doi: 10.3390/nu7125541

[49] Di Sabatino A., Corazza GR. Coeliac disease. The Lancet. 2009;373:1480–93. doi: 10.1016/S0140-6736(09)60254-3

[50] Tatham AS., Shewry PR. Allergy to wheat and related cereals. Clin Exp Allergy. 2008;38:1712–26. doi: 10.1111/j.1365-2222.2008.03101.x

[51] Cianferoni A. Wheat allergy: diagnosis and management. J Asthma Allergy. 2016;9:13–25. doi: 10.2147/JAA.S81550

[52] De Giorgio R, Volta U, Gibson PR. Sensitivity to wheat, gluten and FODMAPs in IBS: facts or fiction? Gut. 2016;65:169–78. doi: 10.1136/gutjnl-2015-309757

[53] Biesiekierski JR., Newnham ED., Shepherd SJ., Muir JG., Gibson PR. Characterization of adults with a self-diagnosis of nonceliac gluten sensitivity. Nutr Clin Pract. 2014;29:504–9. doi: 10.1177/0884533614529163

[54] El-Salhy M., Hatlebakk JG., Gilja OH., Hausken T. The relation between celiac disease, nonceliac gluten sensitivity and irritable bowel syndrome. Nutr J. 2015;14:92. doi: 10.1186/s12937-015-0080-6

[55] Biesiekierski JR., Peters SL., Newnham ED., Rosella O., Muir JG., Gibson PR. No effects of gluten in patients with self-reported non-celiac gluten sensitivity after dietary reduction of fermentable, poorly absorbed, short-chain carbohydrates. Gastroenterology. 2013;145:320–8. doi: 10.1053/j.gastro.2013.04.051

[56] Piacentino D., Rossi S., Alvino V., Cantarini R., Badiali D., Pallotta N., et al. Effects of low-FODMAP and gluten-free diets in irritable bowel syndrome patients: a double-blind randomized controlled clinical study. Gastrointest Endosc. 2014;79:S-82. doi: 10.1016/S0016-5085(14)60294-8

[57] Piacentino D., Rossi S., Alvino V., Di Nunno R., Piretta L., Badiali D., et al. 611 Low-FODMAP diet in irritable bowel syndrome patients offers more benefit than a low-FODMAP gluten-free diet in the medium- and long-term: results from a double-blind randomized controlled clinical study and follow-up. Gastroenterology. 2015;148:S-1–S-1196. doi: 10.1016/S0016-5085(15)30414-5

[58] Zanini B., Basche R., Ferraresi A., Ricci C., Lanzarotto F., Marullo M., et al. Randomised clinical study: gluten challenge induces symptom recurrence in only a minority of patients who meet clinical criteria for non-coeliac gluten sensitivity. Aliment Pharmacol Ther. 2015;42:968–76. doi: 10.1111/apt.13372

[59] Molina-Infante J., Santolaria S., Sanders DS., Fernández-Bañares F. Systematic review: noncoeliac gluten sensitivity. Aliment Pharmacol Ther. 2015;41:807–20. doi: 10.1111/apt.13155

[60] Dore J., Simren M., Buttle L., Guarner F. Hot topics in gut microbiota. United Eur Gastroenterol J. 2013;1:311–8. doi: 10.1177/2050640613502477

[61] Power SE., O'Toole PW., Stanton C., Ross RP., Fitzgerald GF. Intestinal microbiota, diet and health. Br J Nutr. 2014;111:387–402. doi: 10.1017/S0007114513002560

[62] Farrugia G., Simren M., Mawe G., Bradesi S., Bredenoord AJ. Gut microbiota and neurogastroenterology and motility: the good the bad and the ugly. Neurogastroenterol Motil. 2014;26:295. doi: 10.1111/nmo.12322

[63] Distrutti E., Monaldi L., Ricci P., Fiorucci S. Gut microbiota role in irritable bowel syndrome: new therapeutic strategies. World J Gastroenterol. 2016;22:2219–41. doi: 10.3748/wjg.v22.i7.2219

[64] Goulet O. Potential role of the intestinal microbiota in programming health and disease. Nutr Rev. 2015;73:32–40. doi: 10.1093/nutrit/nuv039

[65] Bull MJ., Plummer NT. Part 1: the human Gut Microbiome in health and disease. Integr Med Clin J. 2014;13:17–22.

[66] Kellow JE., Azpiroz F., Delvaux M., Gebhart GF., Mertz HR., Quigley EMM., et al. Applied principles of neurogastroenterology: physiology/motility sensation. Gastroenterology. 2006;130:1412–20. doi: 10.1053/j.gastro.2005.08.061

[67] Rinttilä T., Lyra A., Krogius-Kurikka L., Palva A. Real-time PCR analysis of enteric pathogens from fecal samples of irritable bowel syndrome subjects. Gut Pathog. 2011;3:6. doi: 10.1186/1757-4749-3-6

[68] Ponnusamy K., Choi JN., Kim J., Lee S-Y., Lee CH. Microbial community and metabolomic comparison of irritable bowel syndrome faeces. J Med Microbiol. 2011;60:817–27. doi: 10.1099/jmm.0.028126-0

[69] Williams EA., Nai X., Corfe BM. Dietary intakes in people with irritable bowel syndrome. BMC Gastroenterol. 2011;11:9. doi: 10.1186/1471-230X-11-9

[70] Gibson PR., Shepherd SJ. Evidence-based dietary management of functional gastrointestinal symptoms: the FODMAP approach. J Gastroenterol Hepatol. 2010;25:252–8. doi: 10.1111/j.1440-1746.2009.06149.x

[71] Bull MJ., Plummer NT. Part 2: treatments for chronic gastrointestinal disease and gut dysbiosis. Integr Med (Encinitas). 2015;14:25–33.

[72] Rigsbee L., Agans R., Shankar V., Kenche H., Khamis HJ., Michail S., et al. Quantitative profiling of gut microbiota of children with diarrhea-predominant irritable bowel syndrome. Am J Gastroenterol. 2012;107:1740–51. doi: 10.1038/ajg.2012.287

[73] Carroll IM., Ringel-Kulka T., Ferrier L., Wu MC., Siddle JP., Bueno L., et al. Fecal protease activity is associated with compositional alterations in the intestinal microbiota. PLoS One. 2013;8:e78017. doi: 10.1371/journal.pone.0078017

[74] Carroll IM., Ringel-Kulka T., Keku TO., Chang Y-H., Packey CD., Sartor RB., et al. Molecular analysis of the luminal- and mucosal-associated intestinal microbiota in diarrhea-predominant irritable bowel syndrome. AJP Gastrointest Liver Physiol. 2011;301:G799–807. doi: 10.1152/ajpgi.00154.2011

[75] Si J-M., Yu Y-C., Fan Y-J., Chen S-J. Intestinal microecology and quality of life in irritable bowel syndrome patients. World J Gastroenterol. 2004;10:1802–5. doi: 10.3748/WJG.v10.i12.1802

[76] Lee KJ., Tack J. Altered intestinal microbiota in irritable bowel syndrome. Neurogastroenterol Motil. 2010;22:493–8.

[77] Maukonen J. Prevalence and temporal stability of selected clostridial groups in irritable bowel syndrome in relation to predominant faecal bacteria. J Med Microbiol. 2006;55:625–33. doi: 10.1099/jmm.0.46134-0

[78] Balsari A., Ceccarelli A., Dubini F., Fesce E., Poli G. The fecal microbial population in the irritable bowel syndrome. Microbiologica. 1982;5:185–94.

[79] Rajilić-Stojanović M., Jonkers DM., Salonen A., Hanevik K., Raes J., Jalanka J., et al. Intestinal microbiota and diet in IBS: causes, consequences, or epiphenomena? Am J Gastroenterol. 2015;110:278–87. doi: 10.1038/ajg.2014.427

[80] Camilleri M. Serotonin in the gastrointestinal tract. Curr Opin Endocrinol Diabetes Obes. 2009;16:53–9. doi: 10.1097/MED.0b013e32831e9c8e

[81] Halmos EP., Christophersen CT., Bird AR., Shepherd SJ., Gibson PR., Muir JG. Diets that differ in their FODMAP content alter the colonic luminal microenvironment. Gut. 2015;64:93–100. doi: 10.1136/gutjnl-2014-307264

[82] Camilleri M., Lasch K., Zhou W. Irritable bowel syndrome: methods, mechanisms, and pathophysiology: the confluence of increased permeability, inflammation, and pain in irritable bowel syndrome. AJP Gastrointest Liver Physiol. 2012;303:G775–85. doi: 10.1152/ajpgi.00155.2012

[83] Branum AM., Lukacs SL. Food allergy among children in the United States. Pediatrics. 2009;124:1549–55. doi: 10.1542/peds.2009-1210

[84] Berni Canani R., Gilbert JA., Nagler CR. The role of the commensal microbiota in the regulation of tolerance to dietary allergens. Curr Opin Allergy Clin Immunol. 2015;15:243–9. doi: 10.1097/ACI.0000000000000157

[85] Muir AB., Benitez AJ., Dods K., Spergel JM., Fillon SA. Microbiome and its impact on gastrointestinal atopy. Allergy. 2016; 71:1256-63 doi: 10.1111/all.12943.

[86] Halmos EP., Power VA., Shepherd SJ., Gibson PR., Muir JG. A diet low in FODMAPs reduces symptoms of irritable bowel syndrome. Gastroenterology. 2014;146:67–75. doi: 10.1053/j.gastro.2013.09.046

[87] Shepherd SJ., Lomer MCE., Gibson PR. Short-chain carbohydrates and functional gastrointestinal disorders. Am J Gastroenterol. 2013;108:707–17. doi: 10.1038/ajg.2013.96

[88] Ong DK., Mitchell SB., Barrett JS., Shepherd SJ., Irving PM., Biesiekierski JR., et al. Manipulation of dietary short chain carbohydrates alters the pattern of gas production and genesis of symptoms in irritable bowel syndrome: dietary FODMAPs and IBS symptoms. J Gastroenterol Hepatol. 2010;25:1366–73. doi: 10.1111/j.1440-1746.2010.06370.x

[89] Staudacher HM., Whelan K., Irving PM., Lomer MC. Comparison of symptom response following advice for a diet low in fermentable carbohydrates (FODMAPs) versus standard dietary advice in patients with irritable bowel syndrome. J Hum Nutr Diet. 2011;24:487–95. doi: 10.1111/j.1365-277X.2011.01162

[90] Staudacher HM., Lomer MCE., Anderson JL., Barrett JS., Muir JG., Irving PM., et al. Fermentable carbohydrate restriction reduces luminal bifidobacteria and gastrointestinal symptoms in patients with irritable bowel syndrome. J Nutr. 2012;142:1510–8. doi: 10.3945/jn.112.159285

[91] Böhn L., Störsrud S., Liljebo T., Collin L., Lindfors P., Törnblom H., Simrén M. Diet low in FODMAPs reduces symptoms of irritable bowel syndrome as well as traditional dietary advice: a randomized controlled trialGastroenterology. 2015;149:1399–407.e2. doi: 10.1053/j.gastro.2015.07.054

[92] Koven N., Abry A. The clinical basis of orthorexia nervosa: emerging perspectives. Neuropsychiatr Dis Treat. 2015;11:385–94. doi: 10.2147/NDT.S61665

7

Inflammation as a Potential Therapeutic Target in IBS

Alexandra Chira, Romeo Ioan Chira and
Dan Lucian Dumitrascu

Abstract

The pathogenesis of irritable bowel syndrome (IBS) has been intensively researched, and despite a long journey for unraveling all the structures and the pathways involved, it still remains partially obscure. Inflammation was the first to be hypothesized as a potential pathway for the pathogenesis of IBS. It remains a keystone in the complex machinery of the pathogenesis that is currently considered multifactorial. Elucidating the pathogenesis of IBS is crucial for a targeted therapy of the disease. In this chapter, we review information regarding gut inflammation in IBS, underlining some of the newest data or the cornerstones. Additionally, our aim was also to review treatment currently available and future perspectives regarding anti-inflammatory treatments for IBS. Newer techniques allow detection and research of mediators involved in inflammation, as well as their potential role to be targeted by pharmacological agents. Recent data supports not only further research of the newer agents that are currently being developed but also some of the available ones that do not have sufficient evidence. Emerging therapies that target inflammation are under evaluation, in trials. A multidrug or a multidisciplinary approach needs to be considered in some cases that fail to respond to current treatment.

Keywords: anti-inflammatory, inflammation, irritable bowel syndrome, IBS treatment, postinfectious

1. Introduction

Despite the intensive research on irritable bowel syndrome (IBS) is being conducted, the pathogenesis still remains partially obscure. Since the description of this syndrome, many researchers have questioned the cause of IBS, which is currently being considered as multifactorial [1–3] with increasing evidence that support the concept [4, 5], since there are multiple mechanisms that could trigger the clinical complaints.

Not just one structure or system is involved in the occurrence of IBS, and there is a complex network already described and currently referred to as brain-gut axis [6–9] with multiple directions and ways to communicate or interrelate between these structures and paths [10] that are reflected also in the heterogeneity of the subtypes of IBS.

Although IBS is a functional gastrointestinal disorder [11] with no structural or biochemical abnormalities, there is some evidence suggesting that in some subtypes of IBS, inflammation might play a key role in generating a low-grade inflammatory response and a spectrum of symptoms that sometimes overlap with those of inflammatory bowel diseases in remission [12, 13], leading to difficulties in establishing the diagnosis in clinical practice.

In this chapter, we will review literature data concerning inflammation and its relation to IBS underlining some of the newest data or the key ones. Our aim was also to review treatment currently available and future perspectives regarding anti-inflammatory treatments for IBS.

2. Inflammation in IBS

Inflammation, defined as the answer of the immune system to various triggers, was first described by Celsus [14], who has assigned to it the four signs: *dolor* (pain), *rubor* (redness), *tumor* (swelling), *calor* (heat), and to which Rudolf Virchow [15] added *functio laesa* (functional impairment). All the characteristics that define inflammation are induced by a complex set of mediators [16]. In addition, the triggers that could initiate inflammatory responses are numerous and diverse [17]. The inflammatory responses may be acute or chronic [16, 17].

Inflammation was one of the first hypothesised causes of IBS [18]. Intestinal inflammation was proposed as a potential mechanism involved in the pathogenesis of IBS since 1960s, when Hiatt et al. [18] described mast cells in the muscularis externa of the terminal colon and cecum. Discovered by Paul Ehrlich, mast cells are the precursors of CD34+ hematopoietic stem cells [19]. Due to the diversity of functions of mast cells, they have been a cornerstone in the study of multiple conditions, being intensively researched in the last decades. Mast cells have multiple functions [20], some of them involving the gut: neuroimmune interactions, epithelial secretion and permeability, and visceral sensation [20, 21]. In addition, it can express receptors for several cytokines that are involved in immunity [19] or release key mediators [22]. Numerous studies assessed the presence and/or the role of mast cells in IBS [23–25]. There are also rigorous papers that reviewed studies investigating mast cells and/or the mast cell mediators in IBS [26].

Other types of mediators, such as immunoglobulin (Ig) E and atopia, have been investigated in IBS and linked to mast cells [27, 28]. Degranulation of mast cells and, subsequently, the release of mast cell mediators can also be induced by IgE [28]. There are few data regarding IgE levels in IBS. Vara et al. [29] showed higher levels of IgE in IBS compared with healthy controls.

Besides mast cells, there are data indicating that inflammatory cells are present in colonic mucosa in IBS patients [23]. They showed on colonic biopsies multiple types of cells such as neutrophils and T lymphocytes besides mast cells, all of which may support the role of the immune system in the ethiopathogenesis of IBS [23, 30]. If most of the studies examined mucosa of the rectum [31, 32], there are few studies that assessed also the deeper layers of the enteral wall [33]. There is a complex local response when triggers are detected [16, 34].

The balance of pro-inflammatory and anti-inflammatory responses and the mediators that are involved in the complex interactions have also been the subject of many studies. There is evidence of sustained inflammation in IBS supported by numerous studies that have detected low anti-inflammatory cytokines in IBS patients [35] or others that found high levels of those pro-inflammatory ones or a misbalance of the pro- and anti-inflammatory cytokine proportion [36, 37]. The complex dialogue between the structures involved in maintaining the homeostasis includes interrelation of nervous, immune, and endocrine systems [30, 34], where a pivotal piece is the brain that governs the humoral and neurological systems [34, 38, 39], in a complex network with multidirectional communicating systems [10]. Not only the anatomical integrity but also the functional status of all the systems is of major importance [40].

Psychological factors can participate in this mechanism, maintaining a state of low inflammation [41]. Inflammation in the gut might be responsible also for hyperalgesia [42] present in some patients with IBS contributing to the maintenance of the complaints.

2.1. Postinfectious IBS

Postinfectious IBS (PI-IBS) is a more recently coined type of IBS, initially identified as post-dysenteric IBS (PD-IBS) [43]. PI-IBS is defined as a subset of IBS in which the onset of IBS symptoms develops after an infectious episode and was first described by Chaudhary and Truelove [43]. This entity was confirmed by other studies [44]. The incidence of PI-IBS varies between 4 and 32% [45–47]. More frequently, PI-IBS was described and studied after an enteral infection [44, 48]. Pathogens already recognized to be involved in enteral infections are the following:

- bacteria: *Campylobacter jejuni* [31], *Salmonella enterica* [45], *Shigella* [49], *Escherichia coli* [50–52], *Clostridium difficile* [53]
- viruses: *Norovirus* [50, 54]
- parasites: *Giardia lamblia* [50, 55], *Blastocystis* spp. [56], *Dientamoeba fragilis* [57]

This subset of IBS patients offers a strong support emphasizing the importance of inflammation as one of the main paths to IBS. Enteral pathogens may induce pathological changes [31]. Spiller et al. [31] reported an imbalance of the enteroendocrine cells and of T lymphocytes, these two being assessed by histopathological examination of the rectal biopsies of the PI-IBS when compared with controls. There can be at least three scenarios: a prolonged normal inflammatory response, an augmented pathological inflammatory response in these patients, or there is a certain group of patients with particular characteristics that have a higher susceptibility [44, 58–60]. Anyway, there is not yet a firm conclusion.

2.2. Barrier function

The gut barrier function is important in modulating the gut inflammation [26, 61]. The barrier has multiple roles and its integrity is essential for a normal functionality of the digestive system [61]. An impaired barrier could facilitate the passage of inflammatory triggers that might induce changes in the gut. An increased permeability of the barrier might expose various structures to antigen contact [31].

2.3. Cholinergic system

There is another important piece in the complex domino of Inflammation – the so-called "cholinergic anti-inflammatory pathway" [34, 62, 63]. We did not intend to review the data regarding this system as there are multiple reviews [34] that have already analyzed the evidence, but to find the studies that support the interrelation with inflammation in IBS. Dinan et al. [64] investigated several cytokines, such as interleukin (IL): IL-6, IL-8, IL-10, and the growth hormone in the two arms of the study. They found that only IL-6 and the growth hormone in the group of IBS patients were overproduced when compared with controls after the administration of pyridostigmine that might suggest the implication of the cholinergic system [64].

2.4. Low-grade inflammation

More and more data sustain the hypotheses of a low-grade inflammation in IBS [65–67]. The fine line between normal to a pathological inflammatory response is still difficult to set. There is a low-grade inflammation of the gut that has been already acknowledged and literature data supports the putative role of the low-grade inflammation in IBS [65–68]. Several articles addressed this issue, some authors investigated tissue samples [23], while others assessed blood or stool samples [69–72] in order to detect and determine the inflammation status in IBS patients.

There are already numerous studies that assessed erythrocyte sedimentation rate, C-reactive protein (CRP) from blood sample, fecal calprotectin, and/or lactoferin in order to detect their presence in IBS and/or to calculate their predictive values [71–73]. Valuable information was provided by a meta-analysis, although that assessed their cut-off values in order to exclude inflammatory bowel diseases [74].

There are limited data regarding the presence of high-sensibility CRP [69] in IBS, but results indicate that when compared with healthy subjects, levels of high sensibility CRP are statistically significantly higher in IBS patients ($P < 0.001$) [69]. So literature data supports the presence of low-grade inflammation in IBS since the levels of high-sensibility CRP, though were still within the normal range, were higher in IBS than in controls [69].

A similar situation is for calprotectin, which is used mainly for differential diagnosis of inflammatory bowel diseases [73], but there are also studies that showed increased levels of calprotectin in IBS patients when comparing the values of those of healthy controls [72].

In the search to quantify the levels of inflammation, many authors proposed various biomarkers, and others proposed multiple biomarkers such as a panel or a set of markers [75, 76].

2.5. Genes and inflammation in IBS

Genetic factors have also been suspected as being involved in the inflammation in IBS.

Regarding genes and polymorphism, there are several studies that have assessed gene polymorphism, of which IL-10 and α tumor necrosis factor are some of the ones that are being intensively investigated [77–79].

As for the other studies that addressed IBS, their findings are inconsistent since some of the studies that assessed IL-10 genotypes in IBS patients versus controls showed high-producer genotype for IL-10 had a lower frequency statistically significant in IBS than in controls (P = 0.003) [79], and other studies did not find statistically significant difference of IL-10 polymorphism in IBS patients [78]. Schmulson et al. [78] assessed two polymorphisms: IL-10 (-1082G/A) and α tumor necrosis factor (-308G/A) in IBS patients and compared them with controls. There were no statistically significant differences between IBS and controls regarding either of the two polymorphisms.

There are also other studies besides these that assessed single nucleotide polymorphisms and more complex studies such as genome-wide association studies [80].

2.6. New hypotheses

There is a growing interest in applying the latest techniques used in molecular biology also for the study of IBS, such as the study of microRNA—miRNAs [81], small interfering RNA—siRNAs [82] or new approaches such as meta-omics [83].

Recently, new directions have been proposed in the study of the etiopathogenesis of IBS [81, 84]. The role of stem cells has been already intensively researched [85, 86], even in inflammatory bowel diseases [87], but these potent cells have raised interest about their role or potential use in IBS.

Very recent data advances the hypotheses that intestinal stem cells might be involved in the inflammatory paths discussed in IBS [84, 88]. Due to their properties, stem cells not only are able to respond to pathogens but also may modulate the spectrum of answers by their secretory functions [84, 89]. These stem cells might also represent therapeutic targets [84], but future studies to identify a specific target, either structural or functional, of the stem cells are mandatory.

The scientific community is eager to develop and improve current technologies, both for identifying new therapeutic targets and also for new treatment.

3. Anti-inflammatory treatment

Treatment of IBS still represents a challenge for clinicians. Due to the marked heterogeneity of the IBS subtypes, we will address anti-inflammatory agents used or those with potential use in IBS. Considering the multifactorial etiology, there are authors who propose a treatment determined by the main pathological path that led to IBS [4]. Literature data are limited concerning pharmacological anti-inflammatory classes studied in IBS as well as for the number of the members of these pharmacological classes that were investigated. Since we cannot still establish the main cause that led to IBS, an etiopathogenetic treatment is not possible, and some are currently being developed; a main aim in the treatment of IBS still is to alleviate the symptoms [1]. Though there are few studies that assessed anti-inflammatory classes or members of these classes in IBS, there is an intensive research activity into unraveling new targets and new treatments [90]. There are ongoing trials [91] and research programs and networks [92] that bring valuable information for a deeper understanding of IBS.

4. Aminosalicylic acid agents

Since the discovery of 5-aminosalicylic acid agents (5-ASA) by Svartz [93] and afterward with their active properties being described by Azad et al. [94], these agents were intensively researched as well as used in clinical practice [95]. The 5-ASA derivates have been used in several inflammatory conditions such as the inflammatory bowel disorders [95]. There are already consistent data regarding the efficacy of 5-ASA in ulcerative colitis [95] as well as regarding their safety. The rationale for prescribing 5-ASA agents in IBS is represented by their anti-inflammatory properties and is the result of several mechanisms [96].

Article	Type of article	Conclusions
Min et al. [97]	Letter	In selected subgroups of IBS might be efficient
Törnblom et al. [98]	Commentaries	In selected subgroups of IBS might be efficient
Lazaraki et al. [99]	Review	Inconclusive regarding the use of mesalasine in IBS
Camilleri et al. [100]	Review	Inconclusive, though some studies show a positive effect on pain, results were not replicated by others
Xue et al. [101]	Letter	Inconclusive—analyzed impact of mesalazine on gut microbiota
Hanevik et al. [102]	Letter + pilot CT	Inefficient
Farup et al. [103]	Letter	Inconclusive – authors underline that Andrews et al. [108] did not analyze drop out patients in their study

Table 1. Articles reviewing the use of 5-ASA in IBS.

Though there are few original studies, there are also reviews that analyze the use of 5-ASA in IBS (**Table 1**). Literature data indicate that in certain group of patients such as those with

PI-IBS, especially the IBS with diarrhoea (IBS-D) subtype could benefit, at least for a certain period of the anti-inflammatory effects of this class (see **Tables 1** and **2**). Regarding the length of treatment, dosing, and schemes of treatment, there are few data in the literature, and there is no study to assess all of this. Future studies are required in order to configure an a priori set of features regarding what type of IBS patient is likely to respond to 5-ASA treatment, as well as the regimen and dosing.

Article	Type of article, type of IBS	Dose and time of treatment	Conclusions
Barbara et al. [104]	Placebo-controlled trial (CT), multicentre IBS	800 mg tid, 12 weeks	Mesalazine treatment was not statistically significant or more efficient than placebo (P = 0.870). In certain groups of patients, it might be useful.
Lam et al. [105]	CT, IBS-D	2 g/day—2 weeks, if tolerated 2 g bid—11 weeks	In certain groups of selected IBS-D patients, it might be efficient, although there is no clear evidence of it being useful.
Bafutto et al. [106]	Pilot study, IBS-D	Various dosing—in the fourth groups	May be useful in certain groups of patients.
Tuteja et al. [107]	CT, PI-IBS	1.6 g bid, 12 weeks	No statistically significant improvement of symptoms ($P \geq 0.11$) nor QOL ($P \geq 0.16$).
Andrews et al. [108]	Pilot study, IBS-D	1.5 g bid, 4 weeks	Significant improvement of pain.
Bafutto et al. [109]	CT, IBS-D	800 mg tid, 30 days	Significant improvement of total symptom score, inclusive of pain. ($P < 0.0001$)
Dorofeyev et al. [110]	CT, IBS, all subtypes	500 mg qid, 28 days	Statistical improvement of abdominal pain ($P < 0.01$) as well as some histopathological aspects.
Hanevik et al. [102]	Letter + pilot CT	800 mg bid, 6 weeks	Inefficient.
Corinaldesi et al. [111]	CT, IBS	800 mg tid, 8 weeks	Mesalazine significantly improved only general well-being ($P = 0.038$), having no significant statistic effect regarding bloating ($P = 0.177$), abdominal pain ($P = 0.084$), or bowel habits.
Preobrazhenskii [112]*	Study	4–6 g daily, not shown	Efficient.

*Articles in other languages (Russian) or full text could not be retrieved.

Table 2. Studies assessing 5-ASA agents in IBS.

4.1. Acetylsalicylic acid

Regarding the use of acetylsalicylic acid, we have identified just one study that assessed it in relation to IBS, but the purpose of the study was to determine if certain anti-inflammatory drugs could induce constipation [113]. In fact, the study assessed that the use of some anti-inflammatory drugs among acetylsalicylic acid was related to constipation. [113].

4.2. Mast cell stabilizers

Mast cell stabilizers (cromoglycate and ketotifen) have been tested in IBS, but there are very few literature data concerning this class of drugs. Also, the criteria used for diagnosing IBS were different; therefore, there is no uniformity when comparing these studies. Subsequent studies are mandatory in order to have the answer: which IBS patients are suited to a mast cell stabilizer treatment and what is the dosing, or what is a suitable regimen.

4.3. Ketotifen

Klooker et al. [114] investigated ketotifen, suggesting that it can reduce visceral hypersensitivity and improve the quality of life. Though there is just one study to investigate ketotifen in IBS patients, there has already been questions about its safety [115]. For certain other studies, to assess this class for IBS treatment is mandatory in order to grade the levels of evidence. Although there is just one study with positive results, we also consider encouraging these results [33], and we strongly feel that there are more therapeutic options that have not yet been explored.

4.4. Cromoglycate

Regarding cromoglycate, there are several studies that assessed it in IBS patients. Literature data suggest that they could have a beneficial role in certain groups of patients, especially in those who have also food allergies or intolerances (see **Table 3**). There are methodological issues concerning these studies; so in order to reduce some of the biases, rigorous parallel studies are needed.

Article	Conclusion
Leri et al. [116]	Efficient (in conjunction with dietary exclusions in IBS patients with food intolerance)
Stefanini et al. [117]	Efficient (in IBS patients with food intolerance)
Grazioli et al. [118]	Efficient (in pediatric IBS patients with food intolerance)
Stefanini et al. [119]	Efficient (in IBS patients with food intolerance)
Lunardi et al. [120]	Efficient (in IBS patients with food intolerance)
Paganelli et al. [121]	Inconclusive
Antico et al. [122]*	–
Stefanini et al. [123]	Efficient
Tomecki et al.* [124]	Inefficient

*Article in other languages than English (Polish, Italian) also could not be retrieved.

Table 3. Articles that assessed cromoglycate in IBS.

4.5. Montelukast

There is just one report of the use of montelukast in IBS stating a positive effect [125]. Considering the pathways that are involved in the pathogenesis of IBS, it seems reasonable that the authors proposed and used it. The wonder is that there are so few data regarding it, though there are data regarding IBS and allergies [29]. Montelukast might be an option for the patients who have IBS and allergic conditions, but there is a lack of studies to address this issue. Rigorous trials with such drugs are needed in order to conclude about their use in IBS.

4.6. Corticosteroids

Some authors even proposed corticosteroids as anti-inflammatory agents in IBS [126]. A short course-3 weeks, 30 mg prednisolone/day was administered to PI-IBS patients and compared with placebo. There was no statistically significant difference between the number of enterochromaffin cells between patients treated with prednisolone and those that received placebo ($P = 0.5$). Though for the reduction of the number of T lymphocytes in the lamina propria. Dunlop et al. [126] found a statistically significant difference that favors prednisolone, there was no improvement regarding several symptoms of IBS.

Due to their known side effects, one study investigated the impact of using oral steroids, showing that they do not have a higher risk for inducing IBS symptoms in adults under 40 years [127].

We conducted a search on PubMed search motor between 1–21st July 2016 using multiple strategies as seen in **Table 4**. There is just one study that assessed the corticoid therapy in IBS, though there are several authors who consider corticosteroids as a reasonable treatment option in certain subgroups of IBS patients (**Table 4**).

Strategy	Results	Appropriate	Inappropriate
"Corticosteroids, irritable bowel syndrome"	91	2 [127, 128]	89
"Corticosteroids, IBS"	64	1 [128]	63
"Prednisone, irritable bowel syndrome"	5	0	5
"Prednisolone, irritable bowel syndrome"	12	1 [126]	11
"Prednisolone, IBS"	5	1 [127]	4
"Budesonide, irritable bowel syndrome"	10	1 [128]	9

Table 4. Results retrieved by several search strategies on PubMed search motor.

4.7. Imunglobulin E antibody (Omalizumab)

There is just one study that addresses this issue [28], which presents a case of a patient that had concurrently IBS and asthma. The patient received an IgE antibody with a major improvement of IBS symptoms. These results suggest that in certain subgroups of patients with concurrent diseases as IBS and atopic status, or extra-intestinal symptoms, IgE antibodies might be useful.

5. Conclusions

Inflammation remains an important pathway involved in the pathogenesis of IBS. Despite the high interest in the field of functional gastrointestinal disorders, till now, researchers have not entirely discovered all the pieces of the complex puzzle that is the etiopathogenesis of IBS, or all of the components of the pathways that finally lead to IBS.

Newer techniques allow detection and promote research of mediators that are involved in inflammation, even in low amounts. Also, the new technologies are able to identify new structures, as well as their potential role to be targeted by pharmacotherapeutic agents.

Results suggest that there are potential pharmacological classes, alongside with potential therapeutic targets that deserve to be reassessed for IBS.

Recent data supports further research of the pathways and structures involved, as well as assessment of not only the newer agents that are currently being developed but also of some of the available ones that do not have sufficient evidence. Emerging therapies that target inflammation are under evaluation, in trials. A multidrug or a multidisciplinary approach needs to be considered in cases that fail to respond to current treatment or to a single therapy, heading toward the current trend, of a personalized medicine.

Abbreviations

5-Aminosalicylic acid agents: 5-ASA

Bis in die: bid

C reactive protein: CRP

Irritable bowel syndrome: IBS

IBS with diarrhoea: IBS-D

Immunoglobulin: Ig

Interleukin: IL

Quarter in die: qid

Quality of life: QOL

Placebo-controlled trial: CT

Postinfectious IBS: PI-IBS

Postdysenteric IBS: PD-IBS

Ter in die: tid

Author details

Alexandra Chira[1], Romeo Ioan Chira[2] and Dan Lucian Dumitrascu[1*]

*Address all correspondence to: ddumitrascu@umfcluj.ro

1 - 2nd Medical Clinic, Department of Internal Medicine, "Iuliu Hatieganu" University of Medicine and Pharmacy Cluj-Napoca, Romania

2 - 1st Medical Clinic, Department of Internal Medicine, Div. Gastroenterology, "Iuliu Hatieganu" University of Medicine and Pharmacy Cluj-Napoca, Romania

References

[1] Drossman DA, Camilleri M, Mayer EA, Whitehead WE. AGA technical review on irritable bowel syndrome. Gastroenterology. 2002;123(6):2108–31.

[2] Bellini M, Gambaccini D, Stasi C, Urbano MT, Marchi S, Usai-Satta P. Irritable bowel syndrome: a disease still searching for pathogenesis, diagnosis and therapy. World J Gastroenterol. 2014;20(27):8807–20.

[3] Barbara G, De Giorgio R, Stanghellini V, Cremon C, Corinaldesi R. A role for inflammation in irritable bowel syndrome? Gut. 2002;51 Suppl 1:i41–4.

[4] Malagelada JR, Malagelada C. Mechanism-oriented therapy of irritable bowel syndrome. Adv Ther. 2016;33(6):877–93.

[5] Chumpitazi BP, Shulman RJ. Underlying molecular and cellular mechanisms in childhood irritable bowel syndrome. Mol Cell Pediatr. 2016;3(1):11.

[6] Mayer EA. Gut feelings: the emerging biology of gut-brain communication. Nat Rev Neurosci. 2011;12(8):453–66.

[7] Jones MP, Dilley JB, Drossman D, Crowell MD. Brain-gut connections in functional GI disorders: anatomic and physiologic relationships. Neurogastroenterol Motil. 2006;18(2):91–103.

[8] James W. What is an emotion? Mind. 1884;9:188–205.

[9] Fichna J, Storr MA. Brain-gut interactions in IBS. Front Pharmacol. 2012;3:127.

[10] Koloski NA, Jones M, Talley NJ. Evidence that independent gut-to-brain and brain-to-gut pathways operate in the irritable bowel syndrome and functional dyspepsia: a 1-year population-based prospective study. Aliment Pharmacol Ther. 2016;44(6):592–600.

[11] Longstreth GF, Thompson WG, Chey WD, Houghton LA, Mearin F, Spiller RC. Functional bowel disorders. Gastroenterology. 2006;130(5):1480–91.

[12] Grover M, Herfarth H, Drossman DA. The functional-organic dichotomy: postinfectious irritable bowel syndrome and inflammatory bowel disease-irritable bowel syndrome. Clin Gastroenterol Hepatol. 2009;7(1):48–53.

[13] Berrill JW, Green JT, Hood K, Campbell AK. Symptoms of irritable bowel syndrome in patients with inflammatory bowel disease: examining the role of sub-clinical inflammation and the impact on clinical assessment of disease activity. Aliment Pharmacol Ther. 2013;38(1):44–51.

[14] Celsus AC. De Medicina, praef. iii. 4.

[15] Rather LJ. Disturbance of function (functio laesa): the legendary fifth cardinal sign of inflammation, added by Galen to the four cardinal signs of Celsus. Bull N Y Acad Med 1971;47:303–322.

[16] Baumann H, Gauldie J. The acute phase response. Immunol Today. 1994;15:74–80.

[17] Sell S, editor. Immunology, Immunopathology, and Immunity. 6th ed. Washington, DC: ASM Press; 2001.

[18] Hiatt RB, Katz L. Mast cells in inflammatory conditions of the gastrointestinal tract. Am J Gastroenterol. 1962;37:541–5.

[19] Shea-Donohue T, Stiltz J, Zhao A, Notari L. Mast cells. Curr Gastroenterol Rep. 2010;12(5):349–57.

[20] Zhang L, Song J, Hou X. Mast cells and irritable bowel syndrome: from the bench to the bedside. J Neurogastroenterol Motil. 2016; 22(2):181–92.

[21] Bischoff SC, Kramer S. Human mast cells, bacteria, and intestinal immunity. Immunol Rev. 2007; 217:329–37.

[22] Barbara G, Stanghellini V, De Giorgio R, Cremon C, Cottrell GS, Santini D, et al. Activated mast cells in proximity to colonic nerves correlate with abdominal pain in irritable bowel syndrome. Gastroenterology. 2004;126(3):693–702.

[23] Chadwick VS, Chen W, Shu D, Paulus B, Bethwaite P, Tie A, et al. Activation of the mucosal immune system in irritable bowel syndrome. Gastroenterology. 2002; 122(7): 1778–83.

[24] O'Sullivan M, Clayton N, Breslin NP, Harman I, Bountra C, McLaren A, et al. Increased mast cells in the irritable bowel syndrome. Neurogastroenterol Motil. 2000;12(5):449–57.

[25] Cremon C, Gargano L, Morselli-Labate AM, Santini D, Cogliandro RF, De Giorgio R, et al. Mucosal immune activation in irritable bowel syndrome: gender-dependence and association with digestive symptoms. Am J Gastroenterol. 2009; 104(2):392–400.

[26] Camilleri M, Lasch K, Zhou W. Irritable bowel syndrome: methods, mechanisms, and pathophysiology. The confluence of increased permeability, inflammation, and pain in

irritable bowel syndrome. Am J Physiol Gastrointest Liver Physiol. 2012; 303(7):G775–85.

[27] Coca A, Cooke R. On the classification of the phenomena of hypersensitiveness. J Immunol; 1923 8: 163–182.

[28] Pearson JS, Niven RM, Meng J, Atarodi S, Whorwell PJ. Immunoglobulin E in irritable bowel syndrome: another target for treatment? A case report and literature review. Therap Adv Gastroenterol. 2015;8(5):270–7.

[29] Vara EJ, Valeur J, Hausken T, Lied GA. Extra-intestinal symptoms in patients with irritable bowel syndrome: related to high total IgE levels and atopic sensitization? Scand J Gastroenterol. 2016;51(8):908–13.

[30] Ohman L, Simren M. Pathogenesis of IBS: role of inflammation, immunity and neuroimmune interactions. Nat Rev Gastroenterol Hepatol. 2010;7(3):163–73.

[31] Spiller RC, Jenkins D, Thornley JP, Hebden JM, Wright T, Skinner M, et al. Increased rectal mucosal enteroendocrine cells, T lymphocytes, and increased gut permeability following acute *Campylobacter enteritis* and in post-dysenteric irritable bowel syndrome. Gut. 2000;47(6):804–11.

[32] Goral V, Kucukoner M, Buyukbayram H. Mast cells count and serum cytokine levels in patients with irritable bowel syndrome. Hepatogastroenterology. 2010;57(101):751–4.

[33] O'Sullivan M. Therapeutic potential of ketotifen in irritable bowel syndrome (IBS) may involve changes in mast cells at sites beyond the rectum. Gut. 2011;60(3):423; author reply.

[34] Pavlov VA, Wang H, Czura CJ, Friedman SG, Tracey KJ. The cholinergic anti-inflammatory pathway: a missing link in neuroimmunomodulation. Mol Med. 2003;9(5-8): 125–34.

[35] Schmulson M, Pulido-London D, Rodriguez O, Morales-Rochlin N, Martinez-Garcia R, Gutierrez-Ruiz MC, et al. Lower serum IL-10 is an independent predictor of IBS among volunteers in Mexico. Am J Gastroenterol. 2012;107(5):747–53.

[36] Bashashati M, Rezaei N, Shafieyoun A, McKernan DP, Chang L, Ohman L, et al. Cytokine imbalance in irritable bowel syndrome: a systematic review and meta-analysis. Neurogastroenterol Motil. 2014;26(7):1036–48.

[37] Macsharry J, O'Mahony L, Fanning A, Bairead E, Sherlock G, Tiesman J, et al. Mucosal cytokine imbalance in irritable bowel syndrome. Scand J Gastroenterol. 2008;43(12): 1467–76.

[38] Watkins LR, Maier SF, Goehler LE. Cytokine-to-brain communication: a review and analysis of alternative mechanisms. Life Sci 57:1011–26. 1995.

[39] Elmquist JK, Scammell TE, Saper CB. Mechanisms of CNS response to systemic immune challenge: the febrile response. Trends Neurosci 20:565–9.

[40] Posserud I, Ersryd A, Simren M. Functional findings in irritable bowel syndrome. World J Gastroenterol. 2006;12(18):2830–8.

[41] Tanaka Y, Kanazawa M, Fukudo S, Drossman DA. Biopsychosocial model of irritable bowel syndrome. J Neurogastroenterol Motil. 2011;17(2):131–9.

[42] Farzaei MH, Bahramsoltani R, Abdollahi M, Rahimi R. The role of visceral hypersensitivity in irritable bowel syndrome: pharmacological targets and novel treatments. J Neurogastroenterol Motil. 2016;22(4):558–574.

[43] Chaudhary NA, Truelove SC. The irritable colon syndrome. A study of the clinical features, predisposing causes, and prognosis in 130 cases. Q J Med. 1962;31:307–22.

[44] Gwee KA, Collins SM, Read NW, Rajnakova A, Deng Y, Graham JC, et al. Increased rectal mucosal expression of interleukin 1beta in recently acquired post-infectious irritable bowel syndrome. Gut. 2003;52(4):523–6.

[45] Rodriguez LA, Ruigomez A. Increased risk of irritable bowel syndrome after bacterial gastroenteritis: cohort study. BMJ. 1999;318(7183):565–6.

[46] Thabane M, Kottachchi DT, Marshall JK. Systematic review and meta-analysis: The incidence and prognosis of post-infectious irritable bowel syndrome. Aliment Pharmacol Ther. 2007;26(4):535–44.

[47] McKendrick MW, Read NW. Irritable bowel syndrome—post salmonella infection. J Infect. 1994;29(1):1–3.

[48] Spiller R, Garsed K. Postinfectious irritable bowel syndrome. Gastroenterology. 2009;136(6):1979–88.

[49] Kim HS, Lim JH, Park H, Lee SI. Increased immunoendocrine cells in intestinal mucosa of postinfectious irritable bowel syndrome patients 3 years after acute Shigella infection—an observation in a small case control study. Yonsei Med J. 2010;51(1):45–51.

[50] Grover M. Role of gut pathogens in development of irritable bowel syndrome. Indian J Med Res. 2014;139(1):11–8.

[51] Okhuysen PC, Jiang ZD, Carlin L, Forbes C, DuPont HL. Post-diarrhea chronic intestinal symptoms and irritable bowel syndrome in North American travelers to Mexico. Am J Gastroenterol. 2004;99(9):1774–8.

[52] Andresen V, Lowe B, Broicher W, Riegel B, Fraedrich K, von Wulffen M, et al. Post-infectious irritable bowel syndrome (PI-IBS) after infection with Shiga-like toxin-producing Escherichia coli (STEC) O104:H4: a cohort study with prospective follow-up. United Eur Gastroenterol J. 2016;4(1):121–31.

[53] Wadhwa A, Al Nahhas MF, Dierkhising RA, Patel R, Kashyap P, Pardi DS, et al. High risk of post-infectious irritable bowel syndrome in patients with Clostridium difficile infection. Aliment Pharmacol Ther. 2016;44(6):576–82.

[54] Marshall JK, Thabane M, Borgaonkar MR, James C. Postinfectious irritable bowel syndrome after a food-borne outbreak of acute gastroenteritis attributed to a viral pathogen. Clin Gastroenterol Hepatol. 2007;5(4):457–60.

[55] Wensaas KA, Langeland N, Hanevik K, Morch K, Eide GE, Rortveit G. Irritable bowel syndrome and chronic fatigue 3 years after acute giardiasis: historic cohort study. Gut. 2012;61(2):214–9.

[56] Azizian M, Basati G, Abangah G, Mahmoudi MR, Mirzaei A. Contribution of Blasto-cystishominis subtypes and associated inflammatory factors in development of irritable bowel syndrome. Parasitol Res. 2016;115(5):2003–9.

[57] Borody TJ, Warren EF, Wettstein A, Robertson G, Recabarren P, Fontella A, et al. Eradication of Dientamoeba fragilis can resolve IBS-like symptoms. J Gastroenterol Hepatol 17(Suppl):A103. 2002.

[58] Wouters MM, Van Wanrooy S, Nguyen A, Dooley J, Aguilera-Lizarraga J, Van Brabant W, et al. Psychological comorbidity increases the risk for postinfectious IBS partly by enhanced susceptibility to develop infectious gastroenteritis. Gut. 2016;65(8):1279–88.

[59] Collins SM, Piche T, Rampal P. The putative role of inflammation in the irritable bowel syndrome. Gut. 2001;49(6):743–5.

[60] Spiller RC. Postinfectious irritable bowel syndrome. Gastroenterology. 2003;124(6): 1662–71.

[61] Martinez C, Gonzalez-Castro A, Vicario M, Santos J. Cellular and molecular basis of intestinal barrier dysfunction in the irritable bowel syndrome. Gut Liver. 2012;6(3):305–15.

[62] Tracey KJ. The inflammatory reflex. Nature 2002;420:853–9..

[63] Blalock JE. Harnessing a neural-immune circuit to control inflammation and shock. J Exp Med 2002;195:F25–8.

[64] Dinan TG, Clarke G, Quigley EM, Scott LV, Shanahan F, Cryan J, et al. Enhanced cholinergic-mediated increase in the pro-inflammatory cytokine IL-6 in irritable bowel syndrome: role of muscarinic receptors. Am J Gastroenterol. 2008;103(10):2570–6.

[65] Akiho H, Ihara E, Nakamura K. Low-grade inflammation plays a pivotal role in gastrointestinal dysfunction in irritable bowel syndrome. World J Gastrointest Patho-physiol. 2010;1(3):97–105.

[66] Lee E, Schiller LR, Fordtran JS. Quantification of colonic lamina propria cells by means of a morphometric point-counting method. Gastroenterology. 1988;94(2):409–18.

[67] Sinagra E, Pompei G, Tomasello G, Cappello F, Morreale GC, Amvrosiadis G, et al. Inflammation in irritable bowel syndrome: myth or new treatment target? World J Gastroenterol. 2016;22(7):2242–55.

[68] Barbara G, Cremon C, Carini G, Bellacosa L, Zecchi L, De Giorgio R, et al. The immune system in irritable bowel syndrome. J Neurogastroenterol Motil. 2011;17(4):349–59.

[69] Hod K, Dickman R, Sperber A, Melamed S, Dekel R, Ron Y, et al. Assessment of high-sensitivity CRP as a marker of micro-inflammation in irritable bowel syndrome. Neurogastroenterol Motil. 2011;23(12):1105–10.

[70] Hod K, Ringel-Kulka T, Martin CF, Maharshak N, Ringel Y. High-sensitive C-reactive protein as a marker for inflammation in irritable bowel syndrome. J Clin Gastroenterol. 2015.

[71] Chang MH, Chou JW, Chen SM, Tsai MC, Sun YS, Lin CC, et al. Faecal calprotectin as a novel biomarker for differentiating between inflammatory bowel disease and irritable bowel syndrome. Mol Med Rep. 2014;10(1):522–6.

[72] David LE, Surdea-Blaga T, Dumitrascu DL. Semiquantitative fecal calprotectin test in postinfectious and non-postinfectious irritable bowel syndrome: cross-sectional study. Sao Paulo Med J. 2014:0.

[73] Otten CM, Kok L, Witteman BJ, Baumgarten R, Kampman E, Moons KG, et al. Diagnostic performance of rapid tests for detection of fecal calprotectin and lactoferrin and their ability to discriminate inflammatory from irritable bowel syndrome. Clin Chem Lab Med. 2008;46(9):1275–80.

[74] Menees SB, Powell C, Kurlander J, Goel A, Chey WD. A meta-analysis of the utility of C-reactive protein, erythrocyte sedimentation rate, fecal calprotectin, and fecal lactoferrin to exclude inflammatory bowel disease in adults with IBS. Am J Gastroenterol. 2015;110(3):444–54.

[75] Lembo AJ, Neri B, Tolley J, Barken D, Carroll S, Pan H. Use of serum biomarkers in a diagnostic test for irritable bowel syndrome. Aliment Pharmacol Ther. 2009;29(8):834–42.

[76] Jones MP, Chey WD, Singh S, Gong H, Shringarpure R, Hoe N, et al. A biomarker panel and psychological morbidity differentiates the irritable bowel syndrome from health and provides novel pathophysiological leads. Aliment Pharmacol Ther. 2014;39(4):426–37.

[77] Olivo-Diaz A, Romero-Valdovinos M, Gudino-Ramirez A, Reyes-Gordillo J, Jimenez-Gonzalez DE, Ramirez-Miranda ME, et al. Findings related to IL-

8 and IL-10 gene polymorphisms in a Mexican patient population with irritable bowel syndrome infected with blastocystis. Parasitol Res. 2012;111(1): 487–91.

[78] Schmulson M, Pulido-London D, Rodriguez O, Morales-Rochlin N, Martinez-Garcia R, Gutierrez-Ruiz MC, et al. IL-10 and TNF-alpha polymorphisms in subjects with irritable bowel syndrome in Mexico. Rev Esp Enferm Dig. 2013;105(7):392–9.

[79] Gonsalkorale WM, Perrey C, Pravica V, Whorwell PJ, Hutchinson IV. Interleukin 10 genotypes in irritable bowel syndrome: evidence for an inflammatory component? Gut. 2003;52(1):91–3.

[80] Ek WE, Reznichenko A, Ripke S, Niesler B, Zucchelli M, Rivera NV, et al. Exploring the genetics of irritable bowel syndrome: a GWA study in the general population and replication in multinational case-control cohorts. Gut. 2015;64(11): 1774–82.

[81] Zhou Q, Souba WW, Croce CM, Verne GN. MicroRNA-29a regulates intestinal membrane permeability in patients with irritable bowel syndrome. Gut. 2010;59(6):775–84.

[82] Cenac N, Bautzova T, Le Faouder P, Veldhuis NA, Poole DP, Rolland C, et al. Quantification and potential functions of endogenous agonists of transient receptor potential channels in patients with irritable bowel syndrome. Gastroenterology. 2015;149(2):433–44 e7.

[83] Mondot S, Lepage P. The human gut microbiome and its dysfunctions through the meta-omics prism. Ann N Y Acad Sci. 2016;1372(1):9–19.

[84] Ratanasirintrawoot S, Israsena N. Stem cells in the intestine: possible roles in pathogenesis of irritable bowel syndrome. J Neurogastroenterol Motil. 2016;22(3): 367–82.

[85] Ozkul Y, Galderisi U. The impact of epigenetics on mesenchymal stem cell biology. J Cell Physiol. 2016;231(11):2393–401.

[86] Wang Q, Ding G, Xu X. Immunomodulatory functions of mesenchymal stem cells and possible mechanisms. Histol Histopathol. 2016;31(9):949–59.

[87] De Francesco F, Romano M, Zarantonello L, Ruffolo C, Neri D, Bassi N, et al. The role of adipose stem cells in inflammatory bowel disease: from biology to novel therapeutic strategies. Cancer Biol Ther. 2016;17(9):889–898.

[88] Roostaee A, Benoit YD, Boudjadi S, Beaulieu JF. Epigenetics in intestinal epithelial cell renewal. J Cell Physiol. 2016;231(11):2361–7.

[89] Owens BM. Inflammation, innate immunity, and the intestinal stromal cell niche: opportunities and challenges. Front Immunol. 2015;6:319.

[90] Corsetti M, Whorwell P. Novel pharmacological therapies for irritable bowel syndrome. Expert Rev Gastroenterol Hepatol. 2016;10(7):807–15.

[91] International Foundation for Functional Gastrointestinal Disorders, Inc. (IFFGD) [Internet]. 1998–2016. Available from: http://www.aboutibs.org/take-part-in-online-studies.html [Accessed: 2016-07-21]

[92] GENIEUR.EU [Internet]. 2012. Available from: https://genieur.eu/ [Accessed: 2016-06-12]

[93] Svartz N. Salazopyrin, a new sulfanilamide preparation: A. Therapeutic results in rheumatic polyarthritis. B. Therapeutic results in ulcerative colitis. C. Toxic manifestations in treatment with sulfanilamide preparation. Acta Med Scand 1942;11:557–590.

[94] Azad Khan AK, Piris J, Truelove SC. An experiment to determine the active therapeutic moiety of sulphasalazine. Lancet. 1977;2(8044):892-5.

[95] Bohm SK, Kruis W. Long-term efficacy and safety of once-daily mesalazine granules for the treatment of active ulcerative colitis. Clin Exp Gastroenterol. 2014;7:369–83.

[96] Desreumaux P. Understanding the mechanism of 5-ASA in treating colonic inflammation. Gastroenterol Hepatol (N Y). 2008;4(5):319–20.

[97] Min T, Ford AC. Efficacy of mesalazine in IBS. Gut. 2016;65(1):187–8.

[98] Törnblom H, Simren M. In search for a disease-modifying treatment in irritable bowel syndrome. Gut. 2016;65(1):2–3.

[99] Lazaraki G, Chatzimavroudis G, Katsinelos P. Recent advances in pharmacological treatment of irritable bowel syndrome. World J. Gastroenterol. 2014;20(27):8867–85.

[100] Camilleri M. Pharmacological agents currently in clinical trials for disorders in neurogastroenterology. J Clin Invest. 2013;123(10):4111–20.

[101] Xue L, Huang Z, Zhou X, Chen W. The possible effects of mesalazine on the intestinal microbiota. Aliment Pharmacol Ther. 2012;36(8):813–4.

[102] Hanevik K, Dizdar V, Langeland N, Eide GE, Hausken T. Tolerability and effect of mesalazine in postinfectious irritable bowel syndrome. Aliment Pharmacol Ther. 2011;34(2):259–60.

[103] Farup PG. Questions about mesalazine and the irritable bowel syndrome. Aliment Pharmacol Ther. 2011;34(8):1036–7; author reply 7–8.

[104] Barbara G, Cremon C, Annese V, Basilisco G, Bazzoli F, Bellini M, et al. Randomised controlled trial of mesalazine in IBS. Gut. 2016;65(1):82–90.

[105] Lam C, Tan W, Leighton M, Hastings M, Lingaya M, Falcone Y, et al. A mechanistic multicentre, parallel group, randomised placebo-controlled trial of mesalazine for the treatment of IBS with diarrhoea (IBS-D). Gut. 2016;65(1):91-9.

[106] Bafutto M, Almeida JR, Leite NV, Costa MB, Oliveira EC, Resende-Filho J. Treatment of diarrhea-predominant irritable bowel syndrome with mesalazine and/or *Saccharomyces boulardii*. Arq Gastroenterol. 2013;50(4):304–9.

[107] Tuteja AK, Fang JC, Al-Suqi M, Stoddard GJ, Hale DC. Double-blind placebo-controlled study of mesalamine in post-infective irritable bowel syndrome—a pilot study. Scand J Gastroenterol. 2012;47(10):1159–64.

[108] Andrews CN, Griffiths TA, Kaufman J, Vergnolle N, Surette MG, Rioux KP. Mesalazine (5-aminosalicylic acid) alters faecal bacterial profiles, but not mucosal proteolytic activity in diarrhoea-predominant irritable bowel syndrome. Aliment Pharmacol Ther. 2011;34(3):374–83.

[109] Bafutto M, Almeida JR, Leite NV, Oliveira EC, Gabriel-Neto S, Rezende-Filho J. Treatment of postinfectious irritable bowel syndrome and noninfective irritable bowel syndrome with mesalazine. Arq Gastroenterol. 2011;48(1):36–40.

[110] Dorofeyev AE, Kiriyan EA, Vasilenko IV, Rassokhina OA, Elin AF. Clinical, endoscopical and morphological efficacy of mesalazine in patients with irritable bowel syndrome. Clin Exp Gastroenterol. 2011;4:141–53.

[111] Corinaldesi R, Stanghellini V, Cremon C, Gargano L, Cogliandro RF, De Giorgio R, et al. Effect of mesalazine on mucosal immune biomarkers in irritable bowel syndrome: a randomized controlled proof-of-concept study. Aliment Pharmacol Ther. 2009;30(3):245–52.

[112] Preobrazhenskii VN. Salozinal in the treatment of the irritable bowel syndrome in young persons. Ter Arkh. 1999;71(2):37–9.

[113] Chang JY, Locke GR, Schleck CD, Zinsmeister AR, Talley NJ. Risk factors for chronic constipation and a possible role of analgesics. Neurogastroenterol Motil. 2007;19(11):905-11.

[114] Klooker TK, Braak B, Koopman KE, Welting O, Wouters MM, van der Heide S, et al. The mast cell stabiliser ketotifen decreases visceral hypersensitivity and improves intestinal symptoms in patients with irritable bowel syndrome. Gut. 2010;59(9):1213–21.

[115] Reisinger KW, de Haan JJ, Schreinemacher MH. Word of caution before implementing ketotifen for gastrointestinal transit improvement. World J. Gastroenterol. 2013;19(27):4445–6.

[116] Leri O, Tubili S, De Rosa FG, Addessi MA, Scopelliti G, Lucenti W, et al. Management of diarrhoeic type of irritable bowel syndrome with exclusion diet and disodium cromoglycate. Inflammopharmacology. 1997;5(2):153–8.

[117] Stefanini GF, Saggioro A, Alvisi V, Angelini G, Capurso L, di Lorenzo G, et al. Oral cromolyn sodium in comparison with elimination diet in

the irritable bowel syndrome, diarrheic type. Multicenter study of 428 patients. Scand J Gastroenterol. 1995;30(6):535–41.

[118] Grazioli I, Melzi G, Balsamo V, Castellucci G, Castro M, Catassi C, et al. Food intolerance and irritable bowel syndrome of childhood: clinical efficacy of oral sodium cromoglycate and elimination diet. Minerva Pediatr. 1993;45(6):253–8.

[119] Stefanini GF, Prati E, Albini MC, Piccinini G, Capelli S, Castelli E, et al. Oral disodium cromoglycate treatment on irritable bowel syndrome: an open study on 101 subjects with diarrheic type. Am J Gastroenterol. 1992;87(1):55–7.

[120] Lunardi C, Bambara LM, Biasi D, Cortina P, Peroli P, Nicolis F, et al. Double-blind cross-over trial of oral sodium cromoglycate in patients with irritable bowel syndrome due to food intolerance. Clin Exp Allergy. 1991;21(5):569–72.

[121] Paganelli R, Fagiolo U, Cancian M, Sturniolo GC, Scala E, D'Offizi GP. Intestinal permeability in irritable bowel syndrome. Effect of diet and sodium cromoglycate administration. Ann Allergy. 1990;64(4):377–80.

[122] Antico A, Soana R, Clivio L, Baioni R. Irritable colon syndrome in intolerance to food additives. Minerva Dietol Gastroenterol. 1989;35(4):219–24.

[123] Stefanini GF, Bazzocchi G, Prati E, Lanfranchi GA, Gasbarrini G. Efficacy of oral disodium cromoglycate in patients with irritable bowel syndrome and positive skin prick tests to foods. Lancet. 1986;1(8474):207–8.

[124] Tomecki R. Ineffectiveness of disodium cromoglycate in the treatment of a diarrheal form of irritable bowel syndrome. Pol Tyg Lek. 1985;40(7):181–2.

[125] Fee WH. Irritable bowel syndrome helped by montelukast. Chest. 2002;122(4):1497.

[126] Dunlop SP, Jenkins D, Neal KR, Naesdal J, Borgaonker M, Collins SM, et al. Randomized, double-blind, placebo-controlled trial of prednisolone in post-infectious irritable bowel syndrome. Aliment Pharmacol Ther. 2003;18(1):77–84.

[127] Huerta C, Garcia Rodriguez LA, Wallander MA, Johansson S. Users of oral steroids are at a reduced risk of developing irritable bowel syndrome. Pharmacoepidemiol Drug Saf. 2003;12(7):583–8.

[128] Crentsil V. Will corticosteroids and other anti-inflammatory agents be effective for diarrhea-predominant irritable bowel syndrome? Med Hypotheses. 2005;65(1):97–102.

8

Management of Pediatric Appendicitis

Volkan Sarper Erikci

Abstract

Appendicitis is the most common surgical diagnosis for children who present with abdominal pain to the emergency department. However, there are nonspecific examination findings and variable historical features during its presentation. Diagnosis of appendicitis in the pediatric patient may be challenging for the clinician dealing with these children. It is important to have a high index of suspicion and taking a detailed history and physical examination. In diagnosis of appendicitis, adjunctive studies that may be useful are the white blood cell count, C-reactive protein, urinalysis, ultrasonography and computerized tomography when necessary. When appendicitis is suspected, patients should receive immediate surgical consultation, as well as volume replacement and antibiotics if indicated. The most accurate diagnostic tool is perhaps the serial examinations by the same examiner. With this timely approach, it will be possible to prevent the significant morbidity that is associated with delayed diagnoses in younger patients.

Keywords: appendicitis, children, management

1. Introduction

Acute appendicitis is the most common surgical emergency in children and adolescents. Although uncommon in preschool children, it may be present at any age. The lifetime risk of developing appendicitis is 7–8%, with a peak incidence in the teenage years [1]. There are 250,000 cases in the USA annually and the majority occurs in children with the ages between 6 and 10 years. Nearly one-third of children with appendicitis have perforation at the time of surgical treatment. It affects males more frequently than females with male predominance (M:F ratio 3:2). There is a seasonal variation in the occurrence of appendicitis so that its presentation is increased in the summer months with perforated appendicitis occurring more frequently in the fall and winter seasons [2]. Despite advances and innovations in fluid resuscitation and antibiotics, appendicitis especially in preschool children may be difficult to diagnose and is still associated with significant morbidity even mortality.

2. Embryology and anatomy

As a continuation of the inferior tip of the cecum that becomes visible during the eighth week of gestation, appendix rotates to its final position which is the posteromedial aspect of cecum. According to Treves, there are several variations that can be classified into four types: Type 1, the appendix is of fetal type with a funnel shape; Type 2, the appendix originates from the cecal fundus; Type 3, the appendix originates dorsomedially out of the cecum (most common type); and Type 4, the appendix originates directly beside the ileal orifice [3].

The position of the appendix varies among individuals. According to a study comprising 10,000 cases, 5 positions can be identified: ascending appendix in the retrocecal recess in 65% of cases (most common), descending appendix in the iliac fossa in 31% of cases, transverse appendix in the retrocecal recess in 2.5% of cases, paracecal and preileal ascending appendix in 1% of cases and paracecal and postileal ascending appendix in 0.5% of cases [4]. During surgical treatment, it is important to distinguish if the appendix is non-fixed (appendix libera) or fixed (appendix fixa).

With an average length of 8 cm, the size of appendix varies from 0.3 to 33 cm and its diameter of ranges from 5 to 10 mm. The blood comes from appendiceal branch of the ileocolic artery. There are a few submucosal lymph follicles present at birth and they increase to nearly 200 by the age of 12 and the number of these lymph follicles decreases after the age of 30.

3. Etiology and pathogenesis

Obstruction of the appendiceal lumen is usually the first factor that starts the illness. If unresolved, this obstruction leads to vascular congestion, ischemic necrosis and subsequent infection. Inspissated fecal material or a fecalith are the most common causes that lead to appendiceal luminal obstruction. Other causes of obstruction include lymphoid follicle hyperplasia, foreign bodies, carcinoid or other tumors and rarely parasites. Fecaliths are found in approximately 40% cases of acute appendicitis, 65% cases of gangrenous appendicitis and approximately 90% cases of perforated appendicitis [5].

As the appendiceal mucosa continues to secrete the mucus after occlusion of the appendix lumen, this leads to a rapid increase of intraluminal pressure. Secretion of as little as 0.5 mL leads to an increase of pressure of approximately 45 mm Hg, according to the law of Laplace [5]. This phenomenon also explains the rapid perforation of appendix within a few hours of inflammation. For this reason, all the patients with suspected acute appendicitis, need hospitalization and close clinical monitoring if appendectomy is not to be performed immediately.

Distention stimulates nerve endings of visceral afferent pain fibers and leads to a dull, diffuse mid-abdominal pain that cannot be easily located by the children. As the distention increases, it causes reflex nausea and vomiting and once the inflammatory process has involved the serosal part of the appendix and parietal peritoneum, the characteristic finding of shift of the pain from periumbilical area to the right lower abdominal quadrant occurs. Impaired blood supply leads to compromise of the appendiceal mucosa allowing bacterial invasion of the deeper locations. Absorption of bacterial toxins and necrotic material causes fever, tachycardia and leukocytosis. As the pressure increases, finally perforation occurs usually through the infarcted areas. Although in some patients, the disease may spontaneously resolve, untreated obstruction of the appendiceal lumen usually leads to gangrene and perforation.

4. Clinical presentation

Although appendicitis can affect any age group, it is extremely rare in neonates and infants. It is well known that the clinic of appendicitis in infants is different from older children. Indeed, appendicitis in infants is more violent, extremely dangerous and associated with the clinic of severe intoxication, which is due to the growing phenomena of peritonitis. Defense mechanisms such as inability to limit the inflammation process, decreased amount of omentum in infants, are also important factors that make infants unprotected against the ongoing inflammation process. Older children present clinical signs and symptoms which are quite variable in pattern and order of appearance. As a first symptom, pain usually begins as a dull and vague pattern at the periumbilical area but with time, it may localize to the right lower quadrant. *To be precise, Charles McBurney himself in 1889, localized the pain in the following way: "I affirm that in each case the most severe pain due to finger pressure is exactly localized at a distance of 1.5-2 inches from the anterior superior iliac spine, on the line, conducted from this iliac spine to the navel."* Children usually report a gradual increase in pain intensity as the disease progresses. The anatomical variability in the locations of appendix vermiformis (i.e., retrocecal, pelvic, preileal) is common and may alter pain symptoms accordingly. Pelvic or retrocecal appendicitis may be only present with right lower quadrant pain without periumbilical pain. Flank pain and referred testicular pain are also common symptoms in children with pelvic or retrocecal appendicitis. If the inflamed appendix has a close relationship with ureter or bladder, it may produce symptoms associated with urinary tractus such as urinary frequency, dysuria, urinary retention and bladder distention. It is traditionally known that severe gastrointestinal symptoms that develop prior to the onset of pain usually indicate a diagnosis other than acute appendicitis. On the other hand, mild gastrointestinal symptoms such as decreased appetite, indigestion and changes in bowel habits may develop within a few hours of pain onset.

Typically patients with uncomplicated appendicitis have low-grade fever. Fever above 38.6 degrees, tachycardia and leukocytosis develop as a consequence of mediators released by ischemic tissues, white blood cells and bacteria. Children with appendicitis avoid movement and tend to lie in bed with their knees flexed. Hyperesthesia of the skin can be elicited by touching the skin of the patient. Abdominal tenderness associated with appendicitis varies with the stage of the disease and location of the inflamed vermiform appendix. Classical "McBurney's point" that is the area one-third the distance from anterior superior iliac spine to the umbilicus, is the most common site of maximal tenderness that is found on the abdominal

Gastrointestinal causes-liver, spleen and biliary tract disorders

Gastroenteritis

Mesenteric lymphadenitis

Constipation

Trauma

Peptic ulcer disease

Meckel's diverticulum

Inflammatory bowel disease

Cholecystitis

Intussusception

Neoplasm (carcinoid, lymphoma)

Food poisoning

Intestinal obstruction

Omental torsion

Pancreatitis

Volvulus

Diverticulitis

Perforated viscus

Hepatitis

Cholecystitis

Splenic infarction and splenic rupture

Genitourinary causes

Urinary tract infection

Urinary calculi

Pyelonephritis

Pelvic inflammatory disease

Ectopic pregnancy

Ovarian/testicular torsion

Hematocolpos

Endometriosis

Mittelschmerz

Tubo-ovarian abscess

Ovarian cyst rupture

Metabolic disorders

Diabetic ketoacidosis

Hypoglycemia

Porphyria

Acute adrenal insufficiency

Hematologic disorders

Sickle cell disease

Henoch-Schönlein purpura

Hemolytic uremic syndrome

Pulmonary causes

Pneumonia (right lobe basilar)

Pleuritis

Pulmonary infarction

Drugs and toxins

Erythromycin

Salicylates

Lead poisoning

Other causes

Familial Mediterranean fever

Infantile colic

Parasitic infection

Psoas abscess

Functional pain

Angioneurotic edema

Table 1. Differential diagnosis of pediatric appendicitis.

wall. Rectal tenderness may be observed in patients with pelvic appendicitis. In the case of malrotation, the tenderness due to appendicitis may occur on unusual locations which may be away from the usual site.

There are some clinical signs that should produce high index of suspicion of appendicitis, namely "Rovsings' sign" (palpation of left lower quadrant producing tenderness over the right iliac fossa), and it is a reliable indicator of appendicitis in childhood. The "psoas sign" that is commonly observed in retrocecal appendicitis and the "obturator sign" suggesting pelvic appendicitis are the other useful clinical signs that should prompt clinician to diagnose acute appendicitis early. The physical examination of a patient suspected to have appendicitis (especially pelvic appendicitis) is missing without rectal exam which may reveal a tender palpable mass or abscess.

Differential diagnosis of acute appendicitis has a wide spectrum of diseases and includes gastroenteritis, inflammatory bowel disease such as Crohn's disease, cholelithiasis, mesenteric adenitis, pancreatitis, peptic ulcer disease, Meckel's diverticulitis, constipation, intussusception and many other disease states (**Table 1**). Systemic diseases including diabetic ketoacidosis, lupus erythematosus, hemolytic uremic syndrome, sickle cell crisis, Henoch-Schönlein purpura and parasitic infections may produce symptoms suggesting acute appendicitis. In females with certain situations such as ectopic pregnancy, ovarian torsion, developmental ovarian cysts and pelvic inflammatory disease, a misdiagnosis of acute appendicitis may cause unnecessary surgical interventions. Pneumonia, particularly affecting the right lower lobe of lung, urinary tract diseases such as renal or ureteric stones, pyelonephritis and urinary tract infections can also mimic acute appendicitis. Children with cystic fibrosis have a higher incidence of acute appendicitis. A neonate with appendicitis should increase the suspicion of Hirschsprung's disease in the mind of the clinician.

5. Diagnosis

History and physical examination is important in diagnosing appendicitis in children. The most accurate diagnostic tool is perhaps the serial examinations by the same examiner while the child is cooperative with the clinician. Before starting the palpation of the abdomen, the child should be asked to point out the location of the abdominal pain. Cutaneous hyperesthesia is often an early finding derived from the T10 to L1 nerve roots. There is a mild abdominal pain that cannot be localized at the early stages of the disease. As the disease progresses, localized tenderness is most often found at the McBurney's point. Rectal tenderness may be observed in pelvic appendicitis and tenderness midway between the 12th rib and the posterior superior iliac spine is detected in patients with retrocecal appendicitis. If malrotation accompanies the disease, position of the inflamed appendix has a role in the changing locations of tenderness. Peritonitis ensues as the disease progresses to perforation with generalized abdominal rigidity. Rebound tenderness is seldom necessary for diagnosis and is usually regarded as an unnecessary discomfort for children. Routine rectal examination in diagnosing appendicitis in childhood is a matter of debate and if other signs suggest to the diagnosis of appendicitis, rectal examination may be unnecessary. But it is especially helpful diagnostic tool for patients with pelvic appendicitis with abscess or those with uterine or adnexal pathologic conditions. It should be re-emphasized that when the diagnosis is unclear, with the aid of serial physical examinations, it is possible to decrease the number of unnecessary surgical interventions that may increase risk to the patient if performed. This issue is very important, because in a recent study, among the children undergoing appendectomy, 6.3% in Canada and 4.3% in the USA, are subsequently found to have a normal appendix and it has been reported that a misdiagnosis of appendicitis that leads to negative appendectomy ranges up to 30% [6].

The most often used laboratory aids to diagnose appendicitis are white blood cell (WBC) count, absolute neutrophil count (ANC) and C-reactive protein (CRP) but these tests alone are not helpful or predictive. Leukocyte count above 10,000 is observed in greater than 90% of children with acute appendicitis. But normal WBC count may also be observed in 5% of patients with appendicitis. A shift to left is a usual finding and is of better diagnostic value compared to ANC. A neutrophil-lymphocyte ratio of greater than 3.5 has a greater specificity and sensitivity in diagnosing appendicitis.

There are numerous appendicitis scoring systems that have been suggested as an adjunct to diagnosis of appendicitis. Two systems, namely the Alvarado score and the Pediatric Appendicitis Score (PAS), have been extensively studied but do not have 100% sensitivity and specificity in the diagnosis of appendicitis and they do not replace an experienced pediatric surgeon [7–9]. It has been documented that a pediatric surgeon can differentiate appendicitis from other abdominal disorders with 92% accuracy [10]. Urinalysis is helpful in differentiating urinary tract infections and urolithiasis from appendicitis. However, when inflamed appendix is in close proximity with ureter, hematuria and pyuria may also be detected even if there is no urinary tract infection or urolithiasis.

Imaging studies may be useful in cases where the diagnosis is equivocal and plain film radiography may have a value. The incidence of presence of a fecalith that can be seen on direct roentgenograms ranges from 10 to 20% of cases with appendicitis and this ratio increases accordingly in patients with complicated appendicitis. Other subtle plain film findings are sentinel loop in the right lower quadrant, lumbar scoliosis with a concavity to the right lower quadrant, mass effect due to pelvic abscess, loss of psoas shadow and obliteration of the properitoneal fat stripe. It is necessary to have a chest radiograph for ruling out right lower lobe pneumonia. Although it is usually useful tool in the management of children with intussusception, barium enema may rarely be performed in children suspected of having appendicitis. Barium enema findings in appendicitis include: incomplete filling of the appendix, extrinsic mass effect on the cecum or terminal ileum and irregularities of the appendiceal lumen.

With a sensitivity of 85% and specificity of greater than 90%, ultrasonography (US) is a useful diagnostic tool if performed especially by skilled hands. Sonographic criteria for the diagnosis of appendicitis is demonstration of a noncompressible appendix that is 7 mm or larger in diameter, a wall thicker than 2 mm or an irregular wall that is rigid, and lacks peristalsis [11]. Other findings that may be helpful in diagnosing appendicitis include absence of air in the appendiceal lumen, periappendiceal fat changes, visible appendicolith, complex mass, mesenteric lymph nodes and free fluid [11]. Advantages of US include lack of sedation, contrast agents and radiation during procedure [12]. On the other hand, there are also disadvantages regarding US that include need for operator experience, a lack of regular availability during off hours, difficult visualization especially in obese children [13]. Computed tomography (CT) is also useful for inconclusive cases. It combines the advantages of many other imaging modalities, including rapid acquisition time and a lack of operator dependency [14]. The findings of an enlarged appendix (>6 mm), appendiceal wall thickening (>1 mm) and appendiceal wall enhancement are useful diagnostic criteria that are found in CT. Comparing US and CT in diagnosing appendicitis in children, it has been proposed that US is more specific and CT is more sensitive [15]. Magnetic resonance imaging (MRI) has a high diagnostic accuracy for appendicitis, but it has certain disadvantages including limited utility, lack of availability in many centers, lengthy acquisition time, need for sedation or anesthesia and high cost compared to other imaging modalities [15]. It should be re-emphasized again that these radiological diagnostic modalities, if used routinely, cause hospital resource utilization and delay in surgical treatment. Besides, potential cancer risk associated with ionizing radiation from CT should also be kept in mind and these imaging tools should be reserved for patients with uncertain findings related to appendicitis.

Laparoscopy may be a useful diagnostic tool for patients with inconclusive findings related to appendicitis. It may be a helpful diagnostic aid especially in obese and overweight children. Laparoscopy should be kept in mind when other diagnostic modalities are not enough for diagnosing appendicitis and the attending surgeon should not hesitate to perform laparoscopy.

6. Treatment

There are several treatment modalities of appendicitis with a wide spectrum ranging from nonoperative management to open or laparoscopic surgical interventions. Nonoperative management of appendicitis has been an interest for many scientists and several trials demonstrated successful nonoperative management of acute appendicitis in 70– 85% of cases in the one-year follow-up [16, 17]. On the other hand, it has been stated in another meta-analysis that the combined failure and recurrence rates in nonoperative patients made this approach less effective overall [18]. Regarding the nonoperative management of pediatric appendicitis, children revealed a success rate ranging from 75 to 80%, and in a recent study, up to 89% success rate of nonoperative management has been reported [19, 20]. It has also been demonstrated that as compared to surgically treated patients, nonoperative patients reported higher quality-of-life scores at 30 days [20]. In some situations, nonoperative management of appendicitis may be unsuccessful and one of these predictors of failure of nonoperative management has been reported to be presence of appendicolith on imaging studies [21]. Another study on the nonoperative management of uncomplicated appendicitis demonstrated a failure rate of 60% and was halted early [22]. To sum up, although there are no consensus in which patients should receive nonoperative treatment, it should be emphasized that nonoperative management is permissible only with uncomplicated acute appendicitis for carefully selected children and it is possible and should be kept in mind.

In the surgical management of appendicitis, the goals are to minimize complications and cost, decrease patient anxiety and improve quality of life. Although according to the traditional thinking that emergent appendectomy should be performed at the time of diagnosis, immediate surgical intervention is not considered mandatory for most patients. Many centers dealing with pediatric appendicitis now perform appendectomies in the day time for patients presenting at night time [23]. With this approach, the stress that occurs in the overnight appendectomies for both children, their families and surgeon is avoided. Besides, complication and perforation rates are similar for patients undergoing surgery within 6 hours of admission compared to those undergoing surgery between 6 and 16 hours after admission to the hospital. The majority of pediatric surgeons perform appendectomy within 8 hours after admission. It should be emphasized that the delay in the emergency operation is permissible only with uncomplicated acute appendicitis and after an expedient resuscitation, all the patients with appendicitis must undergo timely surgical exploration.

Initial therapy starts with intravenous fluid resuscitation, broad spectrum antibiotic coverage and keeping the patient nothing per mouth. There is a trend toward decreasing the duration of antibiotic therapy. The recommended duration of antibiotic therapy is preoperative plus 24 hours postoperative period for simple appendicitis and a 10-day course of ampicillin, gentamicin and metronidazole or clindamycin for complicated appendicitis, and these therapies are known as gold standard. On the other hand, it has been documented that both piperacillin/tazobactam and cefoxitin have been shown to be at least as effective as the triple-drug regimen and may also decrease the length of hospital stay and costs [24]. Nevertheless, total length of antibiotic therapy should be determined by the clinical condition of the patient (resolution of fever, pain, bowel function) and WBC count [25].

Surgical treatment modalities include open technique and laparoscopic appendectomy. Except for specific situations including any surgical intervention having right lower quadrant incision such as Meckel's diverticulectomy or intussusception reduction, incidental appendectomy is no longer performed routinely and does not have any benefit. The first appendectomy for acute appendicitis was performed by a British surgeon Lawson Tait in 1880. He removed the gangrenous appendix in a 17-year-old girl. Charles McBurney in 1894 described the muscle splitting incision. In his description, a transverse or oblique right lower quadrant incision is performed and by splitting the muscles, abdominal cavity is entered and mesoappendix is divided followed by excision of the appendix at its base [26]. There are different techniques of management of appendiceal stump including simple ligation, ligation and inversion using a purse-string, or a pure inversion without ligature. The choice of stump management directly relates to attending surgeon.

The world's first complete laparoscopic appendectomy with a stitched mesentery and immersion of stump in the wall of the cecum and Z-stitches was performed in 1981 by the pioneer in minimally invasive surgery, a German gynecologist Kurt Semm. It should be noted that as a gynecologist, he performed only a passing appendectomy for endometriosis of the appendix or chronic appendicitis. Since this first description of endoscopic appendectomy, laparoscopic appendectomies are being performed more and more commonly nowadays and today laparoscopic appendectomies have largely replaced the open surgery by up to 91% [27]. There are several different operative approaches in the laparoscopic management of appendicitis including three-port laparoscopic intervention, transumbilical laparoscopic appendectomy, and single-port/incision techniques. Advantages of laparoscopy include shorter hospital stay, decreased postoperative pain and wound complications, ability to diagnose inconclusive cases, surgical ease in obese patients and faster recovery after surgery. On the other hand, there are disadvantages of laparoscopic approach which are a higher cost of equipment, longer operative time, time needed for learning curve in laparoscopy education, experience required for surgeons and increased incidence of intra-abdominal infection. It has been previously stated that complication rates are lower compared to open appendectomy except that the postoperative intra-abdominal abscess rate is higher with laparoscopic approach [28]. But this topic seems to be changed as it has been found in the meta-analysis and multi-institutional reviews that there are no differences in intra-abdominal abscess rates following laparoscopic surgery compared to open surgical interventions for appendicitis [29, 30]. To sum up, laparoscopy is a safe and effective means of performing an appendectomy in the treatment of pediatric appendicitis.

If a normal appendix is found at laparotomy (5–15% of cases), the abdomen is systematically inspected for evidence of inflammatory bowel disease, a Meckel's diverticulum, mesenteric adenitis and peptic ulcer disease. In females, fallopian tubes and ovaries should be identified and inspected for ovarian cysts or torsion, and for rare occurrence of isolated tubal torsion and pelvic inflammatory disease. Following open surgery or laparoscopic approach, there comes the question of drain usage. Although it has long been stated that irrigating the abdominal cavity is not recommended in patients with simple appendicitis and may have a role in the management of complicated appendicitis, previous studies demonstrated that there was no favoring irrigation for peritoneal contamination in perforated appendicitis [31]. Even an increase in abscesses resulting from the use of irrigation compared to no irrigation following laparoscopic surgical intervention has been reported [32].

Management of children with a palpable abdominal mass who present late (i.e., several days or weeks) is another controversial topic. Some suggest an immediate appendectomy whereas others perform the procedure only when a mass is confirmed either as a result of radiological diagnostic work-up or during the surgery with the patient under anesthesia. In a meta-analysis, evaluating early versus delayed appendectomy for perforated appendicitis concluded that delayed operation was associated with significantly less overall complications, wound infections, intra-abdominal abscesses, bowel obstructions and reoperations [33]. On the other hand, early appendectomy, compared to interval appendectomy, significantly reduced the time away from normal activities [33]. Opponents to interval appendectomy suggest that it is unnecessary because only 14% of patients have recurrent symptoms, and after initial diagnosis, recurrence is uncommon within 2 years. Nevertheless, it is very important that if an operation is to be performed, great care should be taken to avoid damage to adjacent structures such as small intestine, the fallopian tubes, ovaries and ureters. In the case of well-localized periappendiceal abscess or phlegmon, after a prolonged antibiotic therapy (2–3 weeks) CT or sonographic-guided percutaneous abscess drainage may be another option in the treatment of these children. The current standard for patients presenting with a palpable abdominal mass who are usually young children with perforation, is conservative management with interval appendectomy after 8–12 weeks.

7. Complications

Complication rates after appendectomy differ greatly with regard to the severity of the appendicitis. Complications are rarely seen after simple appendicitis but are more often seen in children with complicated appendicitis. Wound infection is the most common complication after appendectomy. With the worldwide usage of antibiotics, the rate of wound infection has fallen from 50% to less than 5%, even in complicated appendicitis. Other complications of appendicitis include intra-abdominal abscess formation, wound dehiscence, postoperative intestinal obstruction, prolonged ileus and rarely enterocutaneous fistula. It has been reported that the postoperative risk of an intra-abdominal abscess is approximately 20% for children with perforated appendicitis, and the risk for children with simple appendicitis to develop an abscess is less than 0.8% [31]. Tubal infertility and pylephlebitis may also be observed after surgical treatment for complicated appendicitis such as pelvic and subhepatic appendicitis, respectively. Sepsis and multisystem organ failure can occur in young children with a prolonged illness before definite diagnosis. As the antibiotics have markedly decreased the incidence of infectious complications, the mortality rate for complicated appendicitis has dropped dramatically to nearly zero. The overall morbidity in children with complicated appendicitis is less than 10%.

8. Conclusion

Appendicitis occurs most commonly between the ages of 10 and 11 years. The classical signs and symptoms of migrating pain to the right lower quadrant and rebound tenderness are present in less than half of the children presenting with appendicitis. When the diagnosis is certain, the combination of evaluation and prompt surgical intervention is all that is needed. If the diagnosis of appendicitis is inconclusive, a period of observation including usage of scoring systems for evaluating the patient followed by radiological imaging modalities becomes a matter of necessity rather than of choice. As CT scans increase radiation exposure, US should be the choice of imaging modality in these patients. Laparoscopic approaches now constitute more than 90% of appendectomies in these patients even in cases with perforated appendicitis. In selected cases, appendicitis can be managed nonoperatively. Although provided that care is given by experienced clinicians and institutions, the best outcome for children with appendicitis may be anticipated, a small number of patients may still develop complications following surgical treatment of appendicitis. Nevertheless, the long-term outcome for the majority of children who undergo appendectomy is very good.

Author details

Volkan Sarper Erikci

Address all correspondence to: verikci@yahoo.com

Department of Pediatric Surgery, Saglık Bilimleri University, İzmir Tepecik Training Hospital, Izmir, Turkey

References

[1] Addis DG, Shaffer N, Fowler BS, et al. The epidemiology of appendicitis and appendectomy in the United States. American Journal of Epidemiology. 1990;**132**(5):910-925

[2] Deng Y, Chang DC, Zhang Y, et al. Seasonal and day of the week variations of perforated appendicitis in US children. Pediatric Surgery International. 2010;**26**(7):691-696

[3] Treves F. Lectures on the anatomy of the intestinal canal and peritoneum in man. British Medical Journal. 1885;**1**(415):527-580

[4] Wakeley CPG. Position of the vermiform appendix as ascertained by analysis of 10,000 cases. Journal of Anatomy. 1933;**67**:277

[5] Arnbjornsson E, Bengmark S. Obstruction of the appendix lumen in relation to pathogenesis of acute appendicitis. Acta Chirurgica Scandinavica. 1985;**42**:184

[6] Cheong LH, Emil S. Outcomes of pediatric appendicitis: An international comparison of the United States and Canada. JAMA Surgery. 2014;**149**(1):50-55

[7] Escriba A, Gamell AM, Fernandez Y, et al. Prospective validation of two systems of classification for the diagnosis of acute appendicitis. Pediatric Emergency Care. 2011; **27**:165-169

[8] Rezak A, Abbas H, Ajemian MS, et al. Decreased use of computed tomography with a modified scoring system in the diagnosis of pediatric acute appendicitis. Archives of Surgery. 2011;**146**:64-67

[9] Goldman RD, Carter S, Stephens S. Prospective validation of the pediatric appendicitis score. The Journal of Pediatrics. 2008;**153**:278-282

[10] Williams RF, Blakely M, Fischer PE, et al. Diagnosing ruptured appendicitis preoperatively in pediatric patients. Journal of the American College of Surgeons. 2009; **208**(5):819-825

[11] Schupp CJ, Klingmuller V, Strauch K, et al. Typical signs of acute appendicitis in ultrasonography mimicked by other disease? Pediatric Surgery International. 2010;**26**:697-702

[12] Binkovitz LA, Unsdorfer KML, Thapa P, et al. Pediatric appendiceal ultrasound accuracy, determinacy and clinical outcomes. Pediatric Radiology. 2015;**45**(13):1934-1944

[13] Yiğiter M, Kantarcı M, Yalçın O, et al. Does obesity limit the sonographic diagnosis of appendicitis in children? Journal of Clinical Ultrasound. 2010;**39**(4):187-190

[14] Bachur RG, Dayan PS, Bajaj L, et al. The effect of abdominal pain duration on the accuracy of diagnostic imaging for pediatric appendicitis. Annals of Emergency Medicine. 2012; **60**(5):582-590.e3

[15] Kulaylat AN, Moore MM, Engbrecht BW, et al. An implemented MRI program to eliminate radiation from the evaluation of pediatric appendicitis. Journal of Pediatric Surgery. 2015;**50**(8):1359-1363

[16] Di SS, Sibilio A, Giorgini E, et al. The NOTA study (non operative treatment for acute appendicitis): Prospective study on the efficacy and safety of antibiotics (amoxicillin and clavulanic acid) for treating patients with right lower quadrant abdominal pain and long-term follow-up of conservatively treated suspected appendicitis. Annals of Surgery. 2014;**260**(1):109-117

[17] Salminen P, Paajanen H, Rautio T, et al. Antibiotic therapy vs appendectomy for treatment of uncomplicated acute appendicitis: The APPAC randomized clinical trial. Journal of the American Medical Association. 2015;**313**(23):2340-2348

[18] Mason RJ, Moazzez A, Sohn H, et al. Meta-analysis of randomized trials comparing antibiotic therapy with appendectomy for acute uncomplicated (no abscess or phlegmon) appendicitis. Surgical Infections. 2012;**13**(2):74-84

[19] Hartwich J, Luks FI, Watson-Smith D, et al. Nonoperative treatment of acute appendicitis in children: A feasibility study. Journal of Pediatric Surgery. 2016;**51**(1):111-116

[20] Minecci PC, Mahida JB, Lodwick DL, et al. Effectiveness of patient choice in nonoperative vs surgical management of pediatric uncomplicated acute appendicitis. JAMA Surgery. 2016;**151**(5):408-415

[21] Svensson JF, Patkova B, Almstrom M, et al. Nonoperative treatment with antibiotics versus surgery for acute nonperforated appendicitis in children. Annals of Surgery. 2015; **261**(1):67-71

[22] Mahida JB, Lodwick DL, Nacion KM, et al. High failure rate of nonoperative management of acute appendicitis with an appendicolith in children. Journal of Pediatric Surgery. 2016;**51**(6):903-911

[23] Pepper VK, Stanfill AB, Pearl RH. Diagnosis and management of pediatric appendicitis, intussusception, and Meckel diverticulum. The Surgical Clinics of North America. 2012; **92**(3):505-526

[24] Goldin AB, Sawin RS, Garrison MM, et al. Aminoglycoside-based triple-antibiotic therapy versus monotherapy for children with ruptured appendicitis. Pediatrics. 2007; **119**:905-911

[25] Lee SL, Islam S, Cassidy LD, et al. Antibiotics and appendicitis in the pediatric population: An American pediatric surgical association outcomes and clinical trials committee systematic review. Journal of Pediatric Surgery. 2010;**45**:2181-2185

[26] McBurney CIV. The incision made in the abdominal wall in cases of appendicitis, with a description of a new method of operating. Annals of Surgery. 1894;**20**:38-43

[27] Jen HC, Shew SB. Laparoscopic versus open appendectomy in children: Outcomes comparison based on a statewide analysis. The Journal of Surgical Research. 2010;**161**(1):13-17

[28] Vegunta RK, Wallace LJ, Switzer DM, et al. Laparoscopic appendectomy in children: Technically feasible and safe in all stages of acute appendicitis. The American Surgeon. 2004;**70**:198-201

[29] Jaschinski T, Mosch C, Eikermann M, et al. Laparoscopic versus open appendectomy in patients with suspected appendicitis: A systematic review of meta-analyses of randomised controlled trials. BMC Gastroenterology. 2015;**15**(1):48

[30] Yau KK, Siu WT, Tang CN, et al. Laparoscopic versus open appendectomy for complicated appendicitis. Journal of the American College of Surgeons. 2007;**205**(1):60-65

[31] St Peter SD, Sharp SW, Holcomb GW III, et al. An evidence-based definition for perforated appendicitis derived from a prospective randomized trial. Journal of Pediatric Surgery. 2008;**43**(12):2242-2245

[32] Hartwich JE, Carter RF, Wolfe L, et al. The effects of irrigation on outcomes in cases of perforated appendicitis in children. The Journal of Surgical Research. 2013;**180**(2):222-225

[33] Simillis C, Symeonides P, Shorthouse AJ, et al. A meta-analysis comparing conservative treatment versus acute appendectomy for complicated appendicitis (abscess or phlegmon). Surgery. 2010;**147**(6):818-829

9

Irritable Bowel Syndrome: Functional Gastrointestinal Disease Regulated by Nervous System

Victor V. Chaban

Abstract

A functional disorder is a medical condition that impairs the normal function, but without major organic cause such as irritation or inflammation and where the organ or part of the body looks completely normal under medical examination. The accumulation of abnormalities that limit body functions is a major risk factor for patients with irritable bowel syndrome (IBS), defined as a gastrointestinal disorder with abdominal pain or discomfort that is associated with a change in bowel habit. Often, this disorder is accompanied by the concomitant decline in cognitive or motor performance. Pain that in some patients is out of proportion to identifiable pathology is the most immediate and dramatic consequence of IBS and is responsible for a highly negative impact on quality of life and substantial workforce loss. For patients with IBS, the most common comorbid diagnoses include painful bladder syndrome (PBS) or chronic pelvic pain (CPP). Cells of the affected tissues may interact in cell-to-cell manner messages through the transfer of hormones, cytokines, and other mediators that influence normal functioning. The complex interplay and balance between these diverse mediators, ageing, genetic background, and environmental factors may ultimately determine the outcome of the progression of the functional disorder. On a cellular level, these responses are highly complex, involving a vast array of enzymes and receptors of virtually every class, directing recruitment of many types of cells to recover the healthy state. Indeed, a balance between the messengers with the inherent redundancy of the different body systems makes therapeutic intervention of functional disorders a considerable challenge.

Keywords: sensory neurons, extrinsic primary afferents, nociception

1. Introduction

The response properties of pelvic extrinsic primary afferent nerves (EPANs) play an important role in etiology of irritable bowel syndrome (IBS). Hypersensitivity of visceral mechanoreceptors could result from excessive production of modulatory neurotransmitters. In addition to direct stimulation of stretch-activated channels on primary afferent neurons located in dorsal root ganglia (DRG), chemicals produced by different target cells (such as smooth muscle cells and interstitial cells of Cajal) in response to stretch or inflammation play an important role in the neuromodulation of nociception. The incidence of persistent, episodic, or chronic visceral pain is more prevalent in females, which also suggests hormonal regulation. Despite extensive research of the properties of pelvic and splanchnic afferent nerves, little is known about the mechanisms underlying normal and pathological signal transduction pathways underlying many functional diseases. Despite considerable efforts by the scientific community and the pharmaceutical industry to develop novel pharmacological treatments aimed at chronic visceral pain, the traditional approaches to identifying and evaluating novel drugs for this target have largely failed to translate into effective IBS treatments [1]. A better understanding of these processes has direct implications for the development of more effective therapies. During the last decade, we identified that DRG neurons can be affected by ATP, NO, estrogen, and other mediators producing neuronal hyper- or desensitization that may unravel the enigma of the development of chronic pelvic pain associated with IBS. Moreover, our recent data that estrogen can gate primary afferent response to modulate nociception support the idea about involvement of peripheral central system in etiology of a wide range of the functional and inflammatory gastrointestinal diseases [2].

2. Role of EPANs in the mechanisms of visceral neurotransduction and modulation

Pelvic nerve afferent fibers innervating the visceral organs of the lower colon have been well characterized (reviewed in Ref. [3]). In general, during colonic distension, a large number of pelvic EPANs show static levels of discharge. Stretches that lead to the opening of stretch-activated (SA) channels on the plasma membrane lead to the selective or nonselective opening of different cation and anion channels in nodose ganglia and DRG neurons. Thus, depending on the cell type and channel type, EPANs activation may result in hyperpolarization, depolarization, or primarily Ca^{2+} influx. The function of SA channels in the plasma membrane differs between various cell types. Influx of Ca^{2+} may repolarize the plasma membrane via activation of K_{ca} channels and inactivating of voltage-gated calcium channels (VGCCs), and thus influence adaptation rates of sensory neurons during ongoing stimulations.

The cell bodies of primary visceral spinal afferent neurons are located in the lumbosacral (L1-S1) DRGs that transmit information about chemical or mechanical stimulation from the periphery to the spinal cord. Nociceptors are small- to medium-size DRG neurons whose peripheral processes detect potentially damaging physical and chemical stimuli. Until recently, ATP release from nonneuronal cells was thought to be exclusively as result of injury. It is now clear that certain integral membrane proteins contain an ATP-binding cassette so this neurotransmitter can act as signaling molecule modulating sensory afferent nerve terminals. Six P2X receptors are expressed in DRGs. Significantly, the P2X3 receptor is found exclusively in a subset of small diameter capsaicin sensitive peripheral sensory neurons (presumably nociceptors) [4]. Today, multiple lines of evidence suggest that ATP signaling via P2X receptors contribute to different pain phenotypes, therefore P2X antagonists may be useful analgesics. The availability of P2X receptor-specific antagonists also holds the promise of revealing the cellular and molecular neurobiology underlying pain states underlying functional diseases [5]. With sufficiently high levels of ATP, P2X and SA channels (which has a greater permeability for Ca^{2+} than Na^{+}) would depolarize nerve terminals directly producing action potentials and leading to sensation of pain. On the other hand, the response of EPANs may be tonically inhibited by NO produced by peripheral nerve terminals. The peripheral sensitization of nerve fibers is transient depending on the duration of stimuli and the presence of visceral (colonic) inflammation.

3. Estrogen receptors and visceral nociception associated with functional diseases

Changes in pain perception and variations of symptoms throughout the menstrual cycle, as well as sexual intercourse triggering symptoms in a significant portion of females diagnosed with irritable bowel syndrome (IBS), painful bladder syndrome (PBS), chronic pelvic pain (CPP), and other function syndromes, points to a connection with sex steroids. Several lines of evidence indicate that 17β-estradiol (E2) directly influence the functions of primary afferent neurons. Both subtypes of estrogen receptors (ERα and ERβ) are present in DRG neurons including the small-diameter putative nociceptors [4]. In vitro, ATP-sensitive DRG neurons respond to E2 [6, 7], which correlated well with the idea that visceral afferents are E2 sensitive: (i) visceral pain is affected by hormonal level in cycling females; (ii) there are sex differences in the prevalence of functional disorders involving the viscera; and (iii) putative visceral afferents fit into the population of DRG neurons that are sensitive to E2 [7]. These data suggest that in addition to the CNS actions, E2 can act in the periphery to modulate nociception [6, 7]. E2 modulates cellular activity by altering ion channel opening, G-protein signaling, and activation of trophic factor-like signal transduction pathways. These effects have been ascribed to membrane-associated receptors [8]. The results from our laboratory and others indicate that E2 acts in DRG neurons to modulate L-type VGCC and through group II metabotropic glutamate receptors [6].

E2 has a significant role in modulating visceral sensitivity, indicating that E2 alterations in sensory processing may underlie sex-based differences in functional pain symptoms [9]. Indeed in most clinical studies, women report more severe pain levels, more frequent pain, and longer duration of pain than men [10]. Little is known about E2-mediated mechanisms in peripheral nervous system, but the fact that DRG neurons express ERs and respond to E2 treatment suggest that they are a potential target for mediating nociception. E2 modulation of nociceptive response depends on the type of pain, its durations, and the involvement of other nociceptive-mediated mechanisms.

E2 (both short-term and long-term exposure) significantly decreased the nociceptive signaling in viscerally labeled DRG neurons [6, 7]. Thus, in addition to central regulation, estrogen may affect nociception associated with IBS peripherally.

4. Primary afferent neurons and viscero-visceral cross-sensitization: emerging model for functional gastrointestinal disorders

Most of the current literature pertains to specific functional syndromes defined by medical subspecialties. These include: IBS (gastroenterology); CPP (gynecology); PBS (urology); fibromyalgia (rheumatology); and others. Many reports described the substantial overlaps between two or more of these syndromes [11, 12]. Moreover, clinical presentations of functional syndromes lack a specific pathology in the affected organ but may respond to a viscero-visceral cross-sensitization in which increased nociceptive input from an inflamed organ (i.e., uterus) sensitizes neurons that receive convergent input from an unaffected organ (i.e., colon or bladder). The site of visceral cross-sensitivity is unknown.

Recent studies from our laboratory demonstrated that hormonal modulation of visceral inputs of primary afferent nociceptors located in the dorsal root ganglia (DRG) is responsible for changes observed in the perception of pain during the etiology of functional pain syndromes [2]. Individuals suffering from CPP frequently have pain emanating from several visceral organs. Viscero-somatic and viscero-visceral hyperalgesia and allodynia lead to the perception of pain spreading from an initial site to adjacent areas. Patients with CPP may at first have only one source of pain in the pelvis, but numerous mechanisms involving the central and peripheral nervous systems may result in the development of painful sensations in adjacent organs, such as IBS being associated with lower colonic pain.

5. Summary

Similar to other chronic diseases, a multicomponent conceptual model of IBS, which involves physiologic, cognitive and behavior factors will be necessary for developing new therapies. The different systems such as neuroendocrine regulation, pain modulation, and autonomic response will affect ascending aminergic systems (**Figure 1**).

From a public health perspective, a substantial impact on our knowledge of nociceptive diseases such IBS will help achieve a deeper understanding of data presented in clinical aspects of these symptoms. Only a thorough understanding of the mechanism implicated in these phenomena can truly contribute to the designing of new and more efficient therapies.

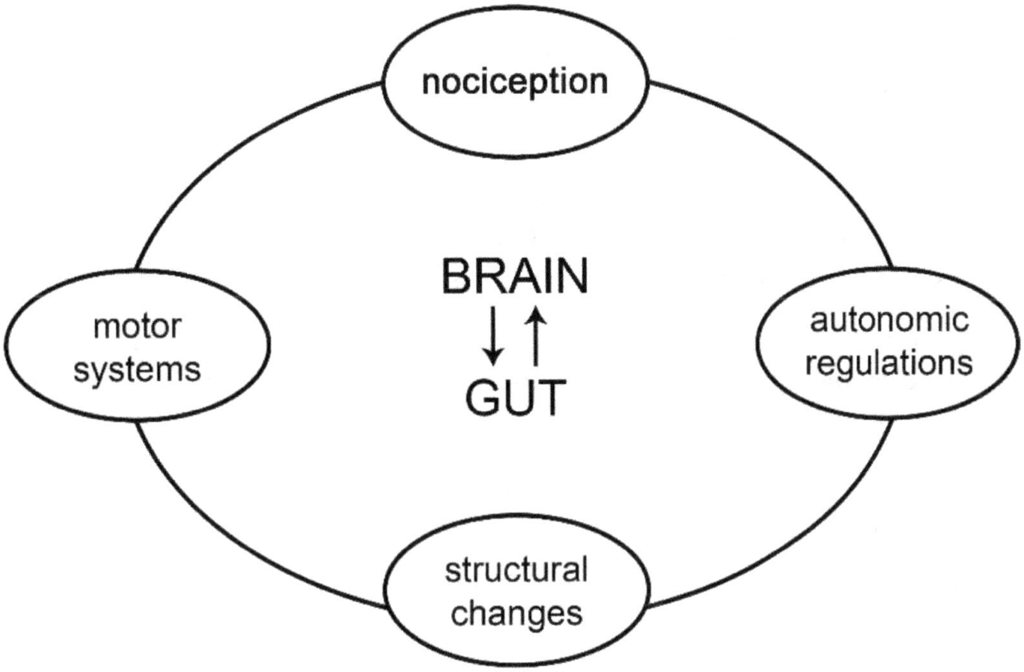

Figure 1. Different regulatory mechanisms involved in irritable bowel syndrome.

Author details

Victor V. Chaban

Address all correspondence to: victorchaban@cdrewu.edu

Department of Internal Medicine, Charles R. Drew University of Medicine and Science, Los Angeles, USA; Department of Medicine, University of California, Los Angeles, USA

References

[1] Holschneider DP, Bradesi S, Mayer EA. The role of experimental models in developing new treatments for irritable bowel syndrome. Expert Review of Gastroenterology and Hepatology, 2011, 5 (1): 43–57.

[2] Chaban V. Unraveling the enigma of visceral pain. Nova Publishers, N.Y. 2016. 77 p. ISBN: 978-63489-430-8. Library of U.S. Congress Control Number: 2015951299.

[3] Mayer EA, Labus JS, Tillisch K, Cole SW, Baldi P Towards a systems view of IBS. Nature Review Gastroenterology and Hepatology 2015, 12 (10): 592–605.

[4] Kobayashi K, Yamanaka H, Noguchi K. Expression of ATP receptors in the rat dorsal root ganglion and spinal cord. Anatomical Science International 2013, 88 (1): 10–16.

[5] Toulme E, Tsuda M, Khakh BS, Inoue K. On the role of ATP-Gated P2X receptors in acute, inflammatory and neuropathic pain. In: Kruger L, Light AR, Editors. Translational pain research: from mouse to man. CRC Press/Taylor & Francis. Chapter 10. Frontiers in Neuroscience. 2010.

[6] Chaban V et al. Estradiol attenuates the adenosine triphosphate-induced increase of intracellular calcium through group II metabotropic glutamate receptors in rat dorsal root ganglion neurons. Journal of Neuroscience Research 2011. 89(11):1707–1710.

[7] Cho, T. and V.V. Chaban, Interaction between P2X3 and ERalpha/ERbeta in ATP-mediated calcium signaling in mice sensory neurons. Journal of Neuroendocrinology 2012. 24(5): 789–97

[8] Srivastava DP et al. Rapid estrogen signaling in the brain: implications for the fine-tuning of neuronal circuitry. Journal of Neuroscience 2011. 31 (45): 16056–16063.

[9] Al-Chaer ED, Traub RJ. Biological basis of visceral pain: recent developments. Pain 2002. 96 (3): 221–225.

[10] Mayer EA. Gut feelings: the emerging biology of gut-brain communication. Nature Review Neuroscience 2011. 12 (8): 453–466.

[11] Malykhina AP. Neural mechanisms of pelvic organ cross-sensitization. Neuroscience 2007. 149(3): 660–672.

[12] Grover M, Herfarth H, Drossman DA. The functional-organic dichotomy: postinfectious irritable bowel syndrome and inflammatory bowel disease-irritable bowel syndrome. Clinical Gastroenterology and Hepatology 2009. 7(1): 48–53.

10

Gastric Antral Vascular Ectasia and Portal Hypertensive Gastropathy

Daryl Ramai, Sandar Linn and Madhavi Reddy

Abstract

Gastric antral vascular ectasia (GAVE) and portal hypertensive gastropathy (PHG) are mucosal lesions that can cause chronic gastrointestinal bleeding in the patients with cirrhosis. While PHG occurs exclusively in patients with liver cirrhosis, GAVE can also present in patients with systemic and autoimmune conditions. The need to accurately characterize these two conditions is dependent on clinical, endoscopic, and histological parameters. The management of GAVE utilizes endoscopic ablation techniques, while medical therapy is directed toward stabilizing portal pressure in patients with PHG. Herein, we review the epidemiology, diagnosis, pathophysiology, and medical, endoscopic, and surgical management of GAVE and PHG.

Keywords: stomach diseases, gastric antral vascular ectasia (GAVE), portal hypertensive gastropathy (PHG), portal hypertension, cirrhosis, management

1. Introduction

Gastric antral vascular ectasia (GAVE) and portal hypertensive gastropathy (PHG) are common gastric mucosal lesions that occur in patients with portal hypertension. These two conditions are responsible for acute on chronic gastrointestinal bleeding. While these two clinical entities share similar clinical presentations, their underlying pathophysiology, endoscopic features, and management options are different. The pathophysiology of GAVE is related to local changes in gastric mucosa, and management is aimed at endoscopic reduction of blood loss using thermal therapies. The pathophysiology of PHG is related to portal hypertension, and management is aimed at reducing portal hypertension using pharmacologic and in some cases portosystemic shunts. Thus, it is important to differentiate GAVE and PHG as their management options are different.

2. Epidemiology

GAVE accounts for approximately 4% of all upper gastrointestinal bleeding [1]. Approximately 40% of GAVE patients have cirrhosis of the liver, and 1 in 40 patients require liver transplantation [2]. Cirrhotic GAVE patients are predominantly males (75%; mean age 65 years), whereas noncirrhotic GAVE patients are predominantly females (71%; mean age of 73 years). GAVE has been associated with autoimmune disorders such as autoimmune connective tissue disorders (62%), Raynaud's phenomenon (31%), and sclerodactyly (20%) [3]. GAVE have also been reported in other medical conditions including scleroderma, bone marrow transplantation, chronic renal failure, ischemic heart disease, hypertension, valvular heart disease, familial Mediterranean fever, and acute myeloid leukemia [3–6].

The prevalence of PHG varies from 20 to 75% in portal hypertensive patients, and from 35 to 80% in patients with cirrhosis [7]. According to the HALT-C trial, approximately 37% of patients (364 of 1011) with biopsy confirmed cirrhosis or bridging fibrosis from hepatitis C had PHG [8]. While PHG can present at any age, its severity can vary from mild to severe. The severity of liver disease and severity of portal hypertension greatly influences the natural progression of PHG [9].

3. Pathophysiology

The pathophysiology of GAVE remains unknown; however, several mechanisms have been proposed including gastric dysmotility or autoimmune reactivity to gastric blood vessels [10–12]. A study on antral motility revealed an increase in antral area transit time with cirrhosis and GAVE when compared to controls [10]. Chronic recurrent trauma can lead to fibromuscular hyperplasia and vascular ectasia. Reduced gastrin levels have also been identified in GAVE patients when compared to patients with severe PTH and normal controls [13]. Prostaglandins E2 (PGE2) levels were found significantly elevated when compared to controls [14]. GAVE is not associated with portal hypertension and treatments aimed to decrease portal pressure have no role in treatment of GAVE [15].

The pathogenesis of PHG is related to increased resistance to portal blood flow in patients with liver disease, and concomitant elevation in portal pressure [16]. In patients with portal hypertension, approximately 70% develop PHG [17]. Resolution of PHG and its recurrence has been observed in patients with cirrhosis posttransjugular intrahepatic portosystemic shunt (TIPS) placement, and in noncirrhotic patients with postsurgical decompression of the portal system [17–19]. However, the linear correlation between the severity of portal hypertension and that of PHG is controversial. In a prospective study of 331 patients, it was reported that severe PHG showed a significantly shorter expected survival time than mild PHG (median survival time, 77.6 ± 9.6 months in severe PHG) [20]. The study concluded that PHG was associated with severity of portal hypertension and prognosis in patients with cirrhosis. However, other studies have been unable to demonstrate a correlation between the severity of portal hypertension and that of PHG [21–23].

Other molecular mediators at the mucosal level have been implicated in the development of PHG including tumor necrosis factor (TNF)-α, endothelin-1 (ET-1), nitric oxide (NO), and prostaglandins [21, 24]. Interestingly, patients with cirrhosis and PHG have abnormal blood circulation, which makes them susceptible to reduced delivery of oxygen to the gastric mucosa [21, 25]. This phenomenon modifies blood circulation which enables reduced resistance of gastric mucosa to irritants in patients with cirrhosis and portal hypertension [26].

4. Diagnostic evaluation

GAVE and PHG can be encountered during upper endoscopy in both symptomatic and asymptomatic patients with liver cirrhosis. GI bleeding is the common significant complication of GAVE and PHG. PHG is responsible for about 8% of nonvariceal upper GI bleeding, while GAVE accounts for up to 4% [27, 28]. Both GAVE and PHG may have similar endoscopic appearances and require further histological analysis. In 1995, Payne et al. established that portal hypertensive gastropathy (PHG) and GAVE are distinct clinical entities that require different forms of treatments [13]. Thus, it is incumbent on clinicians to be able to differentiate both diseases.

GAVE is a disease limited to the stomach and is almost exclusively noted in the gastric antrum on endoscopy [29]. GAVE was first reported in 1984 and initially termed 'watermelon' stomach in three patients with iron deficiency anemia [30]. In their report, they described visible convoluted and tortuous columns of ectatic vessels along rugal folds of the antrum, which converged at the pylorus, resembling stripes of a watermelon. In more severe cases, GAVE can present as more punctate lesions or more diffusely, extending to the gastric body, which is most commonly associated with GAVE in cirrhotics than other etiologies [31]. Interestingly, GAVE patients have been reported to have more severe liver disease, greater blood loss, lower serum gastrin levels, and a higher incidence of previous sclerotherapy [13].

Histologically, GAVE is characterized by dilated mucosal capillaries and venules with intimal thickening, fibrin thrombi, spindle cell proliferation, and fibromuscular hyperplasia of the lamina propria [13, 32]. The presence of these histological features is used to calculate a GAVE score which has 80% diagnostic accuracy. This can be used to distinguish GAVE from PHG with a GAVE score equal or greater than three [13].

PHG lesions are typically seen in the gastric fundus unlike GAVE which is commonly found in the antrum. Endoscopically, PHG appears as a mosaic-like pattern or a diffuse, erythematous, and reticular cobblestone pattern of gastric mucosa consisting of small polygonal areas with superimposed red punctate lesions >2 mm in diameter and a depressed white border [33–35]. Severe PHG is associated with flat or bulging red spots, resembling a scarlatina rash with friability or diffuse hemorrhagic gastropathy [36–38].

5. Management of GAVE

5.1. Endoscopic management

The treatment of choice in managing patients with GAVE is endoscopic ablation of the lesions. Pharmacologic or surgical intervention should be considered when endoscopic therapy has failed. Argon plasma coagulation (APC) has become the method most utilized by endoscopist. APC is a noncontact technique that uses argon gas to equally distribute thermal energy. High-frequency current is applied to the tissue with controllable depth of coagulation (roughly 2–3 mm) [39]. Its efficacy ranges from 90 to 100% [40]. Endoscopic band ligation (EBL) and radiofrequency ablation (RFA) are newer and promising techniques in the treatment of GAVE; however, RFA requires additional training and is not readily available in all endoscopic centers [41].

Compared to older laser therapy methods, APC is more user-friendly, manageable, cheaper, and safer. The risk of perforation is very low and limited to very thin-walled structures [42]. The pooled recurrence rate of bleeding is estimated at 36% [43]. Cryotherapy has also been introduced as another means for managing GAVE. It makes use of nitrous oxide to freeze abnormal mucosa and causes superficial necrosis. A pilot study that assessed 12 patients with GAVE and anemia showed that 50% of patients achieved a complete response after cryotherapy [44]. The remaining patients achieved a partial response with decreased transfusion requirements. However, the optimal delivery mechanism and the number of treatments required remain unclear.

Overall, EBL seems to be the safest and has only been associated with minor complications such as abdominal pain [45]. An observational study of 22 patients (9 patients receiving endoscopic thermal therapy vs. 9 patients receiving EBL) reported fewer bleeding in the EBL cohort (67 vs. 23%), as well as fewer treatment sessions for EBL (4.9 vs. 1.9), and a decrease in EBL-related transfusions (−5.2 vs. −12.7) [46]. A prospective study of 21 patients reported a clinical response that was achieved in 19 patients (91%) after a mean of 2.28 endoscopic sessions and a mean of 16 bands applied [47]. Another study comparing the efficacy of EBL vs. APC reported a lower recurrence rate in the EBL cohort (8.3 vs. 68%) [48].

5.2. Medical treatment

While a variety of drugs have been used to manage GAVE-related bleeding, none has shown to be clinically effective and efficacious as an alternative to invasive methods. Pilot studies with estrogen-progesterone hormone therapy have been shown to control bleeding due to gastrointestinal vascular malformations, including GAVE, with side effects [49–51]. Despite bleeding cessation, GAVE lesions persisted. Reduction of treatment frequency resulted in bleeding relapse, requiring reinstitution of daily therapy for hemostatic control [49, 52, 53]. However, this form of treatment is not well studied and patients are at risk for developing severe side effects, such as menorrhagia and gynecomastia, and increased risk of endometrial and breast cancer [54].

A long acting somatostatin analog, octreotide, has been reported as an effective drug in controlling chronic bleeding due to vascular abnormalities [55]. This may in part be due to the inhibitory effect on neuroendocrine cells, ectatic vessels, and smooth muscle cells [55, 56]. Octreotide also displays antiangiogenic effects and limits the growth of blood vessels [57]. However, octreotide treatment has been unsuccessfully replicated by other authors and thus necessitates further investigation [58]. Success has been reported from the use of corticosteroids, tranexamic acid, thalidomide, and serotonin antagonist [59–63]. However, these treatments have been reported in some case reports and the results have not been confirmed by controlled clinical trials.

5.3. Surgical intervention

Surgical intervention is reserved for patients who do not respond to medical and endoscopic therapies. Surgical approaches include gastrectomy and antrectomy, which may be the only reliable approach to achieving a cure. Antrectomy is more commonly used and has clinical efficacy in eliminating bleeding and transfusion dependency, as patients do not report postoperative recurrence of bleeding was associated with multiorgan failure [64]. Portacaval shunts and TIPS have no role in the management of GAVE [11]. In GAVE patients due to underlying cirrhosis, complete resolution of symptoms has been observed following liver transplant, despite persistent portal hypertension [15].

6. Management of PHG

6.1. Medical treatment

The management of PHG is focused on abating portal pressure, mainly through the use of medical therapy rather than endoscopic means. Similar to esophageal varices, management attempts to reduce hepatic venous pressure gradient (HVPG) to <12 mmHg or by 20% which correlates with a reduction in mortality in some studies [65]. A meta-analysis established that target HVPG is a valid marker to monitor drug efficacy for variceal bleeding and patient prognosis [65]. Beta blockers are first-line drugs used to reduce portal pressure and have the most benefit in patients with mild PHG [66]. Modest effects have been noted in patients with severe PHG [67]. It is unclear whether beta blockers are prophylactically effective in preventing bleeding from PHG [24]. However, in patients receiving propranolol or nadolol for esophageal variceal bleeding prophylaxis, beta blocker therapy showed a reduction in future PHG bleeding [68].

In a randomized controlled trial to investigate the efficacy of propranolol, 26 of 54 patients received propranolol and the rest placebo. Daily doses of 40–320 mg were used. In the cohort receiving propranolol, patients reported significantly lower rates of rebleeding (38 vs. 65%) at 12 months and at 30 months (7 vs. 52%) compared with controls [67]. Similarly, a smaller study using a dose of 24–480 mg/day decreased the incidence of acute bleeding in 16 patients with PHG and also reduced the grade of PHG in 24 asymptomatic patients when given at a dose of 160 mg/day [68].

In unstable patients who have contraindications for beta blockers, other agents have been studied with varying efficacy including somatostatin, octreotide, terlipressin, and vasopressin [69–72]. Somatostatin and its analogs showed complete control of acute bleeding with 11% rebleeding after withdrawing infusion [69]. Octreotide controlled bleeding in 100% of patients within 48 h. Vasopressin controlled bleeding in 64% of patients over the same time [71]. Terlipressin, a vasopressin analog (not available in the United States), was similarly effective as vasopressin [72].

6.2. Endoscopic management

Acute bleeding in the setting of PHG rarely occurs. A large study reported an incidence of acute bleeding from gastropathy in 8 of 315 patients (2.5%), compared to chronic bleeding which occurred in 34 patients (10.8%) [73]; however, if it occurs, such bleeding episodes can be severe and challenging to manage. In addition to intravenous medical therapy with aforementioned agents aimed at reducing portal pressure and hemostatic control, appropriate antibiotic and resuscitation should be initiated and tailored to the patient's needs.

Endoscopic therapy for acute bleeding from PHG remains investigational and may provide temporary control. For patients with refractory bleeding who are not candidates for portosystemic shunting, limited data suggest that endoscopic thermal therapy may be efficacious. Similar to GAVE, APC has proven successful in controlling bleeding and reducing transfusion requirements [74]. Furthermore, hemostatic powder is emerging as a useful means for managing patients with acute bleeding. The powder acts by forming a barrier over the bleeding site and increasing the concentration of clotting factors [75].

6.3. Surgical intervention

In cases of failed medical or endoscopic therapy requiring increase blood transfusions, portosystemic shunt therapy should be considered through the placement of a transjugular intrahepatic portosystemic shunt (TIPS). Shunting works by relieving portal hypertension with the placement of a tube (shunt) between the portal vein which carries blood from the intestines to the liver and the hepatic vein which carries blood from the liver back to the heart. Patients who have the TIPS procedure show significant improvement in endoscopic appearance of PHG and number of transfusion requirements [76].

A prospective study of 30 patients with mild PHG and 10 patients with severe PHG with recurrent GI bleeding had a 75% reduction in endoscopic severity, a Childs-Pugh Score of 11.5, and a mean reduction in portacaval gradient from 20 to 12 mmHg following TIPS [17]. Patients typically show endoscopic improvement in 6 weeks for mild cases and up to 3 months for more severe cases of PHG [77]. A retrospective study of 40 Child-Pugh class A and B cirrhotic patients comparing surgical shunting and TIPS found improved outcomes from surgical shunting with reduced 30-day mortality, reduced rebleeding events, and fewer shunt revisions and hospitalizations [78].

However, surgical shunting carries risks of substantial perioperative morbidity and mortality. In those who survive operation, accelerated hepatic decompensation and neuropsychologic deterioration (portosystemic encephalopathy) significantly diminish the overall benefit of the shunting procedure [78]. Similarly, TIPS carries a potential risk for rapid liver failure necessitating liver transplantation [79].

7. Conclusion

In summary, GAVE and PHG are two clinically distinct entities that present with gastrointestinal blood loss. Majority of patients with portal hypertension and cirrhosis will develop PHG; however, it can also occur in the setting of noncirrhotic portal hypertension. GAVE is associated with gastric dysmotility, autoimmune reactivity, reduced gastrin levels, and elevated prostaglandins. It is not associated with cirrhosis. Therapy of PHG is directed toward lowering and stabilizing portal pressure with beta blockers or shunt procedures. GAVE management mainly involves the use of endoscopic methods to ablate bleeding lesions. When GAVE is complicated by cirrhosis, it is incumbent on clinicians to differentiate it from PHG as GAVE does not respond to treatments aimed at reduction of portal pressure.

Author details

Daryl Ramai[1,2]*, Sandar Linn[1] and Madhavi Reddy[1]

*Address all correspondence to: dramai@sgu.edu

1 Department of Gastroenterology and Hepatology, The Brooklyn Hospital Center – Clinical Affiliate of The Mount Sinai Hospital, Brooklyn, New York, USA

2 Department of Anatomical Sciences, St George's University School of Medicine, True Blue, Grenada, West Indies

References

[1] Dulai GS, Jensen DM, Kovacs TO, et al. Endoscopic treatment outcomes in watermelon stomach patients with and without portal hypertension. Endoscopy. 2004;**36**:68-72

[2] Ward EM, Raimondo M, Rosser BG, et al. Prevalence and natural history of gastric antral vascular ectasia (GAVE) in patients undergoing orthoptic liver transplantation. Journal of Clinical Gastroenterology. 2004;**38**:898-900

[3] Gostout CJ, Viggiano TR, Ahlquist DA, et al. The clinical and endoscopic spectrum of the watermelon stomach. Journal of Clinical Gastroenterology. 1992;**15**:256-263

[4] Tobin RW, Hackman RC, Kimmey MB, et al. Bleeding from gastric antral vascular ectasia in marrow transplant patients. Gastrointestinal Endoscopy. 1996;**44**:223-229

[5] Sebastian S, O'Morain CA, Buckley MJ. Review article: Current therapeutic options for gastric antral vascular ectasia. Alimentary Pharmacology & Therapeutics. 2003;**18**:157-165

[6] Takahashi T, Takuya M, Oki M, et al. Severe hemorrhage from gastric antral vascular ectasia developed in a patient with AML. International Journal of Hematology. 2006;**83**:467-468

[7] Gjeorgjievski M, Cappell MS. Portal hypertensive gastropathy: A systematic review of the pathophysiology, clinical presentation, natural history and therapy. World Journal of Hepatology. 2016;**8**:231-262

[8] Fontana RJ, Sanyal AJ, Ghany MG, et al. Development and progression of portal hypertensive gastropathy in patients with chronic hepatitis C. The American Journal of Gastroenterology. 2011;**106**:884-893

[9] Merli M, Nicolini G, Angeloni S, et al. The natural history of portal hypertensive gastropathy in patients with liver cirrhosis and mild portal hypertension. The American Journal of Gastroenterology. 2004;**99**:1959-1965

[10] Charneau J, Petit R, Cales P, et al. Antral motility in patients with cirrhosis with or without gastric antral vascular ectasia. Gut. 1995;**37**:488-492

[11] Spahr L, Villeneuve JP, Dufresne MP, et al. Gastric antral vascular ectasia in cirrhotic patients: Absence of relation with portal hypertension. Gut. 1999;**44**:739-742

[12] Watson M, Hally RJ, McCue PA, Varga J, Jimenez SA. Gastric antral vascular ectasia (watermelon stomach) in patients with systemic sclerosis. Arthritis & Rheumatology. 1996;**39**:341-346

[13] Payen JL, Cales P, Voigt JJ, et al. Severe portal hypertensive gastropathy and antral vascular ectasia are distinct entities in patients with cirrhosis. Gastroenterology. 1995; **108**:138-144

[14] Saperas E, Perez Ayuso RM, Poca E, et al. Increased gastric PGE2 biosynthesis in cirrhotic patients with gastric vascular ectasia. The American Journal of Gastroenterology. 1990;**85**:138-144

[15] Vincent C, Pomier-Layrargues G, Dagenais M, et al. Cure of gastric antral vascular ectasia by liver transplantation despite persistent portal hypertension: A clue for pathogenesis. Liver Transplantation. 2002;**8**:717-720

[16] Ferraz JG, Wallace JL. Underlying mechanisms of portal hypertensive gastropathy. Journal of Clinical Gastroenterology. 1997;**25**(Suppl 1):S73-S78

[17] Kamath PS, Lacerda M, Ahlquist DA, et al. Gastric mucosal responses to intrahepatic portosystemic shunting in patients with cirrhosis. Gastroenterology. 2000;**118**:905-911

[18] de Melo MR, de Figueiredo JL, AraújoFilho JL, et al. Portal hypertension in mansonic schistosomiasis: Repercussions of surgical treatment on the histomorphometric profile of the gastric mucosa. Revista daSociedadeBrasileirade Medicina Tropical. 2007;**40**:71-75

[19] Soin AS, Acharya SK, Mathur M, et al. Portal hypertensive gastropathy in non-cirrhotic patients. The effect of lienorenal shunts. Journal of Clinical Gastroenterology. 1998;**26**:64-67

[20] Kim MY, Choi H, Baik SK, et al. Portal hypertensive gastropathy: Correlation with portal hypertension and prognosis in cirrhosis. Digestive Diseases and Science. 2010; **55**:3561-3567

[21] Ohta M, Hashizume M, Higashi H, et al. Portal and gastric mucosal hemodynamics in cirrhotic patients with portal-hypertensive gastropathy. Hepatology. 1994;**20**:1432-1436

[22] Sarin SK, Lahoti D, Saxena SP, et al. Prevalence, classification and natural history of gastric varices: A long-term follow-up study in 568 portal hypertension patients. Hepatology. 1992;**16**:1343-1349

[23] Panes J, Bordas JM, Pique JM, et al. Increased gastric mucosal perfusion in cirrhotic patients with portal hypertensive gastropathy. Gastroenterology. 1992;**103**:1875-1882

[24] Cubillas R, Rockey DC. Portal hypertensive gastropathy: A review. Liver International. 2010;**30**:1094-1102

[25] Curvelo LA, Brabosa W, Rhor R, et al. Underlying mechanism of portal hypertensive gastropathy in cirrhosis: A hemodynamic and morphological approach. Journal of Gastroenterology and Hepatology. 2009;**24**:1541-1546

[26] Sarfeh IJ, Soliman H, Waxman K, et al. Impaired oxygenation of gastric mucosa in portal hypertension. The basis for increased susceptibility to injury. Digestive Diseases and Science. 1989;**34**:225-228

[27] Gostout CJ, Viggiano TR, Balm RK. Acute gastrointestinal bleeding from portal hypertensive gastropathy: Prevalence and clinical features. American Journal of Gastroenterology. 1993;**88**:2030-2033

[28] Dulai GS, Jensen DM, Kovacs TO, et al. Endoscopic treatment outcomes in watermelon stomach patients with and without portal hypertension. Endoscopy. 2004;**36**:68-72

[29] Burak KW, Beck PL. Portal hypertensive gastropathy and gastric antral vascular ectasia (GAVE) syndrome. Gut. 2001;**49**:866-872

[30] Jabbari M, Cherry R, Lough JO, et al. Gastric antral vascular ectasia: The watermelon stomach. Gastroenterology. 1984;**87**:1165-1170

[31] Ito M, Uchida Y, Kamano S, et al. Clinical comparisons between two subsets of gastric antral vascular ectasia. Gastrointestinal Endoscopy. 2001;**53**:764-770

[32] Suit PF, Petras RE, Bauer TW, Petrini JL. Gastric antral vascular ectasia. A histologic and morphometric study of the watermelon stomach. The American Journal of Surgical Pathology. 1987;**11**:750-757

[33] Kamath PS, Shah VH. Portal hypertension and bleeding esophageal varices. In: Boyer TD, Manns MP, Sanyal AJ, editors. Zakim and Boyer's Hepatology: A Textbook of Liver Disease. 6th ed. Philadelphia: Elsevier Saunders; 2012. p. 296-326

[34] Feldman M, Lee EL. Gastritis. In: Feldman M, Friedman LS, Brandt LJ, editors. Sleisenger and Fordtran's Gastrointestinal and Liver Disease: Pathophysiology, Diagnosis, Management. 10th ed. Philadelphia: Elsevier Saunders; 2010. p. 868-883

[35] Vigneri S, Termini R, Piraino A, et al. The stomach in liver cirrhosis. Endoscopic, morphological, and clinical correlations. Gastroenterology. 1991;**101**:472-478

[36] Thuluvath PJ, Yoo HY. Portal hypertensive gastropathy. American Journal of Gastroenterology. 2002;**97**:2973-2978

[37] Thuluvath PJ. Management of upper gastrointestinal hemorrhage related to portal hypertension. In: Yamada T, Alpers DH, Kalloo AN, Kaplowitz N, Owyang C, Powell DW, editors. Textbook of Gastroenterology. 5th ed. Oxford, UK: Wiley-Blackwell; 2009. p. 2897-3017

[38] Bhattacharya B. Non-neoplastic disorders of the stomach. In: Iacobuzio-Donahue CA, Montgomery E, Goldblum JR, editors. Gastrointestinal and Liver Pathology. 2nd ed. Philadelphia: Elsevier Saunders; 2012. p. 65-141

[39] Yusoff I, Brennan F, Ormonde D, Laurence B. Argon plasma coagulation for the treatment of watermelon stomach. Endoscopy. 2002;**34**:407-410

[40] Roman S, Saurin JC, Dumortier J, et al. Tolerance and efficacy of argon plasma coagulation for controlling bleeding in patients with typical and atypical manifestations of watermelon stomach. Endoscopy. 2003;**35**:1024-1028

[41] Dray X, Repici A, Gonzalez P, et al. Radiofrequency ablation for the treatment of gastric antral vascular ectasia. Endoscopy. 2014;**46**:963-969

[42] Wahab PJ, Mulder CJ, den Hartog G, Thies JE. Argon plasma coagulation in flexible gastrointestinal endoscopy: Pilot experiences. Endoscopy 1997;**29**:176-181

[43] Jackson CS, Gerson LB. Management of gastrointestinal angiodysplastic lesions (GIADs): A systematic review and meta-analysis. American Journal of Gastroenterology. 2014;**109**:474-483

[44] Cho S, Zanati S, Yong E, et al. Endoscopic cryotherapy for the management of gastric antral vascular ectasia. Gastrointestinal Endoscopy. 2008;**68**:895-902

[45] Zepeda-Gomez S. Endoscopic treatment for gastric antral vascular ectasia: Current options. GE-Portuguese Journal of Gastroenterology. 2017;**24**:176-182

[46] Wells CD, Harrison ME, Gurudu SR, et al. Treatment of gastric antral vascular ectasia (watermelon stomach) with endoscopic band ligation. Gastrointestinal Endoscopy. 2008;**68**:231-236

[47] Zepeda-Gomez S, Sultanian R, Teshima C, et al. Gastric antral vascular ectasia: A prospective study of treatment with endoscopic band ligation. Endoscopy. 2015;**47**:538-540

[48] Sato T, Yamazaki K, Akaike J. Endoscopic band ligation versus argon plasma coagulation for gastric antral vascular ectasia associated with liver diseases. Digestive Endoscopy. 2012;**24**:237-242

[49] Manning RJ. Estrogen/progesterone treatment of diffuse antral vascular ectasia. American Journal of Gastroenterology. 1995;**90**:154-156

[50] Tran A, Villeneuve JP, Bilodeau M, et al. Treatment of chronic bleeding from gastric antral vascular ectasia (GAVE) with estrogen-progesterone in cirrhotic patients: An open pilot study. American Journal of Gastroenterology. 1999;**94**:2909-2911

[51] van Cutsem E, Rutgeerts P, Vantrappen G. Treatment of bleeding gastrointestinal vascular malformations with oestrogen-progesterone. Lancet 1990;**335**:953-955

[52] Schoonbroodt D, Horsmans Y, Hoang P, et al. Vascular gastric anomalies, CREST syndrome and primary biliary cirrhosis: Efficacy of ethinyl estradiol-norethisterone combination. Gastroenterologie Clinique etBiologique. 1994;**18**:649-651

[53] Moss SF, Ghosh P, Thomas DM, Jackson JE, Calam J. Gastric antral vascular ectasia: Maintenance treatment with oestrogen-progesterone. Gut. 1992;**33**:715-717

[54] Grady D, Rubin SM, Petitti DB, et al. Hormone therapy to prevent disease and prolong life in postmenopausal women. Annals of Internal Medicine. 1992;**117**:1016-1037

[55] Nardone G, Rocco A, Balzano T. The efficacy of octreotide therapy in chronic bleeding due to vascular abnormalities of the gastrointestinal tract. Alimentary Pharmacology & Therapeutics. 1999;**13**:1429-1363

[56] Li SC, Martijn C, Cui T, et al. The somatostatin analogue octreotide inhibits growth of small intestine neuroendocrine tumour cells. PloS One. 2012;**7**:e48411

[57] Zalatnai A, Timar F. Vitro antiangiogenic effect of sandostatin (octreotide) on the proliferation of the placental vessels. Anticancer Research. 2002;**22**:4225-4227

[58] Barbara G, De Giorgio R, Salvioli B, et al. Unsuccessful octreotide treatment of the watermelon stomach. Journal of Clinical Gastroenterology. 1998;**26**:345-346

[59] Bhowmick BK. Watermelon stomach treated with oral corticosteroid. Journal of the Royal Society of Medicine. 1993;**86**:52

[60] Suzuki T, Hirano M, Oka H. Long-term corticosteroid therapy for gastric antral vascular ectasia. American Journal of Gastroenterology. 1996;**91**:1873-1874

[61] McCormick PA, Ooi H, Crosbie O. Tranexamic acid for severe bleeding gastric antral vascular ectasia in cirrhosis. Gut. 1998;**42**:750-752

[62] Dunne KA, Hill J, Dillon JF. Treatment of chronic transfusion-dependent gastric antral vascular ectasia (watermelon stomach) with thalidomide. European Journal of Gastroenterology & Hepatology. 2006;**18**:455-456

[63] Cabral JE, Pontes JM, Toste M, et al. Watermelon stomach: Treatment with a serotonin antagonist. American Journal of Gastroenterology. 1991;**86**:927-928

[64] Novitsky YW, Kercher KW, Czerniach DR, Litwin DE. Watermelon stomach: Pathophysiology, diagnosis, and management. Journal of Gastrointestinal Surgery. 2003;**7**: 652-661

[65] Albillos A, Banares R, Gonzalez M, et al. Value of the hepatic venous pressure gradient to monitor drug therapy for portal hypertension: A meta-analysis. American Journal of Gastroenterology. 2007;**102**:1116-1126

[66] Hosking SW, Kennedy HJ, Seddon I, Triger DR. The role of propranolol in congestive gastropathy of portal hypertension. Hepatology. 1987;**7**:437-441

[67] Perez-Ayuso RM, Pique JM, Bosch J, et al. Propranolol in prevention of recurrent bleeding from severe portal hypertensive gastropathy in cirrhosis. Lancet. 1991;**337**:1431-1434

[68] Lo GH, Lai KH, Cheng JS, et al. The effects of endoscopic variceal ligation and propranolol on portal hypertensive gastropathy: A prospective, controlled trial. Gastrointestinal Endoscopy. 2001;**53**:579-584

[69] Kouroumalis EA, Koutroubakis IE, Manousos ON. Somatostatin for acute severe bleeding from portal hypertensive gastropathy. European Journal of Gastroenterology & Hepatology. 1998;**10**:509-512

[70] Panes J, Pique JM, Bordas JM, et al. Effect of bolus injection and continuous infusion of somatostatin on gastric perfusion in cirrhotic patients with portal-hypertensive gastropathy. Hepatology. 1994;**20**:336-341

[71] Zhou Y, Qiao L, Wu J, et al. Comparison of the efficacy of octreotide, vasopressin, and omeprazole in the control of acute bleeding in patients with portal hypertensive gastropathy: A controlled study. Journal of Gastroenterology & Hepatology. 2002;**17**:973-979

[72] Bruha R, Marecek Z, Spicak J, et al. Double-blind randomized, comparative multicenter study of the effect of terlipressin in the treatment of acute esophageal variceal and/or hypertensive gastropathy bleeding. Hepato-Gastroenterology. 2002;**49**:1161-1166

[73] Primignani M, Carpinelli L, Preatoni P, et al. Natural history of portal hypertensive gastropathy in patients with liver cirrhosis. The new Italian endoscopic Club for the study and treatment of esophageal varices (NIEC). Gastroenterology. 2000;**119**:181-187

[74] Herrera S, Bordas JM, Llach J, et al. The beneficial effects of argon plasma coagulation in the management of different types of gastric vascular ectasia lesions in patients admitted for GI hemorrhage. Gastrointestinal Endoscopy. 2008;**68**:440-446

[75] Smith LA, Morris AJ, Stanley AJ. The use of hemospray in portal hypertensive bleeding; a case series. Journal of Hepatology. European Association for the Study of the Liver. 2014;**60**:457-460

[76] Urata J, Yamashita Y, Tsuchigame T, et al. The effects of transjugular intrahepatic portosystemic shunt on portal hypertensive gastropathy. Journal of Gastroenterology & Hepatology. 1998;**13**:1061-1067

[77] Ripoll C, Garcia-Tsao G. The management of portal hypertensive gastropathy and gastric antral vascular ectasia. Digestive and Liver Disease. 2011;**43**:345-351

[78] Helton WS, Maves R, Wicks K, Johansen K. Transjugular intrahepatic portosystemic shunt vs surgical shunt in good-risk cirrhotic patients: A case-control comparison. Archives of Surgery. 2001;**136**:17-20

[79] Qureshi K, Al-Osaimi AM. Approach to the management of portal hypertensive gastropathy and gastric antral vascular ectasia. Gastroenterology Clinics of North America. 2014;**43**:835-847

11

Exclusive and Partial Enteral Nutrition in Crohn's Disease

Darja Urlep, Evgen Benedik and Rok Orel

Abstract

Exclusive enteral nutrition (EEN) is a well-establised primary therapy in active pediatric Crohn's disease (CD). EEN promotes mucosal healing, restores bone mineral density, and improves growth. On the contrary, treatment of active CD with corticosteroids (CS) has a strong negative impact on the linear growth and bone density. Therefore, EEN is recommended as a first-line therapy in children with active CD. EEN has been evaluated in a number of clinical studies including randomized controlled trials. While meta-analyses of adult studies suggest superiority of CS, pediatric studies have shown that EEN is at least as effective as CS in inducing remission. The mechanisms by which EEN suppresses inflammation are not yet fully elucidated. Hypotheses include improvement in nutritional status, decreasing of the inflammatory cascade mechanism, limiting luminal antigen exposure, improving intestinal permeability, and modification of intestinal microbiota.

Keywords: Crohn's disease, exclusive enteral nutrition, partial enteral nutrition, children, adults

1. Introduction

Inflammatory bowel disease (IBD) is an immune-mediated condition, which includes Crohn's disease (CD), ulcerative colitis (UC), and IBD-unclassified (IBD-U) [1]. Nearly 25% of patients are diagnosed before 16 years of age. A number of studies have shown that pediatric-onset IBD presents with a more difficult phenotype when compared to adult-onset IBD and may have the consequences of growth retardation and delayed puberty as well as the psychological consequences of disease onset at a very vulnerable time of psychosocial development [2–5].

Exclusive enteral nutrition (EEN) is successful in the treatment of undernutrition. Moreover, EEN is able to induce remission in CD patients with active inflammation. The European Society of Gastroenterology, Hepatology and Nutrition (ESPGHAN) and the European Crohn's Colitis Organization (ECCO) recommend EEN as a first-line therapy in children with active CD and emphasize the use of EEN over CS in all children with active inflammatory intestinal luminal disease, including colonic involvement [6].

The therapy with EEN provides all of the nutritional needs by a liquid formula either orally or through a nasogastric tube. EEN is usually recommended for 6–8 weeks, and after this period, a normal diet is gradually reintroduced. For EEN therapy, elemental, semi-elemental, or polymeric formulas may be used. Elemental formulas are based on amino acids and contain no whole proteins, while semi-elemental formulas do contain peptides of varying lengths. Polymeric formulas are based on whole proteins and are therefore more palatable [7]. In addition, polymeric formulas usually cost less. The choice of formula most frequently depends on the clinician's experience and local availability [8].

EEN is especially recommended in CD children with stunted growth and in those presenting with low weight and a catabolic state. If EEN is not tolerated orally, a nasogastric tube may be used [6].

Nevertheless, EEN therapy remains underused in clinical practice, especially in adults in whom its efficacy in achieving clinical remission is considered to be less than the standard anti-inflammatory therapies [9].

In current review, different aspects of EEN as well as partial enteral nutrition (PEN) will be addressed, including their efficacy, treatment modalities, impact on mucosal healing, mechanisms of anti-inflammatory effects, and the role of enteral nutrition in maintaining remission.

2. The history of exclusive enteral nutrition

The first report on successful use of enteral feeding was published in 1973 by Voitk et al. It demonstrated improvement in inflammatory indices and weight gain in 13 patients. Nine of them were planned for surgery and two of them were able to avoid it after a period of exclusive elemental formula treatment [10].

In 1981, Logan et al. found a decrease in the number of gut lymphocytes and diminished protein loss when elemental enteral nutrition was used in patients with extensive small bowel CD [11].

Navarro et al. studied the efficacy of continuous elemental EEN on 17 pediatric patients with active CD and demonstrated that EEN was successful in inducing clinical remission. Additionally, therapy with EEN was proven to be safe and well tolerated [12].

Five years later, O'Morain et al. found that elemental EEN was equally successful or even more effective than steroids in inducing clinical remission in adults with active CD [13]. However, in 1995, a meta-analysis by Griffiths et al. demonstrated that therapy with EEN was significantly less effective compared to CS in a mixed population of adult and pediatric patients with CD [14]. But in 1997, in a randomized controlled trial by Zoli et al., EEN with an elemental diet was again shown to be equally effective as CS in inducing remission in a cohort of adult patients with both mild and moderately active CD [15].

3. Elemental versus polymeric enteral feeds

In the 1990s, both elemental and polymeric enteral nutrition were used in the largest pediatric inflammatory centers in United Kingdom as a first line of treatment of active CD. Clinical studies were then conducted to compare elemental versus polymeric enteral formulas [16]. In a randomized controlled trial by Rigaud et al., no significant difference was found in inducing clinical remission in adult CD patients between elemental and polymeric enteral formulas [17]. Ludvigsson et al. conducted a multicentre randomized control trial to compare the efficacy of elemental and polymeric formulas in children with active CD. The efficacy in inducing remission was found not to be different between elemental (E028E; Nutricia) and polymeric formulas (Nutrison Standard; Nutricia). However, patients who were receiving polymeric formula had better weight gain [18].

In a meta-analysis by Griffits et al., the efficacy of EEN therapy with elemental versus nonelemental formulas was compared. They demonstrated that there was no significant difference in the efficacy between the elemental and nonelemental formulas [14].

4. The efficacy of exclusive enteral nutrition versus corticosteroids

EEN has been evaluated in a number of clinical studies including randomized controlled trials (RCTs) that compared EEN with CS in adult and pediatric populations of patients with active CD. To date, eight meta-analyses have been published on the efficacy of EEN versus CS. Among these meta-analyses, three of them were performed exclusively on the pediatric population, whereas others included adult patients as well. While meta-analyses of adult studies have suggested better efficacy of CS, pediatric studies have shown that EEN is at least as effective as CS in inducing remission and is superior to CS in improving nutritional status and growth recovery without adverse side effects [19].

4.1. Efficacy of EEN versus CS in adult and mixed population of CD patients

In the first meta-analysis by Fernandez-Banares et al., the therapy with EEN was significantly less effective compared to CS. The meta-analysis included nine trials with mostly adult CD populations. The overall remission rate was 57.7% for EEN and 79.4% for CS [20]. A meta-analysis by Messori et al. included studies exclusively on the adult CD population which compared the effectiveness of EEN versus CS. The patient-specific end-point of the meta-analysis was occurrence of treatment failure. CS were more effective than EEN for inducing remission in adult active CD. In fact, the relative risk of treatment failure (RTF) was significantly lower in the steroid group than in the EEN group. They concluded that the data examined in this meta-analysis do not support the use of EEN as primary treatment for acute exacerbations of CD in adults [21]. In 1995, Griffiths et al. included eight RCTs (mixed adult and pediatric CD of 413 patients) comparing EEN with CS. Odds ratios (OR) for likelihood of clinical response were calculated. They found that EEN was inferior to CS (OR 0.35; 95% CI 0.23–0.53) [14]. A similar meta-analysis was performed in 2001 by the same team of authors from Toronto. In accordance with the stricter inclusion criteria, only four RCTs were included (130 patients treated with EEN and 123 treated with CS). The meta-analysis yielded a pooled OR for remission of 0.30 favoring CS therapy (95% CI 0.17–0.52) [22]. This meta-analysis was updated in 2007 and included six clinical trials with 192 patients treated with EEN and 160 treated with CS. The pooled OR for remission, after combining all type of enteral diets and comparing them with CS therapy, was 0.33 favoring steroid therapy (95% CI: 0.21–0.53) [23].

4.2. Efficacy of EEN versus CS in pediatric CD population

The first meta-analysis on pediatric population was published in 2000 by Heuschkel et al. The meta-analysis included five RCTs and was composed of 147 pediatric patients with active CD, and it demonstrated that EEN was equally effective as CS in inducing remission (relative risk (RR) = 0.95; 95% CI: 0.67–1.34). EEN was, however, superior in improving growth and pubertal development. Additionally, EEN seemed to be without the side effects. According to the results of this meta-analysis, EEN was then recommended as a first-line therapy in children with active CD [24]. The same results were demonstrated 7 years later in a meta-analysis by Dziechciarz et al. Only four RCTs (144 pediatric CD patients) met the inclusion criteria. No significant difference in remission rates between the patients receiving EEN and CS was found [25].

In the most recent published meta-analysis by Swaminath et al., eight clinical studies (451 pediatric CD patients) were included based on the inclusion criteria and availability of data that could be abstracted into meta-analysis. The efficacy in inducing remission was not different between EEN and CS (OR = 1.26; 95% CI 0.77–2.05). The authors also compared the efficacy between EEN and CS treatment in newly diagnosed CD patients (OR = 1.61; 95% CI 0.87–2.98) with relapsed patients (OR = 0.76; 95% CI 0.29–1.98) [26].

5. Recommendations on exclusive enteral nutrition in adult patients with Crohn's disease

To date, according to the results of meta-analyses on the adult CD population, EEN appears to be less effective than CS. Therefore, therapy with EEN is used as a first-line treatment in active CD only when therapy with CS is contraindicated [27].

In the current ECCO consensus guidelines for medical management of adult CD, therapy with enteral nutrition is regarded as a complementary treatment to improve nutrition and not as a primary therapy. It is still considered appropriate to use EEN in patients who decline all other drug therapies [28]. Further studies on EEN use as a primary therapy to induce remission in adult CD patients are needed to clarify the efficacy of EEN. The reasons for the difference in the efficacy of EEN between the pediatric and adult CD population have still not been elucidated. In adult IBD patients, who have a longer disease course and more frequent complications, EEN may be less effective. EEN may not be so strictly adhered to in adult patients, when compared to children, who are supervised by their parents. Furthermore, children and especially adolescents are generally more motivated to achieve success through this therapy. Most of them refuse CS treatment due to the unpleasant side effects related to appearance such as facies lunata, acne vulgaris, and increased hairiness.

6. Exclusive enteral nutrition and mucosal healing

Mucosal healing is an important therapeutic endpoint that, when achieved early, is associated with fewer hospitalizations, reduced surgical resections, lower risk of fistulizing disease, and less use of biologic drugs [29–32]. It is well established that treatment with EEN is capable of achieving mucosal healing in CD. On the contrary, CS have poor ability to induce mucosal healing. A study made in 1990, on the effects of prednisolone on mucosal healing in patients with active CD, found that 27% of patients still had minor lesions and only 12% achieved complete mucosal healing after 4–7 weeks of CS therapy [33]. Similarly, none out of eight patients with CD, treated with prednisolone for postoperative recurrence, showed mucosal healing after 6–9 weeks, based on the overall endoscopic assessment of the mucosa rather than a detailed endoscopic score [34]. These findings suggest that CS have little or no positive effects on induction of mucosal healing in CD. In a RCT in children with active CD, Borrelli et al. compared not only the efficacy of EEN versus CS in inducing clinical remission but also in achieving mucosal healing. The therapy with EEN was superior in achieving mucosal healing compared to CS. Mucosal healing was found in 14 of 19 CD patients (74%) in the EEN group and in 6 of 18 patients in the CS group (33%, $p < 0.05$) [35]. In a retrospective study by Berni Canani et al., 65% of pediatric CD patients on EEN therapy and 40% on CS ($p < 0.05$) achieved improvement in mucosal inflammation. Seven patients on EEN and none on CS were found to have complete mucosal healing ($p < 0.005$) at the end of treatment. In addition, the duration of clinical remission was longer in the EEN group when compared with the CS group [36]. Recently, Grover et al. had used the Simple Endoscopic Score for CD (SES-CD) to define endoscopic mucosal lesions in 26 children with active CD receiving EEN for 8 weeks. At the end of the EEN therapy, 42% of patients had complete mucosal healing (SES-CD = 0) and the other 58% had complete or near-complete mucosal healing (SES-CD < 3) [37]. Mucosal healing after EEN therapy was also demonstrated in the adult population of active CD patients. In a study by Yamamoto et al., a 4-week therapy with EEN has shown a complete endoscopic remission rate of 44% in the terminal ileum and 39% in the colon [38]. In a recent pediatric meta-analysis by Swaminath et al., two pediatric studies provided data on mucosal healing at the end of induction therapy with EEN versus CS [35, 36]. The occurrence of mucosal healing was significantly more likely in the group of CD children, who were receiving EEN, compared to those receiving CS (OR = 4.5; 95% CI 1.64–12.32) [26]. Furthermore, Rubio et al. compared fractionated oral versus continuous enteral feeding in terms of clinical and mucosal healing and have demonstrated similar rates of mucosal healing in patients receiving ether fractionated or continuous enteral feeding [39].

7. Disease location and efficacy of exclusive enteral nutrition

In the early 2000s, EEN was especially used in CD patients with small bowel disease. That was in accordance with the results of a clinical trial by Afzal et al. which have shown that EEN was less effective in CD patients with colonic disease in comparison with those who had only small bowel involvement or small and large bowel disease [40]. However, recent studies and meta-analyses have not confirmed this negative association [23, 25]. Buchanan et al. found no significant differences in remission rates in terms of disease location [41]. Similar findings were reported in a study by Rubio et al. where the site of disease activity had no impact on response to nutritional therapy [39]. The same results were demonstrated in a study by Gupta et al. where the location of the inflammation in CD did not affect the efficacy of EEN [42].

8. The long-term efficacy of exclusive enteral nutrition

The long-term efficacy of the induction therapy with EEN is not yet well established. Studies comparing the long-term outcomes of EEN versus CS treatment are limited. In a retrospective study by Lambert et al., a lower 1-year (61 versus 77%) and 2-year relapse rate (61 versus 89%) was demonstrated in CD children who were treated with EEN in comparison with those receiving CS [43]. Grover et al. have shown that induction therapy with EEN was superior to CS in reducing growth failure, CS dependency, and loss of response to infliximab over the first 2 years [44]. In a retrospective German study, most of the pediatric patients with active CD, treated with EEN, relapsed during the first year. Fortunately, 66% of them responded to a second course of EEN with remission [45]. In a recent study by Connors et al., both short- and long-term outcomes of EEN and CS induction therapy were examined. Out of 127 patients reviewed, a total of 111 propensity score-matched CD patients receiving EEN (n = 76) or CS (n = 35) were analyzed. Their data showed that clinical remission after EEN was superior to that after CS treatment, with 86.6 versus 58.1% of patients reaching remission within 4–12 weeks of starting treatment. This study supports a more optimistic view toward EEN as an approach to CS avoidance: over 40% of EEN-treated patients in their cohort remained steroid naive for at least 4 years. In addition, patients treated with EEN exhibited significantly greater improvement in height z-scores than patients treated with CS, at 1-year follow-up. The therapy with EEN over CS for induction of remission was associated with avoidance of CS over a 6-year follow-up period. This study showed that long-term steroid avoidance via EEN therapy is feasible without an increased need for escalation to anti-tumor necrosis factor alpha (anti-TNF-α). Most of the patients in the EEN-treated group who remained steroid-naive for 2 and 4 years had also not been exposed to anti-TNF-α, indicating that early anti-TNF-α use could account for only a minor portion of steroid avoidance in this group. They concluded that EEN induction therapy is more effective in achieving early remission and is associated with long-term steroid avoidance without increased use of biologics or need for surgery [46].

9. Current practice

Despite the reported benefits, EEN is not universally used in pediatric centers. Wide differences have been noted in the use of EEN between pediatric gastroenterologists in Europe and North America [47, 48]. A questionnaire-based study by Whitten et al. has shown wide variations in EEN protocols used in different areas of the world. Thirty-five centers were included in the study. The most centers recommend a 6–8 week therapy with polymeric formula and the gradual introduction of food quantity over 4–6 weeks [49].

10. The role of exclusive enteral nutrition in improvement of nutritional status and linear growth

Patients with IBD and especially children and adolescents often present with symptoms of undernutrition [50]. Both inflammation and undernutrition contribute to decreased height velocity [5]. Linear growth patterns correlate with disease activity, and there is strong pathophysiological evidence that inflammation interferes with the growth hormone axis [51, 52]. EEN decreases proinflammatory cytokines, including IL-6 and TNF-α, after which an increase in growth hormones (IGF-1 and IGFBP-3) is observed within 2 weeks of treatment [53]. It is not only that EEN decreases inflammation, it improves malnutrition and other specific nutritional deficiencies as well. Nutritional supplementation plays an important role in linear growth improvement. Importantly, EEN may also influence growth recovery in pediatric CD patients by limiting chronic corticosteroid exposure, which is a significant contributing factor toward growth failure [46, 54].

11. The role of preoperative exclusive enteral nutrition

To date, few experiences have been reported on the role of preoperative EEN in diminishing postoperative complications after bowel resections or other surgical interventions in patients with IBD. Li et al. investigated the influence of preoperative 3-month EEN on the incidence of postoperative intra-abdominal septic complications in CD patients with enterocutaneous fistulas. A retrospective study on 123 CD patients suffering from enterocutaneous fistulas was performed. The patients were divided into an EEN or a non-EEN group. A significantly lower rate of postoperative intra-abdominal septic complications was demonstrated in the EEN group versus the non-EEN group (3.6 versus 17.6%, $p < 0.05$). The results of this study have shown that preoperative EEN is an important factor for reduced risk of postoperative intra-abdominal septic complications [55]. The authors from the same IBD centre conducted another study to evaluate the impact of EEN on the perioperative outcome in CD patients following immunosuppressive therapy. There was a significant difference observed in the incidence of postoperative complications between the groups of CD patients who received and those who did not receive EEN ($p < 0.05$). In addition, the use of EEN decreased the need for urgent surgery and reoperation [56].

12. Mechanisms of action of exclusive enteral nutrition

Therapy with EEN substantially attenuates intestinal inflammation in CD patients. However, the mechanisms by which EEN suppresses inflammation are not yet fully understood. Hypotheses include improvement in nutritional intake and nutritional status, decreasing of the inflammatory cascade mechanism, limiting luminal antigen exposure, improving intestinal permeability, and modification of the intestinal microbiota [57]. Significant progress has been made in understanding mechanisms of how EEN suppresses inflammation. Basic research has demonstrated that EEN has direct anti-inflammatory properties, can correct localization of tight junction proteins and has other important impacts on intestinal permeability, alters micro RNAs expression, and profoundly affects the intestinal microbiota [58].

12.1. Anti-inflammatory effect of EEN

It is clear that EEN suppresses intestinal inflammation. In 1981, Logan et al. found a decrease in the number of gut lymphocytes and diminished protein loss when elemental enteral nutrition was used in patients with extensive small bowel CD [11]. In 1995, Breese et al. demonstrated that therapy with EEN reduced the number of lymphokine-secreting cells in the gut mucosa in CD [59]. Three years later, Beattie et al. reported on different mechanisms of action of EEN in CD. EEN was shown to be able to reduce the number of cytokine-producing cells in the inflamed mucosa of CD patients [16]. In a study by Fell et al., a decline in ileal and colonic interleukin-1beta mRNA was observed after 8 weeks of oral polymeric diet. In addition, a decrease of interferon gamma mRNA with a rise of transforming growth factor beta1 mRNA was demonstrated in the ileum and a fall of interleukin-8 mRNA in the colon [60]. Yamamoto et al. successfully managed acute duodenal CD with a low-speed elemental diet infusion via nasogastric tube in a 28-year-old female and also demonstrated that the duodenal mucosal cytokine levels remarkably decreased compared with those before the treatment [38]. Recently, Nahidi et al. cocultured heat tolerance (HT)-29 colonic epithelial cells with TNF-α in the presence or absence of polymeric formula, as used for EEN. Microarray analysis showed that polymeric formula modulated the expression of genes involved in the nuclear factor kB pathway with consequent downregulation of IL-6 and IL-8 proteins [61]. Alhagamhmad et al. wanted to find out whether the specific components in the polymeric formula drive the demonstrated attenuation of the nuclear factor kB cascade. They used tumor necrosis factor-α-exposed HT-29 colonic epithelial cells to investigate the immunosuppressive activity of the glutamine, arginine, vitamin D3, and α-linolenic acid (ALA), present in polymeric formula, along with curcumin. They found out that glutamine, arginine, and vitamin D3, but not ALA, significantly attenuated IL-8 production. Glutamine and arginine led to a phosphorylation blockade of the signaling components in NF-κB and P38 pathways, reduction in kinase activity, and enhancement in NO production. They concluded that glutamine, arginine, and vitamin D3 can suppress inflammation at concentrations equivalent to those used in polymeric formula. According to these findings, glutamine and arginine-fortified polymeric formulas might be a promising option to enhance the effectiveness of EEN therapy in CD treatment [57]. There is accumulating evidence that microRNAs play an important role in CD pathogenic processes, including regulation of pro and anti-inflammatory pathways. Guo et al. performed a microarray analysis in 25 adult CD patients and 10 healthy individuals treated with EEN. The microarray analysis showed that the mucosal micro RNAs expression profile is significantly altered after EEN therapy compared with the one in inflamed mucosa before EEN treatment [62]. The Australian investigators demonstrated that polymeric formula had a direct anti-inflammatory effect on colonic enterocytes. Polymeric formula was able to reduce interleukin (IL)-8 response to proinflammatory stimuli when it was added to the culture medium. The authors concluded that polymeric formula may modulate gut inflammation by directly reducing the inflammatory response of the intestinal epithelium [63]. Recently, the same team of investigators found that the incubation of human cells (Caco-2 human adenocarcinoma cell line) with a polymeric formula resulted in a dose-dependent increase in the expression of intestinal alkaline phosphatase, which is a recognized marker of enterocyte differentiation. Intestinal alkaline phosphatase is implicated in the innate gut immune response to enteric pathogens. This finding suggests that cell surface-associated intestinal alkaline phosphatase may be an aspect of the gut's innate immune response to pathogenic bacteria that is strengthened by polymeric formula [64].

12.2. Reduction in dietary antigen exposure

In the first years, only elemental formulas were used for the treatment of active CD. It was believed that the effect of EEN was based on exclusion of the dietary antigens which might have a role in inducing and promoting the inflammatory cascade. However, later research has shown that whole protein polymeric formulas were also as effective in inducing remission in patients with active CD [14, 18, 22, 65, 66].

12.3. The role of fats in EN formulas

The influence of the lipid source within the enteral feeds has been examined, but how the lipids composition of enteral nutrition affects its efficacy remains to be elucidated. In a meta-analysis by Zahos et al., the efficacy between the elemental formulas with low fat content (< 20 g/1000 kcal) versus high fat content (> 20 g/1000 kcal) was compared. This meta-analysis did not demonstrate a significant difference in efficacy of the two types of elemental formulas [23]. In the last decades, the impact of the use of fatty acids as potential immune-modulating agents in an inflammatory condition such as CD has been studied [67]. Recently, in a double-blind RCT by Grogan et al., a modest effect on the blood fatty acid composition was seen with both nutritional interventions (with Alicalm and Emsogen). After an intervention with a 6-week therapy with Alicalm, an increase of eicosapentaenoic acid (EPA) and alpha linolenic acid (ALA) was demonstrated with an inverse decrease in arachidonic acid (AA). Arachidonic acid is an important precursor to eicosanoids, which are second messengers in numerous signal transduction processes and have proinflammatory properties. The authors of this study concluded that there may be an advantage of using enteral formula that contains increased levels of ALA, as it is a precursor of anti-inflammatory eicosanoids [68].

12.4. Glutamin and arginine in EN formulas

Glutamine and arginine are conditionally essential amino acids with immunomodulatory properties. Glutamine may be essential in patients with catabolic conditions where the intervention with glutamine-supplements is able to prevent the deterioration of gut permeability and development of intestinal mucosal atrophy [69–71]. Akobeng et al. conducted a RCT, which included 18 pediatric patients with active CD, who were randomly assigned to receive a 4-week course of either: standard polymeric formula with low glutamine content (4% of amino acid composition) or a glutamine-enriched polymeric diet (42% of amino acid composition). They found no significant difference between these two types of formula in terms of clinical efficacy [72]. In a recent meta-analysis of the same authors, only two small RCTs (total 42 patients) met the inclusion criteria. The first study is the aforementioned pediatric study by Akobeng et al. [72]. In the second study, 24 adult CD patients with acute exacerbation of IBD were treated either with glutamine-supplemented or non-supplemented total parenteral nutrition. In both included studies, no statistically significant changes in intestinal permeability were found between patients, who received glutamine supplementation and those who did not [73]. Further randomized controlled clinical studies on the efficacy and safety of glutamin supplementation in patients with active CD are needed.

12.5. The impact of EEN on gut microbiota

While all the pathogenetic mechanisms of action of EEN have not yet been elucidated, EEN is known to cause profound changes in the gut microbiome. Understanding how EEN modifies the gut microbiome to induce remission could provide insight into CD etiopathogenesis and consequently guide the development of microbiome-targeted interventions [74]. In 2005, Lionetti et al. assessed clinical remission and the fecal microbiota in nine children with active CD treated with EEN. Clinical remission was observed in eight of nine children. In all these patients, significant modification of the fecal microbiota was found after EEN therapy. In contrast, control healthy children showed a host-specific and stable microbiota over time [75]. Similarly, Leach et al. demonstrated a significantly different composition of intestinal microbiota in patients with CD treated with EEN in comparison with the microbiota of control subjects. The effect of modificated microbiota remained present for 4 months after EEN [76]. EEN was shown to promote protective species and increase the production of butyrate [77]. Surprisingly, in a Scottish study which included 15 pediatric patients with CD before and after remission with EEN and 21 control subjects, the therapy with EEN was associated with a decrease in diversity of microbiota and not vice versa as was expected. A decrease in specific 'protective' species including *F. prausnitzii* was found as well as a fall in butyrate in fecal samples. These results have challenged the current perception of a protective role of *F. prausnitzii* in CD [78]. Quince et al. have analyzed microbiota in 23 CD children and in 21 healthy controls before, during, and after EEN treatment. They demonstrated lower microbial diversity in CD patients compared with controls before EEN. During the therapy with EEN, the microbial diversity in CD children further decreased and the structure of microbiota became even more dissimilar in comparison with the healthy controls [79]. In another small study, similar results were shown. Fecal microbiota of five children with CD, before, during, and after EEN treatment was analyzed and compared with five healthy controls. It showed a dramatic decrease in the number of operational taxonomic units (OTUs) after therapy with EEN. Inversely, recurrence of inflammation corresponded with an increase in OTUs [80]. In an extension study by Lee et al., fecal samples from patients (n = 86) treated with either PEN, EEN, or anti-TNF-α were analyzed using shotgun metagenomics analysis at four points of time during treatment and compared with healthy controls. After 1 week of treatment, the microbiota composition among the EEN-treated group drifted significantly farther from centroid of the healthy controls compared to anti-TNF-α treated patients who moved closer to the centroid. However, at the end of the study, responders (those with clinical remission and reduction in fecal calprotectin) were closer to the centroid of the healthy controls than nonresponders, regardless of treatment, suggesting that at treatment initiation, the treatment modality is the major determinant affecting gut microbiota, whereas later on, the resolution of inflammation becomes the dominant factor. Still, the resolution of dysbiosis was not complete even among responders at 8 weeks [81].

12.6. Exclusion of specific dietary components

During the 6- to 8-week therapy with EEN, the patients with active CD should not eat any food, and their 100% daily caloric requirements are covered by liquid formula. Therefore, the therapy with EEN automatically involves exclusion of many common dietary components which might have a deleterious effect on the intestinal mucosa. The avoidance of these potentially harmful dietary components might present another potential anti-inflammatory mechanism of EEN [82].

13. Partial enteral nutrition for maintaining remission in Crohn's disease

There are some studies suggesting that nutritional supplementation with liquid formulas may prolong remission in patients with quiescent CD [83–85]. However, the efficacy of partial enteral nutrition (PEN) for maintaining remission in inactive CD has not yet been fully evaluated. On the contrary, the use of immunomodulators and biological medications for maintaining remission in CD is well established. The adverse events of these medications, such as the increased risk of infection and malignancy, have always been concerning [86, 87]. Therefore, we should aim for a safer maintenance regimen, especially in children. Maintenance enteral nutrition (MEN) could be an attractive option for maintaining remission of inactive CD, as it will eliminate serious adverse events associated with the use of immunosuppressive medications and biologics. In 1987, Jones et al. reported their experience with 77 (16–65 years) CD patients in clinical remission who tried to maintain remission by personalized food exclusion diets along with a supplementary elemental diet. Twenty six of 77 (33.7%) patients remained in remission for 2 years and 18 (23.4%) patients for at least 3 years [88]. In a study by Wilschanski et al., pediatric patients with active CD who were successfully treated with EEN were assessed retrospectively according to whether they continued supplementary enteral nutrition or not. Time to relapse and linear growth were compared between the two cohorts. Patients who continued nasogastric supplementary feeding ($n = 28$) after reintroduction of their otherwise normal diet remained in remission longer than those who discontinued nocturnal supplementation ($n = 19$) ($p < 0.02$). Furthermore, continued use of nasogastric supplements before completion of puberty was associated with improved linear growth [85]. In 2000, Verma et al. studied a series of 39 consecutive patients with CD in clinical remission over 12 months. Patients in group 1 ($n = 21$) received oral nutritional supplementation along with their normal diet and patients in group 2 ($n = 18$) had a normal unrestricted diet without the nutritional supplementation. Forty-eight percent of patients in group 1 remained in remission for 12 months compared to the 22% of patients in group 2 ($p < 0.0003$) [89]. In 2007, Akonbeng et al. conducted a systematic review on the efficacy of enteral nutrition for maintenance of remission in CD. Only two studies were included based on the inclusion criteria

[90]. In the first study, a significant lower relapse rate was found in CD patients who received half of their daily nutritional needs from an elemental formula and the remaining half by normal diet compared to patients who only received a normal diet [90]. In the second study, the comparison between elemental and polymeric formulas (providing between 35 and 50% of patients' caloric intake in addition to normal diet) was assessed in terms of maintenance of remission. Both type of formulas were equally effective in maintaining remission and allowing withdrawal of steroid therapy [91, 92]. Recently, Nakahigashi et al. have reviewed the efficacy of EN for the maintenance of remission in patients with quiescent CD. Seven prospective cohort studies were included and three of them were RCTs. In all studies, patients used EN as a supplement or as a nocturnal tube feeding in addition to their normal food. The maintained clinical remission rate at 1 year was significantly higher in patients treated with EN in four of the six studies [93]. Although some studies suggest that PEN may be helpful for the maintenance of remission in the pediatric population [84, 85], data on the long-term usage of PEN for remission maintenance in pediatric CD patients are still lacking. A recent retrospective study by Schulman et al. investigated the efficacy of PEN treatment in the maintenance of remission in the pediatric CD population. In their centre, this approach has been in practice for the last several years. They assessed 42 pediatric CD patients who entered clinical remission on 4–12 weeks of EEN and were maintained on PEN as a supplementary diet (50% of total calories obtained as polymeric formula). The control group consisted of patients who refused PEN. They found that the decrease in the disease activity was greater in the PEN group than in the control group, as was the total increase in body mass index between the time of diagnosis and 8 months after. Laboratory parameters, such as albumin and CRP, also showed better improvement in the PEN group than in the control group. Although PEN was able to maintain short remission in patients initially treated with EEN, most of the patients required concomitant medication at some point after PEN initiation. They conclude that PEN treatment was partially effective in maintaining remission in patients who were initially treated with EEN. To better assess the efficacy of PEN for maintaining remission in children with CD, further prospective studies are required. Recently, El-Matary et al. have published a systematic review on the efficacy of MEN in adult and pediatric patients with CD. Twelve studies (1169 patients, including 95 children) fulfilled the inclusion criteria. As the included studies were significantly heterogeneous, a meta-analysis was not performed. Eleven studies showed that EN was either better than or as effective as its comparator in maintaining remission in patients with inactive CD. Only one adult RCT ($n = 51$), with low risk of bias, compared EN with a regular diet and found a relapse rate of 34% in the EN group versus 64% in the control group ($p < 0.01$) after a mean follow-up of 11.9 months. The authors concluded that EN is more effective than a regular diet and as effective as some medications in maintaining remission for patients with inactive CD. Large, properly designed RCTs of sufficient duration are, however, still required to confirm this outcome regarding EN versus individual medications [94].

14. Partial enteral nutrition in the treatment of active Crohn's disease

In 2006, Jones et al. have published the first RCT on partial enteral nutrition (PEN). Fifty children with active CD (PCDAI >20) were randomly assigned in PEN or EEN group. Children in PEN group had obtained 50% of their caloric requirements from elemental formula and 50% from unrestricted diet, while children in EEN had received 100% of their energy requirements from elemental formula for 6 weeks. This study showed that the conventional treatment with EEN was associated with a significantly higher remission rate in comparison with PEN (42 versus 15%) [95]. The next study on the efficacy of PEN was conducted at The Children's Hospital of Philadelphia (CHOP). The authors retrospectively studied the efficacy of their CHOP protocol of PEN, which allowed patients to consume 10–20% of their daily caloric needs from a normal diet and 80–90% from enteral nutrition. In this study, a remission rate of 65% and response rate of 87% were demonstrated, which is comparable with the remission rate of EEN from literature. The authors concluded that the use of the CHOP protocol may increase compliance in the population of pediatric CD patients by improving quality of life [42]. Recently, Sigall-Boneh et al. treated 47 patients (34 children and 13 young adults) with early mild-to-moderate luminal CD with PEN. Their approach allowed patients to consume 50% of dietary calories from a polymeric formula and remaining calories from a special Crohn's disease exclusion diet (CDED). In the study, a clinical response and remission were achieved in 78.7 and 70.2% patients, respectively. Surprisingly, in six of seven patients who refused PEN and used only the specific exclusion diet for CD, clinical remission was observed. This study has shown for the first time that a combination of PEN with the exclusion diet was successful and led to high remission rates in early mild-to-moderate luminal CD, in children and young adults [96]. Furthermore, the findings of this study suggest that specific dietary products may play a role in the promotion of intestinal mucosal inflammation. The authors of this study hypothesize that the major mechanism leading to response to EEN used in children with active CD is exclusion of specific dietary factors which may have negative impact on the innate immune mechanisms of intestinal mucosa such as the mucous layer, intestinal permeability, or colonization and adherence with adherent-invasive *E. coli* (AIEC). They suggest that specific dietary components such as additives may impair the barrier function of the intestinal epithelium and allow adherence and invasion of nonpathogenic bacteria or bacterial antigens. Adherence of bacteria to the intestinal epithelium, penetration, and replication within epithelial cells, dendritic cells, and macrophages leads to continuous triggering of the adaptive immune system, resulting in inflammation [97]. According to the results of recent epidemiological and animal model studies, they developed CDED based on exclusion of dietary components hypothesized to affect the microbiome or intestinal permeability or other elements of innate immune system involved in CD pathogenesis [82, 97]. CDED is a structured diet that excludes animal fats, milk and dairy, gluten, and all processed and canned foods, which contain additives (especially emulsifiers and maltodextrin) [96]. Although the authors from CHOP and Israel did show that PEN may be effective in inducing the remission in active CD, this approach of treatment is not recommended according to the ESPGHAN/ECCO guidelines on the treatment of active CD in pediatric population [6]. Further studies on the efficacy of PEN are warranted to elucidate the efficacy of this treatment approach.

15. Conclusion

EEN is recommended as a first-line therapy for remission induction in pediatric luminal Crohn's disease. Despite the inconsistent evidence regarding long-term efficacy, EEN has an established advantage over corticosteroids with comparable clinical efficacy but superior mucosal healing effect as well as better safety profile. The exact mechanism by which EEN exerts its beneficial impact is still not established, particularly, whether exclusion of specific potentially harmful dietary components plays an important role. Nevertheless, accumulating evidence suggest a direct anti-inflammatory effect and an effect on the intestinal microbiota. The relationships between these effects and the specific triggers for the observed changes are yet to be elucidated.

Author details

Darja Urlep*, Evgen Benedik and Rok Orel

*Address all correspondence to: darja.urlep@kclj.si

University Children's Hospital, University Medical Centre Ljubljana, Ljubljana, Slovenia

References

[1] Conrad MA, Rosh JR. Pediatric inflammatory bowel disease. Pediatric Clinics of North America. 2017;**64**:577-591. DOI: 10.1016/j.pcl.2017.01.005

[2] Vernier–Massouille G, Balde M, Salleron J, Turck D, Dupas JL, Mouterde O, et al. Natural history of pediatric Crohn's disease: A population-based cohort study. Gastroenterology 2008;**135**:1106-1113. DOI: 10.1053/j.gastro.2008.06.079

[3] Van Limbergen J, Russell RK, Drummond HE, Aldhous MC, Round NK, Nimmo ER, et al. Definition of phenotypic characteristics of childhood-onset inflammatory bowel disease. Gastroenterology. 2008;**135**:1114-1122. DOI: 10.1053/j.gastro.2008.06.081

[4] Pigneur B, Seksik P, Viola S, Viala J, Beaugerie L, Girardet J-P, et al. Natural history of Crohn's disease. Inflammatory Bowel Diseases. 2010;**16**:953-961. DOI: 10.1002/ibd.21152

[5] Griffiths AM. Growth retardation in early-onset inflammatory bowel disease: Should we monitor and treat these patients differently? Digestive Diseases. 2009;**27**:404-411. DOI: 10.1159/000228581

[6] Ruemmele FM, Veres G, Kolho KL, Griffiths A, Levine A, Escher JC, et al. Consensus guidelines of ECCO/ESPGHAN on the medical management of pediatric Crohn's disease. Journal of Crohn's and Colitis. 2014;**8**:1179-1207. DOI: 10.1016/j.crohns.2014.04.005

[7] Malchow H, Steinhardt HJ, Lorenz-Meyer H, Strohm WD, Rasmussen S, Sommer H, et al. Feasibility and effectiveness of a defined-formula diet regimen in treating active Crohn's disease. European cooperative Crohn's disease study III. Scandinavian Journal of Gastroenterology 1990;**25**:235-244

[8] Critch J, Day AS, Otley A, King-Moore C, Teitelbaum JE, Shashidhar H, et al. Use of enteral nutrition for the control of intestinal inflammation in pediatric Crohn's disease. Journal of Pediatric Gastroenterology and Nutrition. 2012;**54**:298-305. DOI: 10.1097/MPG.0b013e318235b397

[9] Kansal S, Wagner J, Kirkwood CD, Catto-Smith AG. Enteral nutrition in Crohn's disease: An underused therapy. Gastroenterology Research and Practice. 2013;**2013**:1-11. DOI: 10.1155/2013/482108

[10] Voitk AJ, Echave V, Feller JH, Brown RA, Gurd FN. Experience with elemental diet in the treatment of inflammatory bowel disease. Is this primary therapy? Archives of Surgery 1973;**107**:329-333

[11] Logan RF, Gillon J, Ferrington C, Ferguson A. Reduction of gastrointestinal protein loss by elemental diet in Crohn's disease of the small bowel. Gut. 1981;**22**:383-387

[12] Navarro J, Vargas J, Cezard JP, Charritat JL, Polonovski C. Prolonged constant rate elemental enteral nutrition in Crohn's disease. Journal of Pediatric Gastroenterology and Nutrition. 1982;**1**:541-546

[13] O'Morain C. Elemental diets and Crohn's disease. Acta Gastroenterologica Belgica. 1987;**50**:574-578

[14] Griffiths AM, Ohlsson A, Sherman PM, Sutherland LR. Meta-analysis of enteral nutrition as a primary treatment of active Crohn's disease. Gastroenterology. 1995;**108**:1056-1067

[15] Zoli G, Carè M, Parazza M, Spanò C, Biagi PL, Bernardi M, et al. A randomized controlled study comparing elemental diet and steroid treatment in Crohn's disease. Alimentary Pharmacology & Therapeutics. 1997;**11**:735-740

[16] Beattie RM, Bentsen BS, MacDonald TT. Childhood Crohn's disease and the efficacy of enteral diets. Nutrition 1998;**14**:345-350

[17] Rigaud D, Cosnes J, Le Quintrec Y, René E, Gendre JP, Mignon M. Controlled trial comparing two types of enteral nutrition in treatment of active Crohn's disease: Elemental versus polymeric diet. Gut. 1991;**32**:1492-1497

[18] Ludvigsson JF, Krantz M, Bodin L, Stenhammar L, Lindquist B. Elemental versus polymeric enteral nutrition in paediatric Crohn's disease: A multicentre randomized controlled trial. Acta Paediatrica. 2004;**93**:327-335

[19] Levine A, Turner D, Pfeffer Gik T, Amil Dias J, Veres G, Shaoul R, et al. Comparison of outcomes parameters for induction of remission in new onset pediatric Crohn's disease. Inflammatory Bowel Diseases. 2014;**20**:278-285. DOI: 10.1097/01.MIB.0000437735.11953.68

[20] Fernández-Bañares F, Cabré E, Esteve-Comas M, Gassull MA. How effective is enteral nutrition in inducing clinical remission in active Crohn's disease? A meta-analysis of the randomized clinical trials. Journal of Parenteral and Enteral Nutrition. 1995;**19**:356-364. DOI: 10.1177/0148607195019005356

[21] Messori A, Trallori G, D'Albasio G, Milla M, Vannozzi G, Pacini F. Defined-formula diets versus steroids in the treatment of active Crohn's disease: A meta-analysis. Scandinavian Journal of Gastroenterology. 1996;**31**:267-272

[22] Zachos M, Tondeur M, Griffiths A. Enteral nutritional therapy for induction of remission in Crohn's disease. In: Zachos M, editor. Cochrane Database of Systematic Reviews. Chichester, UK: John Wiley & Sons, Ltd; 2001. p. CD000542. DOI: 10.1002/14651858.CD000542

[23] Zachos M, Tondeur M, Griffiths AM. Enteral nutritional therapy for induction of remission in Crohn's disease. In: Zachos M, editor. Cochrane Database of Systematic Reviews. Chichester, UK: John Wiley & Sons, Ltd; 2007. p. CD000542. DOI: 10.1002/14651858.CD000542.pub2

[24] Heuschkel RB, Menache CC, Megerian JT, Baird AE. Enteral nutrition and corticosteroids in the treatment of acute Crohn's disease in children. Journal of Pediatric Gastroenterology and Nutrition. 2000;**31**:8-15

[25] Dziechciarz P, Horvath A, Shamir R, Szajewska H. Meta-analysis: Enteral nutrition in active Crohn's disease in children. Alimentary Pharmacology & Therapeutics. 2007;**26**:795-806. DOI: 10.1111/j.1365-2036.2007.03431.x

[26] Swaminath A, Feathers A, Ananthakrishnan AN, Falzon L, Li Ferry S. Systematic review with meta-analysis: Enteral nutrition therapy for the induction of remission in paediatric Crohn's disease. Alimentary Pharmacology & Therapeutics. 2017;**46**:645-656. DOI: 10.1111/apt.14253

[27] Lochs H, Dejong C, Hammarqvist F, Hebuterne X, Leon-Sanz M, Schütz T, et al. ESPEN guidelines on enteral nutrition: Gastroenterology. Clinical Nutrition. 2006;**25**:260-274. DOI: 10.1016/j.clnu.2006.01.007

[28] Esser D, Cornillie F, Diamond RH, Spiegel RJ. On the updated ECCO consensus guidelines for medical management of Crohn's disease. Journal of Crohn's and Colitis. 2011;**5**:165-166. DOI: 10.1016/j.crohns.2010.02.002

[29] Baert F, Moortgat L, Van Assche G, Caenepeel P, Vergauwe P, De Vos M, et al. Mucosal healing predicts sustained clinical remission in patients with early-stage Crohn's disease. Gastroenterology. 2010;**138**:463-468. DOI: 10.1053/j.gastro.2009.09.056

[30] Schnitzler F, Fidder H, Ferrante M, Noman M, Arijs I, Van Assche G, et al. Mucosal healing predicts long-term outcome of maintenance therapy with infliximab in Crohn's disease. Inflammatory Bowel Diseases. 2009;**15**:1295-1301. DOI: 10.1002/ibd.20927

[31] D'Haens G, Baert F, van Assche G, Caenepeel P, Vergauwe P, Tuynman H, et al. Early combined immunosuppression or conventional management in patients with newly diagnosed Crohn's disease: An open randomised trial. Lancet. 2008;**371**:660-667. DOI: 10.1016/S0140-6736(08)60304-9

[32] Neurath MF, Travis SPL. Mucosal healing in inflammatory bowel diseases: A systematic review. Gut. 2012;**61**:1619-1635. DOI: 10.1136/gutjnl-2012-302830

[33] Modigliani R, Mary JY, Simon JF, Cortot A, Soule JC, Gendre JP, et al. Clinical, biological, and endoscopic picture of attacks of Crohn's disease. Evolution on prednisolone. Groupe d'Etude Thérapeutique des Affections Inflammatoires Digestives. Gastroenterology 1990;**98**:811-818

[34] Olaison G, Sjödahl R, Tagesson C. Glucocorticoid treatment in ileal Crohn's disease: Relief of symptoms but not of endoscopically viewed inflammation. Gut. 1990;**31**:325-328

[35] Borrelli O, Cordischi L, Cirulli M, Paganelli M, Labalestra V, Uccini S, et al. Polymeric diet alone versus corticosteroids in the treatment of active pediatric Crohn's disease: A randomized controlled open-label trial. Clinical Gastroenterology and Hepatology. 2006;**4**:744-753. DOI: 10.1016/j.cgh.2006.03.010

[36] Berni Canani R, Terrin G, Borrelli O, Romano MT, Manguso F, Coruzzo A, et al. Short- and long-term therapeutic efficacy of nutritional therapy and corticosteroids in paediatric Crohn's disease. Digestive and Liver Disease. 2006;**38**:381-387. DOI: 10.1016/j.dld.2005.10.005

[37] Grover Z, Muir R, Lewindon P. Exclusive enteral nutrition induces early clinical, mucosal and transmural remission in paediatric Crohn's disease. Journal of Gastroenterology. 2014;**49**:638-645. DOI: 10.1007/s00535-013-0815-0

[38] Yamamoto T, Nakahigashi M, Umegae S, Kitagawa T, Matsumoto K. Impact of elemental diet on mucosal inflammation in patients with active Crohn's disease: Cytokine production and endoscopic and histological findings. Inflammatory Bowel Diseases. 2005;**11**:580-588

[39] Rubio A, Pigneur B, Garnier-Lengliné H, Talbotec C, Schmitz J, Canioni D, et al. The efficacy of exclusive nutritional therapy in paediatric Crohn's disease, comparing fractionated oral vs. continuous enteral feeding. Alimentary Pharmacology & Therapeutics. 2011;**33**:1332-1339. DOI: 10.1111/j.1365-2036.2011.04662.x

[40] Afzal NA, Davies S, Paintin M, Arnaud-Battandier F, Walker-Smith JA, Murch S, et al. Colonic Crohn's disease in children does not respond well to treatment with enteral nutrition if the ileum is not involved. Digestive Diseases and Sciences. 2005;**50**:1471-1475

[41] Buchanan E, Gaunt WW, Cardigan T, Garrick V, McGrogan P, Russell RK. The use of exclusive enteral nutrition for induction of remission in children with Crohn's disease demonstrates that disease phenotype does not influence clinical remission. Alimentary Pharmacology & Therapeutics. 2009;**30**:501-507. DOI: 10.1111/j.1365-2036.2009.04067.x

[42] Gupta K, Noble A, Kachelries KE, Albenberg L, Kelsen JR, Grossman AB, et al. A novel enteral nutrition protocol for the treatment of pediatric Crohn's disease. Inflammatory Bowel Diseases. 2013;**19**:1374-1378. DOI: 10.1097/MIB.0b013e318281321b

[43] Lambert B, Lemberg DA, Leach ST, Day AS. Longer-term outcomes of nutritional management of Crohn's disease in children. Digestive Diseases and Sciences. 2012;**57**:2171-2177. DOI: 10.1007/s10620-012-2232-2

[44] Grover Z, Lewindon P. Two-year outcomes after exclusive enteral nutrition induction are superior to corticosteroids in Pediatric Crohn's disease treated early with Thiopurines. Digestive Diseases and Sciences. 2015;**60**:3069-3074. DOI: 10.1007/s10620-015-3722-9

[45] Frivolt K, Schwerd T, Werkstetter KJ, Schwarzer A, Schatz SB, Bufler P, et al. Repeated exclusive enteral nutrition in the treatment of paediatric Crohn's disease: Predictors of efficacy and outcome. Alimentary Pharmacology & Therapeutics. 2014;**39**:1398-1407. DOI: 10.1111/apt.12770

[46] Connors J, Basseri S, Grant A, Giffin N, Mahdi G, Noble A, et al. Exclusive enteral nutrition therapy in paediatric Crohn's disease results in long-term avoidance of corticosteroids: Results of a propensity-score matched cohort analysis. Journal of Crohn's and Colitis. 2017;**11**:1063-1070. DOI: 10.1093/ecco-jcc/jjx060

[47] Van Limbergen J, Haskett J, Griffiths AM, Critch J, Huynh H, Ahmed N, et al. Toward enteral nutrition for the treatment of pediatric Crohn disease in Canada: A workshop to identify barriers and enablers. Canadian Journal of Gastroenterology and Hepatology. 2015;**29**:351-356

[48] Stewart M, Day AS, Otley A. Physician attitudes and practices of enteral nutrition as primary treatment of paediatric Crohn disease in North America. Journal of Pediatric Gastroenterology and Nutrition. 2011;**52**:38-42. DOI: 10.1097/MPG.0b013e3181e2c724

[49] Whitten KE, Rogers P, Ooi CKY, Day AS. International survey of enteral nutrition protocols used in children with Crohn's disease. Journal of Digestive Diseases. 2012;**13**:107-112. DOI: 10.1111/j.1751-2980.2011.00558.x

[50] Vasseur F, Gower-Rousseau C, Vernier-Massouille G, Dupas JL, Merle V, Merlin B, et al. Nutritional status and growth in pediatric Crohn's disease: A population-based study. The American Journal of Gastroenterology. 2010;**105**:1893-1900. DOI: 10.1038/ajg.2010.20

[51] Ley D, Duhamel A, Behal H, Vasseur F, Sarter H, Michaud L, et al. Growth pattern in paediatric Crohn disease is related to inflammatory status. Journal of Pediatric Gastroenterology and Nutrition. 2016;**63**:637-643. DOI: 10.1097/MPG.0000000000001177

[52] DeBoer MD, Scharf RJ, Leite AM, Férrer A, Havt A, Pinkerton R, et al. Systemic inflammation, growth factors, and linear growth in the setting of infection and malnutrition. Nutrition. 2017;**33**:248-253. DOI: 10.1016/j.nut.2016.06.013

[53] Shamir R, Phillip M, Levine A. Growth retardation in pediatric Crohn's disease. Inflammatory Bowel Diseases. 2007;**13**:620-628. DOI: 10.1002/ibd.20115

[54] Sanderson IR. Growth problems in children with IBD. Nature Reviews. Gastroenterology & Hepatology. 2014;**11**(10):601. DOI: 10.1038/nrgastro.2014.102

[55] Li G, Ren J, Wang G, Hu D, Gu G, Liu S, et al. Preoperative exclusive enteral nutrition reduces the postoperative septic complications of fistulizing Crohn's disease. European Journal of Clinical Nutrition. 2014;**68**:441-446. DOI: 10.1038/ejcn.2014.16

[56] Li Y, Zuo L, Zhu W, Gong J, Zhang W, Gu L, et al. Role of exclusive enteral nutrition in the preoperative optimization of patients with Crohn's disease following immunosuppressive therapy. Medicine (Baltimore). 2015;**94**:e478. DOI: 10.1097/MD.0000000000000478

[57] El-Matary W. Enteral nutrition as a primary therapy of Crohn's disease: The Pediatric perspective. Nutrition in Clinical Practice. 2009;**24**:91-97. DOI: 10.1177/0884533608329660

[58] Alhagamhmad MH, Day AS, Lemberg DA, Leach ST. Exploring and enhancing the anti-inflammatory properties of polymeric formula. Journal of Parenteral and Enteral Nutrition. 2017;**41**:436-445. DOI: 10.1177/0148607115625627

[59] Breese EJ, Michie CA, Nicholls SW, Williams CB, Domizio P, Walker-Smith JA, et al. The effect of treatment on lymphokine-secreting cells in the intestinal mucosa of children with Crohn's disease. Alimentary Pharmacology & Therapeutics 1995;**9**:547-552

[60] Fell JM, Paintin M, Arnaud-Battandier F, Beattie RM, Hollis A, Kitching P, et al. Mucosal healing and a fall in mucosal pro-inflammatory cytokine mRNA induced by a specific oral polymeric diet in paediatric Crohn's disease. Alimentary Pharmacology & Therapeutics. 2000;**14**:281-289

[61] Nahidi L, Corley SM, Wilkins MR, Wei J, Alhagamhmad M, Day AS, et al. The major pathway by which polymeric formula reduces inflammation in intestinal epithelial cells: A microarray-based analysis. Genes & Nutrition. 2015;**10**:29. DOI: 10.1007/s12263-015-0479-x

[62] Guo Z, Gong J, Li Y, Gu L, Cao L, Wang Z, et al. Mucosal MicroRNAs expression profiles before and after exclusive enteral nutrition therapy in adult patients with Crohn's disease. Nutrients. 2016;**8**:519. DOI: 10.3390/nu8080519

[63] de Jong NSH, Leach ST, Day AS. Polymeric formula has direct anti-inflammatory effects on enterocytes in an in VitroModel of intestinal inflammation. Digestive Diseases and Sciences 2007;**52**:2029-2036. DOI: 10.1007/s10620-006-9449-x

[64] Budd GR, Aitchison A, Day AS, Keenan JI. The effect of polymeric formula on enterocyte differentiation. Innate Immunity. 2017;**23**:240-248. DOI: 10.1177/1753425916689333

[65] Giaffer MH, North G, Holdsworth CD. Controlled trial of polymeric versus elemental diet in treatment of active Crohn's disease. Lancet (London, England). 1990;**335**:816-819

[66] Verma S, Brown S, Kirkwood B, Giaffer MH. Polymeric versus elemental diet as primary treatment in active Crohn's disease: A randomized, double-blind trial. The American Journal of Gastroenterology. 2000;**95**:735-739. DOI: 10.1111/j.1572-0241.2000.01527.x

[67] Turner D, Zlotkin S, Shah P, Griffiths A. Omega 3 fatty acids (fish oil) for maintenance of remission in Crohn's disease. In: Turner D, editor. Cochrane Database of Systematic Reviews. Chichester, UK: John Wiley & Sons, Ltd; 2007. p. CD006320. DOI: 10.1002/14651858.CD006320.pub2.

[68] Grogan JL, Casson DH, Terry A, Burdge GC, El-Matary W, Dalzell MA. Enteral feeding therapy for newly diagnosed Pediatric Crohn's disease: A double-blind randomized controlled trial with two years follow-up§. Inflammatory Bowel Diseases. 2012;**18**:246-253. DOI: 10.1002/ibd.21690

[69] Alhagamhmad MH, Day AS, Lemberg DA, Leach ST. An update of the role of nutritional therapy in the management of Crohn's disease. Journal of Gastroenterology. 2012;**47**:872-882. DOI: 10.1007/s00535-012-0617-9

[70] Coëffier M, Marion-Letellier R, Déchelotte P. Potential for amino acids supplementation during inflammatory bowel diseases. Inflammatory Bowel Diseases 2010;**16**:518-524. DOI: 10.1002/ibd.21017

[71] Lecleire S, Hassan A, Marion-Letellier R, Antonietti M, Savoye G, Bole-Feysot C, et al. Combined glutamine and arginine decrease proinflammatory cytokine production by biopsies from Crohn's patients in association with changes in nuclear factor-B and p38 mitogen-activated protein kinase pathways. The Journal of Nutrition. 2008;**138**:2481-2486. DOI: 10.3945/jn.108.099127

[72] Akobeng AK, Miller V, Stanton J, Elbadri AM, Thomas AG. Double-blind randomized controlled trial of glutamine-enriched polymeric diet in the treatment of active Crohn's disease. Journal of Pediatric Gastroenterology and Nutrition. 2000;**30**:78-84

[73] Akobeng AK, Elawad M, Gordon M. Glutamine for induction of remission in Crohn's disease. In: Akobeng AK, editor. Cochrane Database of Systematic Reviews. Vol. 2. Chichester, UK: John Wiley & Sons, Ltd; 2016. p. CD007348. DOI: 10.1002/14651858.CD007348.pub2

[74] Lewis JD, Chen EZ, Baldassano RN, Otley AR, Griffiths AM, Lee D, et al. Inflammation, antibiotics, and diet as environmental stressors of the gut microbiome in pediatric Crohn's disease. Cell Host & Microbe. 2015;**18**:489-500. DOI: 10.1016/j.chom.2015.09.008

[75] Lionetti P, Callegari ML, Ferrari S, Cavicchi MC, Pozzi E, de Martino M, et al. Enteral nutrition and microflora in pediatric Crohn's disease. Journal of Parenteral and Enteral Nutrition. 2005;**29**:S173-S178. DOI: 10.1177/01486071050290S4S173

[76] Leach ST, Mitchell HM, Eng WR, Zhang L, Day AS. Sustained modulation of intestinal bacteria by exclusive enteral nutrition used to treat children with Crohn's disease. Alimentary Pharmacology & Therapeutics. 2008;**28**:724-733

[77] Day AS, Lopez RN. Exclusive enteral nutrition in children with Crohn's disease. World Journal of Gastroenterology. 2015;**21**:6809-6816. DOI: 10.3748/wjg.v21.i22.6809

[78] Gerasimidis K, Bertz M, Hanske L, Junick J, Biskou O, Aguilera M, et al. Decline in presumptively protective gut bacterial species and metabolites are paradoxically associated with disease improvement in pediatric Crohn's disease during enteral nutrition. Inflammatory Bowel Diseases. 2014;**20**:861-871. DOI: 10.1097/MIB.0000000000000023

[79] Quince C, Ijaz UZ, Loman N, Eren AM, Saulnier D, Russell J, et al. Extensive modulation of the fecal metagenome in children with Crohn's disease during exclusive enteral nutrition. The American Journal of Gastroenterology. 2015;**110**:1718-1729. DOI: 10.1038/ajg.2015.357

[80] Kaakoush NO, Day AS, Leach ST, Lemberg DA, Nielsen S, Mitchell HM. Effect of exclusive enteral nutrition on the microbiota of children with newly diagnosed Crohn's disease. Clinical and Translational Gastroenterology. 2015;**6**:e71. DOI: 10.1038/ctg.2014.21

[81] Lee D, Baldassano RN, Otley AR, Albenberg L, Griffiths AM, Compher C, et al. Comparative effectiveness of nutritional and biological therapy in north American children with active Crohn's disease. Inflammatory Bowel Diseases. 2015;**21**:1786-1793. DOI: 10.1097/MIB.0000000000000426

[82] Sarbagili-Shabat C, Sigall-Boneh R, Levine A. Nutritional therapy in inflammatory bowel disease. Current Opinion in Gastroenterology. 2015;**31**:303-308. DOI: 10.1097/MOG.0000000000000178

[83] Harries AD, Jones LA, Danis V, Fifield R, Heatley RV, Newcombe RG, et al. Controlled trial of supplemented oral nutrition in Crohn's disease. Lancet (London, England). 1983;**1**:887-890

[84] Belli DC, Seidman E, Bouthillier L, Weber AM, Roy CC, Pletincx M, et al. Chronic intermittent elemental diet improves growth failure in children with Crohn's disease. Gastroenterology. 1988;**94**:603-610

[85] Wilschanski M, Sherman P, Pencharz P, Davis L, Corey M, Griffiths A. Supplementary enteral nutrition maintains remission in paediatric Crohn's disease. Gut. 1996;**38**:543-548

[86] Kotlyar DS, Lewis JD, Beaugerie L, Tierney A, Brensinger CM, Gisbert JP, et al. Risk of lymphoma in patients with inflammatory bowel disease treated with azathioprine and 6-Mercaptopurine: A meta-analysis. Clinical Gastroenterology and Hepatology. 2015;**13**:847-858.e4. DOI: 10.1016/j.cgh.2014.05.015

[87] Dulai PS, Thompson KD, Blunt HB, Dubinsky MC, Siegel CA. Risks of serious infection or lymphoma with anti-tumor necrosis factor therapy for pediatric inflammatory bowel disease: A systematic review. Clinical Gastroenterology and Hepatology. 2014;**12**:1443-1451. DOI: 10.1016/j.cgh.2014.01.021

[88] Jones VA. Comparison of total parenteral nutrition and elemental diet in induction of remission of Crohn's disease. Long-term maintenance of remission by personalized food exclusion diets. Digestive Diseases and Sciences. 1987;**32**:100S-107S

[89] Verma S, Kirkwood B, Brown S, Giaffer MH. Oral nutritional supplementation is effective in the maintenance of remission in Crohn's disease. Digestive and Liver Disease. 2000;**32**:769-774

[90] Akobeng AK, Thomas AG. Enteral nutrition for maintenance of remission in Crohn's disease. In: Akobeng AK, editor. Cochrane Database of Systematic Reviews. Chichester, UK: John Wiley & Sons, Ltd; 2007. p. CD005984. DOI: 10.1002/14651858.CD005984.pub2

[91] Takagi S, Utsunomiya K, Kuriyama S, Yokoyama H, Takahashi S, Iwabuchi M, et al. Effectiveness of an "half elemental diet" as maintenance therapy for Crohn's disease: A randomized-controlled trial. Alimentary Pharmacology & Therapeutics. 2006;**24**:1333-1340. DOI: 10.1111/j.1365-2036.2006.03120.x

[92] Verma S, Holdsworth CD, Giaffer MH. Does adjuvant nutritional support diminish steroid dependency in Crohn disease? Scandinavian Journal of Gastroenterology. 2001;**36**:383-388

[93] Nakahigashi M, Yamamoto T, Sacco R, Hanai H, Kobayashi F. Enteral nutrition for maintaining remission in patients with quiescent Crohn's disease: Current status and future perspectives. International Journal of Colorectal Disease 2016;**31**:1-7. DOI: 10.1007/s00384-015-2348-x

[94] El-Matary W, Otley A, Critch J, Abou-Setta AM. Enteral feeding therapy for maintaining remission in Crohn's disease: A systematic review. Journal of Parenteral and Enteral Nutrition. 2017;**41**:550-561. DOI: 10.1177/0148607115621051

[95] Johnson T, Macdonald S, Hill SM, Thomas A, Murphy MS. Treatment of active Crohn's disease in children using partial enteral nutrition with liquid formula: A randomised controlled trial. Gut. 2006;**55**:356-361. DOI: 10.1136/gut.2004.062554

[96] Sigall-Boneh R, Pfeffer-Gik T, Segal I, Zangen T, Boaz M, Levine A. Partial enteral nutrition with a Crohn's disease exclusion diet is effective for induction of remission in children and young adults with Crohn's disease. Inflammatory Bowel Diseases. 2014;**20**:1353-1360. DOI: 10.1097/MIB.0000000000000110

[97] Pfeffer-Gik T, Levine A. Dietary clues to the pathogenesis of Crohn's disease. Digestive Diseases. 2014;**32**:389-394. DOI: 10.1159/000358143

12

The Purview of Phytotherapy in the Management of Gastric Ulcer

Sabiu Saheed, Ajani Emmanuel Oladipo,
Taofik Olatunde Sunmonu,
Fatai Oladunni Balogun and
Anofi Omotayo Tom Ashafa

Abstract

Stomach/gastric ulcer is a debilitating disease affecting more than 10% of the global population. Sufferers often have chronic pains with life-threatening gastrointestinal haemorrhage or perforation. Since the first diagnosis of stomach ulcer (SU) in the 19th century, excessive gastric juice that eroded the mucosa of the stomach was opined as its major cause. Efforts were channelled toward effective control of the resulting acid build-up through the use of antiulcer medications and reduction in stress-induced activities, which may aggravate gastric hyperacidity. An intense treatment option involved vagotomy (surgically severing the nerves surrounding an ulcer) to prevent hyperacidity and further perforation of the stomach epithelium. Despite these interventions, SU disease remained an impediment to clinical practice. Literatures revealed that many botanicals have been used to treat SU and this is hinged on their being endowed with antiulcerogenic phytonutrients of therapeutic significance. In this review, attempts have been made to highlight the main mechanisms of action and limitations of the conventional antiulcerogenic drugs, various antiulcerogenic experimental models, as well as compile selected medicinal plants and their implicated phytonutrients that will ultimately and eventually present effective and globally competitive exciting opportunities for the development of new lead therapeutics for the management of SU disorders.

Keywords: antiulcerogenic, gastric ulcer, gastropathy, hemorrhage, *Helicobacter pylori*, pepsin, perforation, phytonutrients, vagotomy

1. Introduction

Ulcer is an open sore of the biological membrane characterized by sloughing of inflamed dead tissue [1]. More specifically, it could either occur as a lesion on the surface of the skin or a mucous membrane with significant superficial loss of tissue. Although, ulcers may be encountered at almost any part of the body, they are mostly found on the skin of the lower extremities and in the gastrointestinal tract [2]. There are many types of ulcer including mouth, esophageal, peptic and genital ulcer. Of these, peptic ulcer (PU) is the most prevalent [2]. The PUs are erosion of lining of either the stomach or duodenum [3] and this has availed the two most common types of PU as the gastric/stomach ulcer (SU) and duodenal ulcer. A person may have both gastric and duodenal ulcers at the same time. SUs are located in the stomach and mainly characterized by hemorrhage and pain. Other symptoms may include nausea, vomiting, and weight loss. Although patients with SU have normal or diminished acid production, yet ulcers may occur even in complete absence of acid [3]. Generally, pain occurs when the stomach is empty and relieves after eating. In some cases, SU can be life threatening with symptoms like bloody stool, severe abdominal pain, and cramps coupled with blood vomiting [4].

Under normal conditions, a physiologic balance exists between gastric acid secretion and mucosal defense. The epithelial cells of the stomach secrete mucus in response to irritation of the epithelial lining and as a result of cholinergic stimulation [5]. Ordinarily, the superficial portion of the gastric mucosa is jelly-like and impermeable to acid and pepsin. Other gastric cells secrete bicarbonate, which buffers acid that lies penultimate to the mucosa. Also, the prostaglandins of the E (PGE) type of the epithelia offered significant protection by increasing the bicarbonate content and consequently strengthening the mucous layer. However, when the acid and pepsin enters the epithelial cells, further fortifying mechanisms are triggered to ameliorate injury [5]. This may be best observed within the epithelial cells, where ion pumps in the basolateral cell membrane aids intracellular pH regulation through removal of excess H^+ and subsequent migration of healthy cells to the site of injury. By so doing, the acid that diffused through the injured mucosa is effectively removed by the flow of blood in the mucosa. This also provides bicarbonate to the superficial epithelial cells. However, when there is disequilibrium between offensive (acid, pepsin, and *Helicobacter pylori*) and defensive factors (mucin, prostaglandin, bicarbonate, nitric oxide, and growth factors), the pathophysiological features of SU become evident [6]. Although, SU was once believed to be caused by spicy food and stress, they have however been established to be mere aggravating factors while the real causes include reaction to various medications, particularly nonsteroidal anti-inflammatory drugs (NSAIDS) and *H. pylori* infection [7]. *H. pylori*, NSAIDS, emotional stress, alcohol abuse, and smoking are the principal etiological factors associated with SU [8]. Usually, SU occur as breaks across the entire length of the stomach epithelia and in some cases, the deeper layers of the muscle wall are considerably affected. This disruption of the mucosal integrity may potentiate perforation, bleeding, obstruction, pain and death, if proficient treatments are not timely administered. The exclusive production of urease by *H. pylori* renders its microenvironment alkaline and allows its long-lasting survival in the hostile acidic environment of the stomach, where it either worsens the severity of SU disease or merely causes mucosal inflammation. More often in SU cases, inflammation is secondary to the colonizing action of *H. pylori* on the gastric mucosa [5]. In patients infected with *H. pylori*, high levels of gastrin and pepsinogen and reduced levels of somatostatin have been measured [5]. Most patients with SU have impaired gastric bicarbonate secretion, which has also proven to be caused by *H. pylori* because its eradication reverses the defect [9]. Similarly, pepsin (a proteolytic enzyme) and HCl are both essential for food digestion but at the same time have the tendency to erode the cell linings of the digestive system if secreted in excess. Although, the stomach defends itself from these aggravating factors by creating a mucus coating and producing bicarbonates, *H. pylori* infection and NSAIDS can impair the protective functions and make the linings of the gastrointestinal tract susceptible to HCl and pepsin action and consequently results in the formation of ulceration [10].

Globally, SU is the most prevalent gastrointestinal disorder ever known, affecting more than 10% of people and accounting for an estimated 15,000 mortality yearly [11]. The annual incidence of SU perforation and hemorrhage were 3.8–14.0 and 19.4–57.0 per 100,000 persons, respectively and this is anticipated to further worsen if no practical and viable alternatives are sought [12]. Specifically in the United States, PU disease affects approximately 4.5 million people annually and about 10% of the US population has evidence of a SU at some point in their life time [5]. Initially, PU diseases were more prevalent in the male populations but the current statistics suggest quite similar figures in both males and females with the overall lifetime prevalence tending toward 8–11% and 11–14% in women and men, respectively [5]. The age trends for the occurrence of PU show appreciably declining rates in younger males, while it is increasing steadily in older women. The statistics for SU disease in other countries is variable and is hinged primarily on the major causes of the disease: *H. pylori* and NSAIDs [13].

Although, orthodox medicine has provided succor in the management of SU disease over the years, a significant percentage of the global population still use traditional systems of medicine to manage and treat SU due to better cultural acceptability, improved compatibility, affordability, and lesser side effects [14]. The present study was conducted to review medicinal plants considered as gastroprotective and healing agents on SUs with particular focus on selected antiulcerogenic botanicals and their implicated phytonutrients. To achieve this, information were retrieved from online databases (Google, Pubmed, MEDLINE, Science Direct, Scopus and SID) in form of published articles, books, conference proceedings and other high profile intellectual resources. The retrieved studies either showed effectiveness of these plants or indirectly their efficacy on the involved mechanisms in the treatment of SU.

2. The conventional therapy for stomach ulcer management

SU therapy has witnessed many strides over the last decades and a number of drugs are now available for its treatment. Since the occurrence of SU disease is attributable to either pepsin action and hyperacidity or inadequate mucosal resistance, hence, its effective management lies exclusively in stemming the aggressive factors or fortify the defensive mechanisms. A corner stone in this approach was the advent of histamine H_2-receptors and the respective antagonist [15], which signified a landmark achievement in the management of disorders characterized by gastric hypersecretion. The H_2-antagonists were instantaneously identified as potent and safe agents which may replace the previously used drugs. For instance, the appearance of cimetidine (an H_2-antagonist agent), led to the virtual disappearance of drugs of unknown mechanism like gefarnate, sulphoglycopeptide, amilopectine, zolimidine, xylamide, etc. Despite the inherent improvement witnessed with the use of the H_2-antagonist over the previously used drugs, their untoward reactions have undermined their appreciable application. Generally, the antiulcer drugs may be classified according to the site and/or mechanism of action as: (a) antacids; (b) gastric muscle stimulants; (c) agents which protect the mucosa, increase mucosal resistance or coat ulcer craters; (d) antisecretory drugs, which may be anticholinergic agents; (e) corticohypothalamic drugs; and (f) proton pump inhibitors.

2.1. Antacids

It is noteworthy that either antacid mixtures or combinations of antacids with other compounds are more commonly used than single-entity antacids [15]. These kinds of formulation have been made to elicit a better neutralizing effect and to extenuate side effects associated with single constituent entities. The calcium and aluminium combinations reduce diarrhea while magnesium caters well for constipation. Similarly, a combination of slow- and fast-acting agents could increase the total buffering time. More improved benefits are claimed for mixtures having alginic acid (a foam-forming agent), which floats above the gastric juice with eventual aiding of contact between the antacid and the mucosa. In the event of gastroesophageal reflux, the alginic acid appears to prevent reflux by being the first to come in contact with the esophagus. By so doing, further erosion by the gastric acid is effectively prevented. Also, when simethicone (dimethylpolysiloxanes with characteristics antifoaming and water-repellant properties) is used, defoaming the gastric juice to reduce flatulence and gastroesophageal reflux is achieved. However, the resulting contributory adverse effects of the respective constituent in the antacid especially gastric irritation are a major challenge consistent with the use of antacids.

2.2. Gastric muscle stimulants

In individuals with stomach atony where there is consequential prolonged contact time between acid and mucosa due to the delay in gastric emptying, stimulants of gastric motility produce satisfactory outcomes. Domperidone and metoclopramide are the two most widely used compounds in this category. While both accelerates gastric emptying in experimental animals and humans, the metoclopramide still acts via other four important mechanisms that have made it more potent: (i) a cholinergic effect on muscarinic receptors; (ii) a direct effect on smooth muscle; (iii) an effect on specific centers regulating gastrointestinal motility; and (iv) a release of motilin which could be strongly responsible for the effects on the proximal bowel [15].

2.3. Mucosa protecting agents

Compounds like sucralfate, carbenoxolone and chelated bismuthate belong to this class of drugs. The sucralfate (a complex of sucrose and aluminium hydroxide) potentiates its action by inhibiting gastric hydrolysis with significant affinity for ulcerated mucosa. It forms a complex with susceptible proteins (fibrinogen, albumin etc) that adhere to the ulcerated area, thereby shielding against acid, pepsin action and penetration of bile acid. The merits of sucralfate over other antiulcer drugs relate to a lack of systemic effect due to the poor absorption of the compound [16]. The disadvantages include a certain delay in gastric emptying and constipation which affects almost 2% of the sufferers. Furthermore, compliance is another issue of concern as sucralfate must be taken four times daily (q.i.d.) and at least one hour before meals to be optimally effective. While chelated bismuthate and carbenoxolone works quite similar to sucralfate, appreciable incidence of aldosterone-like adverse effects (sodium and fluid retention, hypertension etc) have hampered their use.

2.4. Drugs with antisecretory effect

2.4.1. Anticholinergics

Despite that the drugs in this class have been used for many years, information on their ulcer healing capacity is still elusive. This may be attributable to the radiological method that was initially used but later found not to be very effective in wound healing assessment. Hyoscyamine, atropine, phentonium, propantheline and methantheline with characteristic ganglion-blocking and antimuscarinic effects are the classical examples of anticholinergics. Subsequent to the discovery and acceptance of the H_2-antagonists, the anticholinergics virtually disappeared due to inherent adverse effects of dry mouth, blurring of vision, delay in gastric emptying, tachycardia, possible constipation, and urinary retention.

2.4.2. H_2-antagonists

Undoubtedly, the H_2-antagonists are the most significant agents for the management and treatment of SU and for pathological conditions characterized by hyperacidity. Burimamide (the prototype of H_2-antagonists) was faced-out because of low oral activity and toxicological concerns. Similarly, metiamide (the 2nd agent in the series), was orally active but potentiated significant bone marrow toxicity in clinical trials. Cimetidine (still the most widely used antiulcer drug), is the 3rd drug in this class and well over 70 million sufferers have so far benefitted from its pharmacological efficacy till date. This was closely followed by ranitidine, which was the first agent with an alkyl furan ring, which substituted the imidazole ring of the preceding H_2- antagonists. More recent reports however suggest that optimum H_2-antagonism may also be achieved also with other different agents. For this class of drugs, not only could potency and efficacy be optimized, the pharmacokinetics could also be modified with the known duration of action of 4–6 h, exclusive to the 'short-acting' H_2-blockers [17], optimized to and beyond 24–48 h to have 'long-acting' H_2-blockers. Generally, over the last three decades, the most frequently used H_2-antagonists in clinical practice are cimetidine, ranitidine and famotidine [2]. However, many adverse reactions such as effects on the endocrine, cardiovascular and central nervous systems (CNS) have been associated with these drugs.

2.5. Corticohypothalamic drugs

A role has been established for the CNS in the regulation of gastric secretion and in the pathogenesis of peptic ulcer, although clarification is required in many areas. It is not surprising that drugs which act specifically on the CNS may exert a beneficial effect on SU, which sometimes is significantly better than other drugs. Trimipramine is a tricyclic antidepressant which causes a slight decrease in gastric secretion that is apparently not connected with its anticholinergic action. Like other traditional tricyclic antidepressants, it may have some H_2-antagonistic effects and may also act on α-adrenoceptors enhancing catecholamine availability at central synapses [18], or may depress central vagal function. However the use of trimipramine in non-depressed ulcer patients is questionable.

2.6. Proton pump inhibitors (PPIs)

At present, PPIs are the most commonly prescribed class of antiulcer drugs. Their mode of action involves blockage of the site of gastric acid secretion in the parietal cell of the stomach [19]. However, because the parietal cells are constantly reproducing in millions, effective inhibition of gastric acid secretion is almost unachievable and this partly explains their relative safety compared to other groups of antiulcer drugs. In general, the incidence of short-term adverse effects subsequent to PPI usage is relatively low and this may be the reason for their being well tolerated. Their long-term use has not been frequently studied and the dearth of information in this regards has made it difficult to make definitive statements [20]. For all the PPIs (omeprazole, lansoprazole, dexlanprazole, esomeprazole, pantoprazole, rabeprazole and ilaprazole), the occurrence of adverse effects are similar, though they have been reported more frequently with omeprazole. This may be due to its longer availability. The common adverse effects with PPIs include headache, nausea, diarrhea, abdominal pain, fatigue and dizziness. Infrequent adverse effects may also include rash, itch, flatulence, constipation, anxiety, depression, myopathies and rhabdomyolysis [21].

3. Ulcer inducing agents/models

The pathological mechanisms of SU disease that compromises its functional capability and the structural integrity has been established to arise mainly through either production of too much acid and pepsin, or weakening of the gastric epithelia that consequently results in too little mucosal resistance [2]. **Table 1** shows some of the known ulcerogenic agents/models and the pathological mechanism involved in their ulcer pathogenesis. A good understanding of the pathogenic mechanism of action of these models is crucial to spotting and either managing or preventing ulceration and the associated disorders.

Agent/model	Underlying mechanism	Reference(s)
NSAIDs (aspirin, indomethacin and ibuprofen)	Gastric acid secretion and inhibition of prostaglandin synthetase activity	[22]
Water-immersion/cold-restraint stress	Release of histamine resulting in increased acid secretion, decreased mucus production and poor flow of gastric blood	[23, 24]
Ethanol	Solubilizes mucous membrane and renders it vulnerable to the proteolytic and hydrolytic actions of HCl and pepsin	[25]
Acetic acid	Induces round, deep ulcers in the stomach through over production of acid secretion	[26]
Histamine	Acid stimulating and vasodilating effect that results to increased vascular permeability of the gastric mucosa	[27]
Reserpine	Degranulation of gastric mast cells consequent to histamine liberation that is facilitated by cholinergic system	[28]
Serotonin	Causes vasoconstriction thereby reducing gastric mucosal blood flow resulting to acute mucosal injury	[29]
Pylorous-ligation	Accumulation of gastric acid that consequently produces ulcer subsequent to the breakdown of gastric mucosal barriers	[30]
Ischemia-reperfusion	Causes erosion of the gastric epithelia due to free radicals formation	[31]
Acetic acid-*H. pylori*	Increased acid secretion and decreased mucus production	[32]
Iron-ascorbic acid	Linked with lipid peroxidation mediated by oxygen radicals	[33]

Table 1. Commonly used experimental models for ulcer induction.

4. Some scientifically validated antiulcerogenic medicinal plants

Despite the rapidly changing concept of SU disease management from conventional vagotomy, H_2-receptor antagonists and antacids to proton pump inhibitors, gastrointestinal toxicity and other inherent adverse effects remain significant impediments to their application in clinical practice. Investigation on the phytotherapeutic applications of medicinal plants that are highly valued and widely used in the traditional systems of medicine have been and still providing efficient formulation for better management of SU [2, 22].

The under-listed medicinal plants have been pharmacological reported to possess antiulcer activity as previously compiled [34–39]. They are:

Acacia arabica (Family: Mimosaceae); *Abutilon indicum* L. (Family: Malvaceae); *Adansonia digitate; Aegle marmelos* (Family: Rutaceae); *Allium sativum* (Family: Liliaceae); *Allophylus serratus* Kurz (Family: Sapindaceae); *Aloe vera* (Family: Liliaceae); *Alstonia scholaris; Annona squamosa* (Family: Annonaceae); *Asparagus racemosus; Azadirachta indica* (Family: Meliaceae); *Bacopa monnieri; Benincasa hispida; Bauhinia purpurea* (Family: Leguminosae); *Bauhinia variegate* (Family: Caesalpiniaceae); *Berberis aristata; Beta vulgaris; Buchanania lanzan* Spreng. (Family:

Anacardiaceae); *Butea frondosa* Roxb. (Family: Fabaceae); *Boswellia serrata* (Family: Burseraceae); *Careya arborea* (Family: Myrtaceae); *Carica papaya* (Family: Caricaceae); *Capsicum annuum* L. (Family: Solanaceae); *Centella asiatica; Cissus quadrangularis* L. (Family: Vitaceae); *Curcuma longa* L. (Family: Zingiberaceae); *Desmostachya bipinnata* (L.) Stapf (Family: Gramineae); *Desmodium gangeticum; Emblica officinalis* (Family: Euphorbiaceae); *Excoecaria agallocha* (Family: Euphorbiaceae); *Garcinia cambogia; Glycyrrhiza glabra* (Family: Leguminosae); *Ficus arnottiana; Ficus religiosa* (Family: Urticaceae); *Hemidesmus indicus; Hibiscus rosa sinensis* (Family: Malvaceae); *Ipomoea batatas* L. (Family: Convolvulaceae); *Ixora pavetta* (Family: Rubiaceae); *Kielmeyera coriacea* Mart (Family: Guttiferae); *Lagenaria siceraria* (Family: Cucurbitaceae); *Leucas lavandulifolia* Sm. (Family: Labiatae); *Mangifera indica* (Family: Anacardiaceae); *Mimosa pudica* (Family: Fabaceae); *Mentha arvensis* L. (Family: Lamiaceaea); *Momordica charantia* (Family: Cucurbitaceae); *Momordica cymbalaria* Hook. (Family: Cucurbitaceae); *Morinda citrifolia; Moringa oleifera* (Family: Moringaceae); *Musa sapientum; Myrtus communis* (Family: Myrtaceae); *Ocimum sanctum* (Family: Lamiaceae); *Oryza sativa* (Family: Gramineae); *Phyllanthus niruri* (Family: Euphorbiaceae); *Plectranthus amboinicus; Polyalthia longifolia* (Family: Annonaceae); *Psidium guyava* (Family: Myrtaceae); *Rhus coriaria* (Family: Anacardiaceae); *Rhizophora mangle* L. (Family: Rhizophoraceae); *Sapindus trifoliatus* L. (Family: Sapindaceae); *Sesbania grandiflora* (Fabaceae); *Shorea robusta* (Family: Dipterocarpaceae); *Solanum nigrum* (Family: Solanaceae); *Tamarindus indica* (Family: Caesalpiniaceae); *Tamarindus indica* (Family: Caesalpiniaceae); *Tecomaria capensis* (Family: Bignoniaceae); *Terminalia chebula* (Family: Combretaceae); *Terminalia pallida; Utleria salicifolia Bedd.* Ex.Hook. F. (Family: Periplocaceae); *Vinca minor* L. (Family: Apocynaceae). A comprehensive list of some selected plants being embraced as antiulcerogenic agents is presented in **Table 2**.

Plant	Family	Plant used	Phytonutrients	Reference(s)
Acacia arabica	Mimosaceae	Gum, leaves	Arabic acid, malate, sugar, mineral elements, tannins	[40, 41]
Achyranthus aspera	Amaranthaseae	Root, seeds	Saponin, glycosides	[42]
Adansonia digitata	Malvaceae	Leaves	Mucilage, glucose, albuminoids, adansonin, tannin	[43]
Aegle marmelos	Rutaceae	Leaves	Flavonoid, tannins, saponin	[44]
Aleo vera	Liliaceae	Whole plant	Aloin, isobarbaloin, emodin, saponin	[45]
Alhagi maurorum	Fabaceae	Root	Terpenes, saponin, tannins	[46]
Allium sativum	Liliaceae	Bulb	Mucilage, starch, albumen, vitamins, sugar, allicin, alliin	[47]
Annona squamosa	Annonaceae	Leaves	Alkaloids, flavonoids, saponini, tannins	[48]
Azadirachta indica	Meliaceae	Leaves	Saponin, flavonoids, phenolics, tannin	[49]
Bauhinia variegate	Caesalpiniaceae	Stem-bark, root	Rutin, quercetin, apigenin, tannin	[50]
Berberis aristata	Berberidaceae	Root	Alkaloids	[51]
Bata vulgaris	Chenopodiaceae	Root	Betin	[52]
Carica papaya	Caricaceae	Fruit, seeds	Papain, pectin, carpaine, carposide	[53]

Plant	Family	Plant used	Phytonutrients	Reference(s)
Centella asiatica	Apiaceae	Whole plant	Flavonoids, narigin, alkaloids, saponin, asiatic acid	[54]
Cordial myxa		Fruit	Tannins, carbohydrate, saponin	[55]
Ficus exasperata	Moraceae	Leaves, stem-bark	Flavonoids, saponin, alkaloids, glycosides, tannins	[2]
Ficus religiosa	Urticaceae	Stem-bark	Tannins, wax, cochtone	[56]
Gossypium barbadense	Malvaceae	Leaves	Gossypol, saponin, steroids, cardiac glycosides	[22]
Gossypium herbaceous	Malvaceae	Flowers	Flavonoids, phenolics, saponin	[57]
Hibiscus rosa sinensis	Malvaceae	Root	Phenolics, cyanidin, hydrocitrate	[58]
Langeneria breviflora	Cucurbitaceae	Fruit, leaves	Saponin, phenolics, cucurbitacin	[59]
Langeneria siceraria	Cucurbitaceae	Fruit	Flavonoids, steroids, phenols, saponin	[42]
Mangifera indica	Anacardiaceae	Leaves	Alkaloids, sterols, saponin, tannins, flavonoids, mangiferin	[60]
Momordica tuberose	Cucurbitaceae	Tubers	Alkaloids, tannins, saponin	[61]
Moringa oleifera	Moringaceae	Leaves	Quercetin, β-sitoterol, β-carotene, alkaloids, tannins, saponin	[62]
Musa paradisiacal	Musaceae	Root, leaves, trunk	Tannins, starch, vitamin C, albuminoids	[42]
Myrtus communis	Myrtaceae	Leaves	Resin, tannins, citrate, malate, sugar	[63]
Nerium indicum	Apocynaceae	Flowers	Alkaloids, glycosides, flavonoids, phenolics, tannins	[64]
Ocimum sanctum	Lamiaceae	Leaves	Alkaloids, tannins, saponin, flavonoids, sterols	[65]
Oryza sativa	Gramineae	Grain, bran	Starch, mineral matter, protein	[66]
Phyllanthus niruri	Euphorbiaceae	Whole plant	Alkaloids, tannins, flavonoids, carbohydrate, glycosides	[67]
Prunus amygdalus	Rosaceae	Seeds, fruit	Ursolic acid, quercetin, flavonoids	[42]
Psidium guyava	Myrtaceae	Leaves, stem-bark	Resin, tannins, cellulose, flavonoids, quercetin, quajaverin	[68]
Rhus coriaria	Anacardiaceae	Whole plant	Tannins, flavonoids	[69]
Sesbania grandiflora	Fabaceae	Leaves	Saponin, tannins, triterpenes	[70]
Smilax china	Smilacaceae	Root	Tannins, resin, saponin, flavonoids	[71]
Solanum nigrum	Solanaceae	Leaves	Flavonoids, saponin, alkaloids, phytosterols	[72]
Spondias mombin	Anacardiaceae	Leaves	Tannins, saponin, flavonoids, phenolics, glycosides	[73]
Tamarindus indica	Caesalpiniaceae	Leaves, seeds	Albuminoids, fiber, pectin, tannins	[74]
Terminalia chebula	Combretaceae	Leaves	Gallic acid, sorbitol, tannins, mucilage	[75]

Table 2. Some selected medicinal plants with antiulcerogenic properties.

Following the experimental demonstration that many medicinal plants are endowed with good antiulcerogenic activity with relatively lesser adverse effect compared with the conventional drugs, further steps have been taken in presenting a good number of them for clinical trials. Despite this giant stride, not many of the medicinal plants have passed market entry stage. To the best of our knowledge, of the many presented for developmental evaluations in 2004, only *Azadirachta indica* (Family: Meliaceae) received remarkable attention at its advance stage of clinical trial. It exhibited significant therapeutic potency by reducing gastric hypersecretion, gastroesophageal and gastroduodenal ulcers [76].

5. Phytonutrients associated with antiulcerogenic activity

Several phytonutrients have proven health benefits and have been reported to elicit significant antiulcerogenic potential in both humans and experimental animal models [73]. While steroid glycosides, tannins, terpenoids and flavonoids have been shown to preserve gastric mucosal against oxidative insults of reactive metabolites and oxidative stress [22, 59], the tendency of phenolic compounds and alkaloids to regulate gastric acid secretion and protect the gastric mucosal epithelia against erosion and other aggressive factors in different ulcer models have been demonstrated [77]. While **Table 1** also presents some of these phytonutrients as being responsible for the elicited antiulcerogenic properties of the plants, several others have also been identified and isolated from diverse plants. Some of these include; saponins, phobaphenes, glucose, luvangetin, tartarate, potash, nimbidin, quercetin, apigenin, papain, chymopapain, pectin, carposide, carotenoids, antheraxanthin, carpaine, resin, euphorbon, caoutchouc, rutin, anthocyanins, cyanindin, kaempferol, sterols, mucilage, terpenoids, kaepferom, ash, starch, fats, proteins, glycosides, ellagic acid, beta sitosterol, gallic acid, limonene, pinene, albuminous matter, cellulose, chlorophyll, mineral salts, myricitin, triterpenes, and sorbitol [37]. These compounds have either been elucidated to decrease acid/pepsin secretion or confer cytoprotection via effective modulation on mucosal defensive factors.

6. Some selected medicinal plants with antiulcerogenic properties in Nigeria

In Nigeria, SU remains a significant public health challenge affecting people of all ages. While its management through orthodox medicine has recorded substantial successes over the years, a considerable proportion of the populace still rely exclusively on complementary and alternative medicine (CAM) in seeking aid to treat and manage SU. This may be due to the ease of accessibility, affordability and minimal side effect associated with the use of medicinal plants [22]. A compilation of selected antiulcerogenic medicinal plants in Nigeria revealed that the most widely used plants in the management of SU are *Occimum basillicum, M. paradisiaca, Aloe vera, Azadiracter indica, Brassica oleracae* and *Carica papaya* [78]. Others include but not limited to the following: *Diodia sarmentosa, Cassia nigricans, Ficus exasperate, Synclisia scabrida, Artocarpus heterophyllus* Lam., *Blighia sapida* Konig., *Dialium guineense* Willd., *Emblica officinalis* Gaertn., *Gongronema latifolium, Ageratum conyzoides, Aloe vera, Artocarpusaltilis, Aspilia africana, Bryophyllum pinnatum, Fluerya aestuans, Musa paradiasiaca, Musa sapientum, Persea Americana, Talinum triangulare, Fluerya aetuans, Brassica oleracae, Acacia nilotica* L., *Alchornea cordifolia Schum & thonn, Anacardium occidentale* L., *Balanites aegyptiaca* L., *Bridelia ferruginea* Benth, *Carica papaya* Linn, *Ficus thonningii* Blume, *Guiera senegalensis* J. F. Gmel, *Hibiscus sabdariffa* L., *Mangifera indica* L., *Momordica charantia* L., *Ocimum gratissium* L., *Piliostigma reticulatum* (DC) Hochst, *Pisidium guajava* L., *Scoparia dulcis, Vernonia kotschyana* Sch. Bip., *Zingiber officinale* Rosc [79].

7. The role of medicinal plants in oxidative gastropathy

Reactive oxygen species (ROS) are a by-product of normal metabolism and have roles in cell signaling and homeostasis [80]. Mechanisms exist that regulate cellular levels of ROS, as their reactive nature may otherwise cause damage to key cellular components including DNA, protein, and lipids [81]. A good number of NSAIDS have been implicated in cellular toxicity leading to oxidative gastropathy [82]. Despite the use of NSAIDS as antipyretic and anti-inflammation agents, and in the treatment of rheumatic, musculoskeletal, and cardiovascular diseases [83], gastrointestinal toxicity through ROS formation has limited their application [84, 85]. It has been proposed that NSAID-mediated gastrointestinal lesions involve the uncoupling of oxidative phosphorylation and inhibition of electron transport chain causing incomplete reduction of oxygen [82]. This they do by tenaciously binding to a site near complex I and ubiquinone, thus facilitating events leading to ROS generation [86, 87]. Subsequently, when the gastric antioxidant capacity is overwhelmed, the epithelia mitochondrial aconitase is inhibited, resulting in the release of iron that reacts with H_2O_2, producing hydroxyl radical. These cascades of event amplify gastric oxidative stress whose consequential effect is manifested as gastropathy [88]. Oxidative stress-induced functional loss is well correlated with numerous disease states including cardiovascular, neurological, cancer, aging processes and gastropathy [83] and is also implicated in a variety of drug-induced toxicities such as SU [2]. Antioxidative and free radical scavenging mechanisms play an important role in the protection against ROS mediated toxicities [89]. Over the past decades, interests in medicinal plants, especially the antioxidative ones, have increased appreciably and they have been elucidated to significantly either protect against or ameliorate ROS-mediated oxidative gastropathy [22, 90]. Such annihilation of ROS in SU diseases have been achieved through induction of enzymic antioxidants (superoxide dismutase, catalase, glutathione reductase and peroxidase) and optimization of reduced glutathione (GSH) contents [2, 22, 59]. Harmonizing the foregoing, a probable mechanism of antioxidative and gastroprotective activities of medicinal plants may be idealized as illustrated in **Figure 1**. This ultimately involves induction and optimization of preventive (catalase, glutathione peroxidase) and chain-breaking (superoxide dismutase, glutathione reductase) antioxidants that subsequently improve gastric GSH level, annihilate liberated reactive metabolite and effectively scavenge ROS (O_2^-, OH^-) (**Figure 1**). This may also be opined to regulate mucosal fluidity and strengthens defensive mechanisms against oxidative gastric damage.

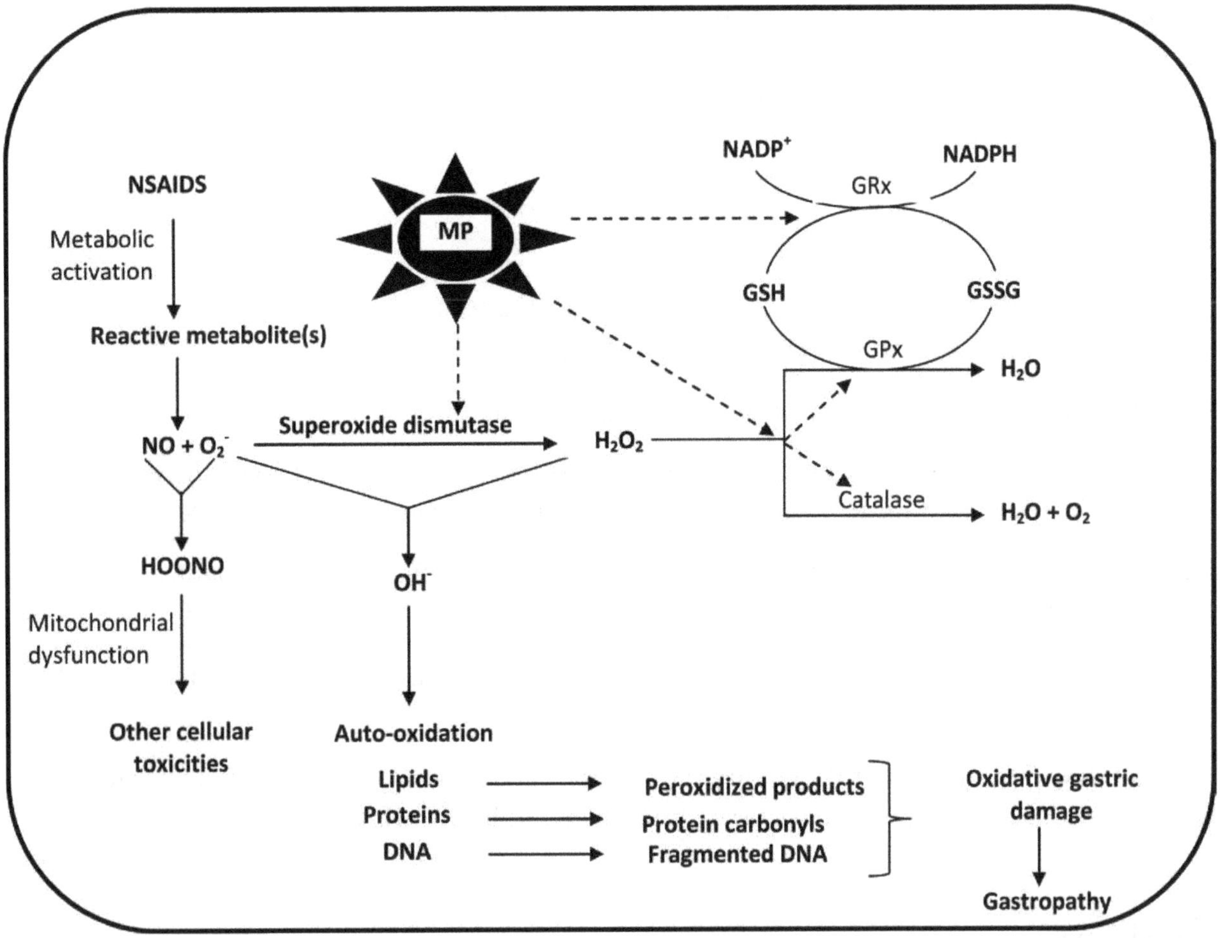

Figure 1. Probable mechanism of antioxidative and gastroprotective capabilities of medicinal plants. The dotted arrows represent sites of induction and optimization by the plants that consequently promote scavenging of O_2^- and OH^-. This will normalize and increase gastric reduced glutathione (GSH) content and promotes its mobilization toward detoxification of the liberated reactive metabolites. NSAIDS, nonsteroidal anti-inflammatory drugs; MP, medicinal plants; GPx, glutathione peroxidase; GRx, glutathione reductase; GSSG, oxidized glutathione.

8. Conclusion

Globally, SU is a devastating disease posing serious threat to the quality of life of humans. It affects significant proportion of the populace in both developed and developing countries. Although, conventional drugs have been used to manage and treat SU sufferers, affordability and inherent side effects have limited their application. Consequently, alternatives are being sought in medicinal plants, which provide a potential source of antiulcerogenic drugs and are widely used in traditional systems of medicine. Several medicinal plants have been investigated for their proven health benefits in SU management with their phytonutrients playing significant roles. Of the phytonutrients, tannins seem to top the list and has suggested probable focus on their characterization for antiulcer therapy. In spite of the impressive experimental evaluation of medicinal plants for the treatment of SU, very few have reached clinical trials and not very many have been marketed. This indicates that the intended benefits of CAM research are not yet having far-reaching effect. Nevertheless, the continuous search for antiulcerogenic agents of plant origin (available as gifts of nature) is imperative. This will ultimately and eventually present effective and globally competitive exciting opportunities for the development of new lead therapeutics for SU and other related disorders.

Author details

Sabiu Saheed[1,2,3*], Ajani Emmanuel Oladipo[1], Taofik Olatunde Sunmonu[4], Fatai Oladunni Balogun[2] and Anofi Omotayo Tom Ashafa[2]

*Address all correspondence to: saeed.sabiu@gmail.com

1 Phytomedicine, Food Factors and Toxicology Research Laboratory, Biochemistry Department, School of Basic Medical Sciences, Kwara State University, Ilorin, Nigeria

2 Phytomedicine and Phytopharmacology Research Group, Plant Sciences Department, University of the Free State, Phuthaditjhaba, South Africa

3 Department of Microbial, Biochemical, and Food Biotechnology, University of the Free State, Bloemfontein, South Africa

4 Phytomedicine and Plant Biochemistry Research Laboratory, Biochemistry Unit, Department of Biological Sciences, Al-Hikmah University, Ilorin, Nigeria

References

[1] Chan FKL, Graham DY. Review article: prevention of non-steroidal anti-inflammatory drug gastrointestinal complications—Review and recommendations based on risk assessment. Alimentary Pharmacology and Therapeutics. 2004;**19**(10):1051-1061

[2] Sabiu S, Sulyman AO, Garuba T, Sunmonu TO, Abdulrahaman AA. Combined administration of *Spondias mombin* and ficus exasperata leaf extracts stall indomethacin-mediated gastric mucosal onslaught in rats. African Journal of Traditional Complementary Alternative Medicine. 2015;**12**:45-51

[3] Debjit B, Chiranjib C, Tripathi KK, Pankaj J, Sampath KP. Recent trends of treatment and medication peptic ulcerative disorder. International Journal of PharmTech Research. 2010;**2**(1):970-980

[4] Vyawahare NS, Deshmukh VV, Godkari MR, Kagathara VG. Plants with anti-ulcer activity. Pharmacognosy Review. 2009;**3**:108-115

[5] Anand BS. Peptic ulcer diseases. Gastroenterology. 2017;**1**:23-35

[6] Hoogerwerf WA, Pasricha PJ. Agents Used for Control of Gastric Acidity and Treatment of Peptic Ulcers and Gastro Esophageal Reflux Disease, 10th ed. New York, NY, USA: McGraw-Hill; 2001. pp. 1005-1019

[7] Marshall BJ, Warren JR. Unidentified curved bacilli in the stomach of patients with gastritis and peptic ulceration. The Lancet. 1984;**1**(8390):1311-1315

[8] Malfertheiner P, Chan FK, McColl KE. Peptic ulcer disease. The Lancet. 2009;**374**(9699):1449-1461

[9] Sung JJ, Tsoi KK, Ma YK, Yung MY, Lau JY, Chiu PW. Causes of mortality in patients with peptic ulcer diseases: A prospective cohort study of 10428 cases. American Journal of Gastroenterology. 2010;**105**(1):84-89

[10] Bansal, et al. Herbal approach to peptic ulcer disease: Review. Journal of Bioscience Technology. 2009;**1**:52-58

[11] Shristi B, Neha J, Indu BP, Rajesh G. A review on some Indian medicinal plants for anti-ulcer activity. Journal of Science Research and Pharmacy. 2012;**1**:6-9

[12] Lau JY, Sung J, Hill C, Henderson C, Howden CW, Metz DC. Systematic review of the epidemiology of complicated peptic ulcer disease: Incidence, recurrence, risk factors and mortality. Digestion. 2011;**84**(2):102-113

[13] Cai S, Garcia RLA, Masso-Gonzalez EL, Hernande-Diaz S. Uncomplicated peptic ulcer disease in the United Kingdom: Trends from 1997 to 2005. Alimentary Pharmacology Therapeutics. 2009;**30**(10):1039-1048

[14] Kumar R. A review on medicinal plants for peptic ulcer. Der Pharmacia Lettre. 2011;**3**(3):414-420

[15] Bertaccini G, Coruzzi G. Pharmacology of the treatment of peptic ulcer disease. Digestive Diseases and Sciences. 1985;**30**(11):43s-51s

[16] Martin F, Farley A, Gagnon M, Bensemana D. Comparison of healing capacities of sucralfate and cimetidine in short treatment of duodenal ulcer. Double blind randomized trial. Gastroenterology. 1982;**82**:401-405

[17] Buyniski JP, Cavanagh RL, Pircio AW, Agieri AA, Crenshaw RR. In: Melchiorre C, Gianella M, editors. Highlights in Receptor Chemistry. Amsterdam: Elsevier; 1984. pp. 195-213

[18] Pendleton RG, McCafferty JP, Roesler JM, Hieble JP. Mechanism for gastric antisecretory effects of desmethylimipramine in rats. European Journal of Pharmacology. 1981;**75**:171-178

[19] Sachar H, Vaidya K, Laine L. Intermittent vs continuous proton pump inhibitor therapy for high-risk bleeding ulcers: a systematic review and meta-analysis. JAMA Internal Medicine. 2014;**174**(11):1755-1762

[20] Corleto VD. Proton pump inhibitor therapy and potential long-term harm. Current Opinion in Endocrinology, Diabetes and Obesity. 2016;**21**(1):3-8

[21] Rossi S, editor. Australian Medicines Handbook 2006. Adelaide: Australian Medicines Handbook 2006

[22] Sabiu S, Ajani EO, Ajao AA, Sunmonu TO, Ibraheem AS, Ibrahim R, Mustapha H, Adekeye AO. Biomembrane stabilization and antiulcerogenic properties of aqueous leaf extract of *Gossypium barbadense* L. (Malvaceae). Beni-Suef University Journal of Basic and Applied Sciences. 2017. http://dx.doi.org/10.1016/j.bjbas.2017.05.007

[23] Senay EC, Levine RJ. Synergism between cold and restraint for rapid production of stress ulcers in rats. Proceedings of the Society for Experimental Biology and Medicine. 1967;**124**(4):1221-1223

[24] Kitagawa H, Fujiwara M, Osumi Y. Effects of water immersion stress on gastric secretion and mucosal blood flow in rats. Gastroenterology. 1979;**77**(2):298-302

[25] Oates PJ, Hakkinen JP. Studies on the mechanism of ethanol-induced gastric damage in rats. Gastroenterology. 1988;**94**(1):10-21

[26] Okabe S, Amagase K. An overview of acetic acid ulcer models: The history and state of the art of peptic ulcer research. Biological and Pharmaceutical Bulletin. 2005;**28**(8):1321-1341

[27] Cho CH, Pfeiffer CJ. Gastrointestinal ulceration in the guinea pig in response to dimaprit, histamine, and H_1- and H_2-blocking agents. Digestive Diseases and Sciences. 1981;**26**(4):306-311

[28] Singh S. Evaluation of gastric anti-ulcer activity of fixed oil of *Ocimum basilicum Linn.* and its possible mechanism of action. Indian Journal of Experimental Biology. 1999;**37**(3):253-257

[29] LePard KJ, Stephens RL. Serotonin inhibits gastric acid secretion through a 5-hydroxy-tryptamine1-like receptor in the rat. Journal of Pharmacology and Experimental Therapeutics. 1994;**270**(3):1139-1147

[30] Shay H, Komarov SA, Fels SS, Meranze D, Gruenstein M, Siplet H. A simple method for the uniform production of gastric ulceration in the rat, Gastroenterology. 1945;**5**:43-61

[31] Wada K, Kamisaki Y, Kitano M, Kishimoto Y, Nakamoto K, Itoh T. A new gastric ulcer model induced by ischemia reperfusion in the rat: Role of leukocytes on ulceration in rat stomach. Life Sciences. 1996;**59**(19):295-301

[32] Konturek PC, Brzozowski T, Kania J. Pioglitazone, a specific ligand of peroxisome proliferator-activated receptorgamma, accelerates gastric ulcer healing in rat. European Journal of Pharmacology. 2003;**472**(3):213-220

[33] Naito Y, Yoshikawa T, Yoneta T. A new gastric ulcer model in rats produced by ferrous iron and ascorbic acid injection. Digestion. 1995;**56**(6):472-478

[34] Kaur D, Rana AC, Sharma N, Kumar S. Herbal drugs with antiulcer activity. Journal of Applied Pharmaceutical Science. 2012;**2**(3):160-165

[35] Srinivas TL, Lakshmi SM, Shama SN, Reddy GK, Prasanna KR. Medicinal plants as anti-ulcer agents. Journal of Pharmacognosy and Phytochemistry. 2013;**2**(4):91-97

[36] Schmeda-Hirschmann, G, Yesilada E. Traditional medicine and gastroprotective crude drugs. Journal of Ethnopharmacology. 2005;**100**(1-2):61-66

[37] Vimala G, Shoba GF. A Review on antiulcer activity of few Indian medicinal plants. International Journal of Microbiology. 2014;Article ID 519590, 14 pages

[38] Priyanka A. Some of the medicinal plants with anti-ulcer activity: A review. Journal of Pharmaceutical Science and Research. 2015;**7**(9):772-775

[39] Mehta D. Ulcer-Review on types, anti-ulcer drugs, anti-ulcer medicinal plants, anti-ulcer drug market, diagnostics and current global clinical trials status. Invention and Rapid Pharmacy Practice. 2016;**2**:1-8

[40] Nadkarni's KM. Indian Materia Medica. Popular Prakashan, Mumbai, India. 1976;**1**:9-10

[41] Abd El-Mawla AMA, Osman HEH. Effects of *Gum acacia* aqueous extract on the histology of the intestine and enzymes of both the intestine and the pancreas of albino rats treated with meloxicam. Pharmacognosy Research. 2011;**3**(2):114-121

[42] Maury PK, Jain SK, Lal N, Alok S. A review on antiulcer activity. International Journal of Pharmaceutical Science Research. 2012;**3**(8):2487-2493

[43] Nadkarni's KM. Indian Materia Medica. Popular Prakashan, Mumbai, India. 1976;**1**:38-39

[44] Ilavarasan JR, Monideen S, Vijayalakshmi M. Antiulcer activity of *Aegle marmelos*. Ancient Science of Life. 2002;**21**(4):23-26

[45] Borra SK, Lagisetty RK, Mallela GR. Anti-ulcer effect of *Aloe vera* in non-steroidal anti-inflammatory drug induced peptic ulcers in rats. African Journal of Pharmacy and Pharmacology. 2011;**5**(16):1867-1871

[46] Shaker E, Mahmoud H, Mnaa S. Anti-inflammatory and anti-ulcer activity of the extract from *Alhagi maurorum* (camelthorn). Food and Chemical Toxicology. 2010;**48**:2785-2790

[47] Azamthulla M, Asad M, Prasad VS. Antiulcer activity of *Allium sativum* bulb juice in rats. Saudi Pharmaceutical Journal. 2009;**17**(1):70-77

[48] Mohamed TSS, Pradeep RK, Priyanka N, Madhuri M, Sravanti V, Sarala K. Anti-ulcerogenic effect of aqueous extract of *Annona squamosa* (Linn). International Journal of Research in Phytochemistry and Pharmacology. 2012;**2**(3):157-159

[49] Divakar MC, Rao SB, Nair GRN, Hisham A. The role of fatty acids on the ulcer healing property of the nimbidin fraction of the neem oil. Journal of Medicinal and Aromatic Plants Science. 2001;**23**(3):404-408

[50] Kumar YR, Rajani GP. Analgesic and anti-ulcer activities of ethanol and aqueous extracts of root of *Bauhinia variegate* Linn. International Journal of Pharmacology. 2011;**7**(5):616-622

[51] Nadkarni's KM. Indian Materia Medica. Popular Prakashan, Mumbai, India. 1976; **1**:187-188

[52] Nadkarni's KM. Indian Materia Medica. Popular Prakashan, Mumbai, India. 1976;**1**:197

[53] Indran M, Mahmood AA, Kuppusamy VR. Protective effect of *Carica papaya* L leaf extract against alcohol induced acute gastric damage and blood oxidative stress in rats. West Indian Medical Journal. 2008;**57**(4):323-326

[54] Sairam K, Rao CHV, Goel RK. Effect of *Centella asiatica* Linn on physical and chemical factors induced gastric ulceration and secretion. Indian Journal of Experimental Biology. 2001;**39**:137-142

[55] Inas ZA, Abdallah-Hala AH, Khattab H, Gehan HH. Gastroprotective effect of *Cordia Myxa* L. fruit extract against indomethacin-induced gastric ulceration in rats. Life Sciences Journal. 2011;**8**:433-445

[56] Gregory M, Divya B, Mary RA, Hipolith MMV, Kalaichelvan VK, Palanivel V. Anti-ulcer activity of *Ficus religiosa* leaf ethanolic extract. Asian Pacific Journal of Tropical Biomedicine. 2013;**3**(7):554-556

[57] Khalid MS, Hassan SK, Suresh DK, Hasan R, Saleem MA, Farooqui Z. Antiulcer activity of ethanolic extract of *Gossypium herbaceous* flowers. RGUH. Journal of Pharmaceutical Sciences. 2011;**1**:79S-84S

[58] Srivastava JJ, Gautam H, Sharma S, Rao CV. Anti-ulcer activity of methanol extract of *Hibiscus rosa sinensis* leaves. International Journal of Pharmacy and Pharmaceutical Sciences. 2013;**5**(3):829-830

[59] Ajani EO, Sabiu S, Bamisaye FA, Salami MR, Nurain IO. Ethanolic leaf extract of *Lagenaria brevifolia* (Bitter gourd) inhibits gastric onslaught in indomethacin ulcerated rats. Journal of Applied Biosciences. 2015;**85**:7871-7880

[60] Neelima MS, Patil MB, Lakshmi BVS. Anti-ulcer activity and HPTLC analysis of *Mangifera indica* leaves. International Journal of Pharmaceutical and Phytopharmacological Research. 2012;**1**(4):146-155

[61] Pramod K, Devala RG, Lakshmayya A, Ramachandra SS. GC-MS analysis and antiulcer activity of ethanol extract of tubers of *Momordica tuberosa* Cogn. (cucurbitaceae) in rats. Journal of Applied Pharmacy. 2011;**4**:359-369

[62] Verma VK, Singh N, Saxena P, Singh R. Anti-ulcer and anti-oxidant activity of *Moringa oleifera* (Lam) leaves against aspirin and ethanol induced gastric ulcer in rats. International Research Journal of Pharmacy. 2002;**2**:46-57

[63] Sumbul S, Ahmad MA, Asif M, Saud I, Akhtar M. Evaluation of *Myrtus communis* Linn. berries in experimental ulcer models in rats. Human and Experimental Toxicology. 2010;**29**(11):935-944

[64] Kamble RD, Maske KS, Shaikh HM, Balghare KC, Shikare ON. A review of antiulcer medicinal plants. International Journal of Pharmacy. 2013;**4**(1):78-81

[65] Singh S, Majumdar DK. Evaluation of the gastric antiulcer activity of fixed oil of *Ocimum sanctum* (Holy Basil). Journal of Ethnopharmacology. 1999;**65**(1):13-19

[66] Panchal S, Goswami SS, Shan MB, Santani DD. Effect of *Oryza sativa* bran oil in various experimental ulcer models. Indian Journal of Pharmacology. 2008;**40**(2):146-148

[67] Okoli CO, Ezike AC, Akah PA. Studies on wound healing and antiulcer activities of extract of aerial parts of *Phyllanthus niruri* L. (Euphorbiaceae). American Journal of Pharmacology and Toxicology. 2009;**4**(4):118-126

[68] Umana EU, Timbuak JA, Musa SA, Ikyembe DT, Abdurrashid S, Hamman WO. Ulceroprotective effect of methanol extract of *Psidium guajava* leaves on ethanol induced gastric ulcer in adult wistar rats. Asian Journal of Medical Sciences. 2012;**4**(2):75-78

[69] Ahmad H, Wadud A, Jahan N, Khazir M, Sofi G. Evaluation of anti-ulcer activity of hydro alcoholic extract of Post Sumaq (*Rhus coriaria* Linn.) in ethanol induced gastric ulcer in experimental rats. International Research Journal of Medical Sciences. 2013;**1**(10):7-12

[70] Bhalke RD, Giri MA, Anarthe SJ, Pal SC. Antiulcer activity of the ethanol extract of leaves of *Sesbania grandiflora* (Linn.). International Journal of Pharmacy and Pharmaceutical Sciences. 2010;**2**(4):206-208

[71] Khan I, Nisar M, Ebad F, Nadeem S, Saeed M, Khan H. Anti-inflammatory activities of sieboldogenin from *Smilax china* Linn.: Experimental and com putational studies. Journal of Ethnopharmacology. 2009;**121**:175-177

[72] Kavitha GGS, Parvathi S, Ramkumar PSS, Shanmuga SP. Pharmacological and phytochemical evaluation of anti-ulcerogenic potential of *Solanum nigrum.* Indian Journal of Pharmaceutical Science and Research. 2012;**3**(8):2837-2840

[73] Saheed S, Taofeeq G, Taofik OS, Emmanuel OA, Abdulhakeem S, Ismaila NI, Abdulazeez B. Indomethacin-induced gastric ulceration in rats: Protective roles of *Spondias mombin* and *Ficus exasperate*. Toxicology Report. 2015;**2**:261-267

[74] Kumar S, Suman S, Sharma S, Kalra P. Antiulcer effect of the methanolic extract of *Tamarindus indica* seeds in different experimental models. Journal of Pharmacy and Bioallied Sciences. 2011;**2**(3):236-241

[75] Raju D, Ilango K, Chitra V, Ashish K. Evaluation of antiulcer activity of methanolic extract of *Terminalia chebula* fruits in experimental rats. Journal of Pharmaceutical Sciences and Research. 2009;**1**(3):101-107

[76] Bandyopadhyay U,Biswas K, Sengupta A, Moitra P, Dutta P, Sarkar D, Debnath P, Ganguly CK, Banerjee RK. Clinical studies on the effect of Neem (*Azadirachta indica*) bark extract on gastric secretion and gastroduodenal ulcer. Life Sciences. 2004;**75**(24):2867-2878

[77] Michael BA, Charles A, Isaac G, Alexander N. *In vivo* models used for evaluation of potential antigastroduodenal ulcer agents. *Ulcers*, 2013. Article ID 796405, 12 pages

[78] Kadiri M, Ojewumi AW, Kokumo YO. Ethnobotanical study of plants used in managing ulcer in Abeokuta metropolis, Ogun State, Nigeria. Journal of Natural Science, Engineering and Technology. 2013;**12**:76-88

[79] Alebiosu CO, Ugwah OM, Ugwah-Oguejiofor CJ, Njan AA. Ethno botanical studies of medicinal plants used in the management of Peptic ulcer disease in Sokoto State, North Western Nigeria. International Research Journal of Pharmacy and Pharmacology. 2012;**2**(9):225-230

[80] Sabiu S, O'neill FH, Ashafa AOT. *Zea mays, Stigma maydis* prevents and extenuates acetaminophen-perturbed oxidative onslaughts in rat hepatocytes. Pharmaceutical Biology, 2016;**54**(11): 2664-2673. DOI: http://dx.doI.org/10.1080/13880209.20161178307

[81] Ajani EO, Sabiu S, Bamisaye FA, Adenigba BV, Awomoyi DD, Adeyanju MM. Hepatoprotective and antioxidative effect of ethanolic leaf extract of *Langenaria breviflora* (bitter gourd) on indomethacin-ulcerated rats. IOSR Journal of Pharmacy and Biological Science. 2014;**9**(5 V I):61-68

[82] Hong Y, Xingchang P, Zhixiu S, Shaokang W, Ligang Y, Guiju S. Protective effect of wheat peptides against indomethacin-induced oxidative stress in IEC-6 cells. Nutrients. 2014;**6**:564-574

[83] Dae YC, Jin IK, Soo-Heon P, Jae KK. Proanthocyanidin from grape seed extracts protects indomethacin-induced small intestinal mucosal injury. Gastroenterology Research Practice. 2014;**14**:618-626

[84] Bjornsson E. Review article: Drug-induced liver injury in clinical practice. Alimentary Pharmacology Therapeutics. 2013;**32**:3-13

[85] Jarupongprapa S, Ussavasodhi P, Katchamart W. Comparison of gastrointestinal adverse effects between cyclooxygenase-2 inhibitors and non-selective, non-steroidal anti-inflammatory drugs plus proton pump inhibitors: A systematic review and meta-analysis. Journal of Gastroenterology. 2013;**48**:830-838

[86] Kang HS, Ock J, Lee HJ, Lee YJ, Kwon BM, Hong SH. Early growth response protein-1-upregulation and nuclear translocation by 2'-benzoyloxycinnamaldehyde induces prostate cancer cell death. Cancer Letter. 2013;**329**:217-227

[87] Vaish V, Piplani H, Rana C, Vaiphei K, Sanyal SN. NSAIDs may regulate EGR-1- mediated induction of reactive oxygen species and non-steroidal anti-inflammatory drug-induced gene (NAG)-1 to initiate intrinsic pathway of apoptosis for the chemoprevention of colorectal cancer. Molecular Cell Biochemistry. 2013;**378**:47-64

[88] Valko M, Leibfritz D, Moncol J, Cronin MTD, Mazur M, Telser J. Free radicals and antioxidants in normal physiological functions and human disease. International Journal of Biochemistray and Cell Biology. 2007;**39**:44-84

[89] Sabiu S, Wudil AM. Comparative effects of *Telfaira occidentalis* and *Vernonia amygdalina* on garlic-induced hepatotoxicity in rats. Biological and Environmental Sciences Journal for the Tropics. 2011;**8**(4):193-197

[90] Shu YZ. Recent natural products based drug development: A pharmaceutical industry perspective. Journal of Natural Product. 1998;**61**:1053-1107

13

Nutritional Therapy for Inflammatory Bowel Disease

Rok Orel, Evgen Benedik, Janez Eržen,
Anija Orel and Darja Urlep

Abstract

The components of a diet influence intestinal microbiota, epithelial barrier function, immune system, and many other factors that play important role in both development and treatment of inflammation in gastrointestinal tract. We briefly review potential role of specific dietary compounds as a risk or protective factor, but we predominantly concentrate on nutritional status and nutritional intervention in patients with inflammatory bowel disease. Besides exclusive enteral nutrition as a potential first-line treatment in active Crohn's disease, other nutritional therapeutic modalities such as partial enteral nutrition, parenteral nutrition, diets based on carbohydrate modifications, anti-inflammatory diet, and the use of specific dietary compounds with anti-inflammatory properties, known as pharmaconutrition, are presented.

Keywords: inflammatory bowel disease, Crohn's disease, ulcerative colitis, nutrition, nutritional therapy

1. Introduction

The exact etiology and pathophysiologic mechanisms of inflammatory bowel diseases (IBD) are not completely explained, but the complex interplay among genetic background, environmental factors, intestinal microbiota, and immune system seems to be implemented. The incidence and prevalence of both types of IBD, Crohn's disease (CD) and ulcerative colitis (UC), has dramatically increased in western countries and in developed Asian countries in the last 50 years [1]. In addition, several epidemiologic studies revealed that the incidence of IBD in descendants of immigrants from the parts of the world with low incidence to the countries with high incidence resembles the one of the native population and not of the county of their origin [2, 3]; these points to the crucial role of environmental factors/changes in IBD epidemics. The potential influences of specific factors such as changes in hygiene/sanitation, decreased exposure to infectious agents, smoking, water and air pollution, psychological stress, and an increased use of certain drugs have all been proposed and are reviewed elsewhere [4, 5]. An increasing body of evidence is linking IBD with diet.

Dietary constituents and their proportions can affect human physiology directly. However, intestinal microbiota, recently recognized as an essential component of metabolism, immune and neuroendocrine regulation, is also importantly influenced by diet. For example, intestinal microbiota of African children, whose diet is based on fiber-rich, plant-derived diet, was found to be vastly different to microbiota of their European peers, who consume diet rich in sugar, diary, fat, and protein [6]. Animal studies revealed that change from low-fat, high-fiber diet to "Western style" diet rich in fat and sugar resulted in substantial shift in microbiota within a single day [7]. Changes in composition and function of intestinal microbiota because of specific dietary patterns may lead to a state not favorable for host organism, defined as dysbiosis. Numerous studies have shown that gut microbiota of IBD patients substantially differs from the one of healthy individuals and that these changes may play a crucial role in the development and activity of the disease [8]. Enteric microbiota plays an essential role in metabolizing nutrients, especially those not completely digestible by human digestive enzymes, such as fiber, resulting in production of diversity of biologically active components, such as short chain fatty acids (SCFAs) and intestinal gases. A study from Japan showed that people living in rural areas consuming traditional Japanese food have more abundant Bifidobacteria, which are recognized as an important producer of SCFAs, than urban population eating western-type diet [9]. Western-type diets, rich in saturated fat and protein and poor in plant fiber, result in depletion of Firmicutes, which are involved in metabolism of plant polysaccharides, and decrease in SCFA production [10]. On the other hand, this kind of diet promotes growth of proteolytic bacteria, such as Bilophila wadsworthia and other bile tolerant microbes, which use proteins and bile acids as a source of organic sulfur and produce hydrogen sulfide (H2S). H2S can be genotoxic, modulate expression in cell cycle progression, trigger inflammatory response, and impair DNA repair [8].

Direct effects of relative abundancy/deficiency of specific nutrients and changes in composition and functioning of intestinal microbiota can lead to impairment of intestinal barrier function, including decreased resistance to invasion of pathobionts, dysfunction of innate, and adaptive immune system that finally results in chronic inflammation and tissue damage characteristic for IBD.

In this chapter, we try to review current knowledge about the effects of specific food components on IBD concentrating on clinical evidence about efficacy of different dietary interventions in IBD patients.

2. Role of specific food constituents

Most of our knowledge about the influence of specific food ingredients on intestinal function, development of inflammation, and IBD in particular originates either from animal model experiments or from epidemiological studies.

2.1. Fats

There is a growing evidence that some types of fat act pro-inflammatory, while the others protect against development of intestinal inflammation. Several big epidemiologic studies, such as European Investigation into Cancer and Nutrition Study (EPIC) and the Nurses' Health Study have pointed to an increased risk of IBD among people who consume greater amounts of meat and fats, particularly polyunsaturated fatty acids and omega-6 fatty acids [11–13]. The EPIC study revealed an association between greater consumption of an omega-6 polyunsaturated fatty acid (PUFA), linoleic acid, present in high concentrations in red meat, cooking oils, and margarine and higher incidence of UC. In contrast, people who consumed higher levels of omega-3 PUFA docosahexaenoic acid (DHA) were less likely to develop UC [11–13]. Similarly, consumption of large quantities of nuts and fish, which are rich in omega-3 PUFA such as DHA, eicosapentaenoic acid (EPA), and docosapentaenoic acid (DPA), was shown to lower the risk for CD [14]. Omega-3 fatty acids were shown to have an anti-inflammatory, antithrombotic, antiarrhythmic, and hypolipemic effect [15]. There was also a significantly reduced risk for CD when ratio of long-chain omega-3/arachidonic acid was high in the consumed food [14].

In conclusion, it seems that diet rich in animal fats and particularly omega-6 PUFA promotes dysbiosis and intestinal inflammation that may lead to development of IBD in genetically susceptible hosts. On the other hand, omega-3 PUFA seems to play a protective role and may even promote anti-inflammatory mechanisms.

2.2. Proteins

As already mentioned, several epidemiologic studies revealed an association between consumption of large quantities of meat and increased risk for IBD [11–13]. It is not clear whether this association was only due to increased intake of fats or also of proteins, as the results of the studies regarding the role of proteins in IBD were conflicting [13]. In one study, high intake of proteins found in meat but not in dairy products was found to be positively associated with IBD [16].

Among the specific proteins and peptides, the effects of gluten-derived proteins were particularly attentive. In animal model, gluten-fortified experimental diet induced chronic ileitis [17]. They found reduced occludin expression levels, and these findings suggest a negative role of gluten on intestinal barrier integrity. Experiments on intestinal epithelial cell lines showed that gliadin induces an increase in intestinal permeability due to zonulin release by binding to the chemokine receptor CXCR3 [18]. Zonulin is the physiologic modulator of tight junctions that regulate intestinal permeability through the epithelial paracellular pathway. Its upregulation in genetically susceptible individuals may lead to different immune-mediated diseases [19]. It was observed that intestinal permeability increased after gliadin exposure not only in patients with celiac disease or nonceliac gluten sensitivity but, although to a lesser extent, also in healthy subjects [20].

2.3. Carbohydrates

Many epidemiological studies pointed out that excessive consumption of simple carbohydrates, refined sugars, sweet carbonized drinks, or even artificial sweeteners might represent a risk factor for the development of IBD; however, as many others failed to prove this association [21]. Individual studies even showed that low complex carbohydrates and low refined sugar intake significantly improved laboratory inflammatory markers and fecal calprotectin in patients with IDB [22].

On the other hand, consummation of vegetables and fruits rich in both soluble and insoluble fiber has been shown to be negatively associated with IBD [14, 23, 24]. Animal studies confirmed that plant polysaccharides and poorly digestible fibrous plant components have reduced features of experimental colitis [25]. Fermentable fiber is fermented by saccharolytic gut microbiota, resulting in increased production of SCFAs. SCFAs, especially butyrate, are utilized not only as fuel sources for colonocyte that results in enhancement of the intestinal barrier, but also possess anti-inflammatory effect, mainly through inhibition of the production and release of inflammatory mediators [26, 27]. In addition, some vegetables like broccoli and cabbage are thought to activate the aryl hydrocarbon receptor (AhR), which is highly expressed by intestinal intraepithelial lymphocytes and is involved in immune regulation and defense against attacks of luminal microorganisms [28]. Overall, refined and processed carbohydrates and intake of sweetened beverages are thought to be risk factors for developing IBD, while complex carbohydrates like vegetables, fruit, and fiber showed to be protective.

2.4. Food additives

It has been hypothesized that emulsifiers, detergent-like molecules that are a ubiquitous component of processed foods, can disrupt intestinal mucus layer, increase intestinal permeability, and enable bacterial translocation across epithelia [29]. In mice, relatively low concentrations of two commonly used emulsifiers, carboxymethylcellulose and polysorbate-80, induced low-grade inflammation in wild-type hosts and promoted robust colitis in mice predisposed to IBD [30].

Maltodextrin, a polysaccharide derived from starch hydrolysis, was found to promote adherent-invasive E coli (AIEC) biofilms and increase adhesion of AIEC strains to intestinal epithelial cells and macrophages [31]. Strains of AIEC have been isolated from the ileum and the colon of CD patients [32, 33].

Therefore, consumption of maltodextrin and emulsifiers may possibly support growth of intestinal pathobionts, such as AIEC and their translocation across epithelial barrier, where they could survive in macrophages and lead to chronic inflammation.

3. Nutritional status of IBD patients

According to available data, malnutrition affects 65–75% of patients with CD and 18–62% of patients with UC [34, 35]. In pediatric IBD patients, malnutrition frequently results not only in weight loss but also in growth retardation [36, 37].

Main reason for malnutrition in IBD patients is insufficient food intake due to the loss of appetite and avoidance of certain foods presumably worsening the symptoms, resulting in prolonged restrictive diets [38, 39]. Intestinal inflammation and inflammatory cytokines released from immune cells can damage epithelial integrity and impair absorption of nutrients. In addition, bacterial overgrowth and increased intestinal mobility may contribute to malabsorption [40, 41]. Fat and fat-soluble vitamin absorption may be especially impaired in CD patients when terminal ileum is seriously affected due to the biliary salt malabsorption [42]. Some of the medications used for IBD treatment, such as glucocorticoids, sulfasalazine, and immune system suppressants, could have a negative impact on micronutrient absorption and utilization [34, 42]. It should be noted that IBD patients with active inflammation have increased metabolic rate, which leads to increased energy expenditure [36, 37, 43].

An important aspect of malnutrition in IBD patients is alteration of body composition. Fat mass (FM) consists of adipose tissues (both visceral and subcutaneous) while fat-free mass (FFM) consists of water, proteins, minerals, and other components [35]. Clinical studies revealed an important reduction of both FM and FFM in active phase of IBD. However, it was also reported that FM was frequently recovered during remission phase, while FFM remained depleted [35].

Malnutrition, immobility, low protein synthesis, and increased proteolysis due to inflammation are the main mechanisms leading to sarcopenia, a progressive and generalized loss of skeletal muscle mass and strength with risk of poor quality of life and physical disability [44]. Sarcopenia has various negative health consequences such as pathological fractures due to bone demineralization, cardiovascular disease, and higher probability of hospitalization [44].

Several studies reported that despite aforementioned causes leading to malnutrition in IBD, one-third of the patients are obese, the proportion is similar in CD and UC patients [45, 46]. Obese IBD patients do not have worst long-term clinical outcome than normal weight patients [47]. However, simultaneous presence of sarcopenia and obesity, so-called sarcopenic obesity, is related to a fast functional decline of patient's status, with a high risk of morbidity, disability, and mortality [44].

Micronutrient and vitamin deficiencies are common in IBD patients. Preventions of those deficiencies are mandatory for avoidance of possible clinical complications. The most common micronutrient deficiencies described in IBD patients are known for iron, calcium, selenium, zinc, magnesium, and vitamins, in particular B12, folic acid, A, D, and K [34, 42].

One of the important features of IBD is anemia. Its prevalence in pediatric patients is up to 70% and in adult patients up to 50% [48]. The most frequent cause of anemia in IBD patients is iron deficiency (prevalence estimated in 36–90% of CD and UC patients), following vitamin B12 (prevalence estimated in 22% of CD and 3% of UC patients) [34, 49], and folic acid (vitamin B9) deficiencies (prevalence estimated in 29% of CD and 9% of UC patients) [50]. These deficiencies are the consequence of bleeding from mucosal lesions, inadequate dietary intake, impaired absorption and utilization, surgery (ileal resection greater than 60 cm will develop B12 deficiency), systemic inflammation, and medications [37, 50, 51].

Calcium and Vitamin D deficiency are often in IBD patients, especially in those with duodenal and jejunal disease, when their absorption is disturbed [34, 42]. Their prevalence is 70% in CD and 40% in UC patients. Besides its influence on bone metabolism, vitamin D have important role in preserving mucosal integrity and mucosal healing capacity. In case of its deficiency, the risk for mucosal damage and for IBD is higher [34, 42]. It was shown that high levels of active vitamin D not only reduce the risk of developing CD, but also the risk of developing UC [52, 53].

Vitamin A deficiency in IBD patients is high up to 90%. Vitamin A deficiency results in impaired wound healing, night blindness, and xerophthalmia [34, 42].

Vitamin K deficiency in IBD patients is also reported, but the prevalence is unknown. Most important source of vitamin K is intestinal production by gut microbiota. Dysbiosis, use of antibiotics, and malabsorption may contribute to this deficiency [34, 42].

Inadequate dietary intake and chronic loss because of diarrhea are the main reasons for selenium, zinc, and magnesium deficiencies in IBD patients for which the exact prevalence is not known. Symptoms associated with deficiencies include bone health impairment, cartilage degeneration, fatigue, and poor wound healing [34, 42].

4. Nutritional intervention

EEN has been evaluated in a number of clinical studies including randomized controlled trials (RCTs) that compared EEN to CS in adult and pediatric populations of patients with active CD. To date, eight meta-analyses have been published on the efficacy of EEN versus CS. Among these meta-analyses, three of them were performed exclusively on the pediatric population while others included adult patients as well. While meta-analyses of adult studies have suggested better efficacy of CS, pediatric studies have shown that EEN is at least as effective as CS in inducing remission and is superior to CS in improving nutritional status and growth recovery without adverse side effects [54].

The main goals of nutritional intervention in IBD patients are treatment and prevention of malnutrition, treatment of active inflammation and maintaining remission in Crohn's disease, and symptomatic treatment in specific situations [55].

Regular evaluation of nutritional status, early detection of specific deficits and specific risk factors are crucial for adequate nutritional treatment. Anthropometric measurements and basic laboratory tests, such as hemoglobin concentration and markers of inflammation, should be checked regularly at every visit, while the frequency of albumin, ferritin, vitamin, and trace element concentration checkout depends on the activity of the disease, but should be done at least once a year when the disease is quiescent [55]. Periodical evaluation of detailed body composition and bone mineral density is recommended. Bioimpedance (BIA) and dual-energy X-ray absorptiometry (DEXA) are considered as the gold standard for measuring body composition [56]. A dietary history and, sometimes, prospective dietary record are necessary to get a good estimate of food intake. We should be aware that many patients develop special dietary habits due to their belief that consumption of specific foods (e.g., dairy, meat, fruit, and vegetables) results in symptoms or even worsen the disease course, which may additionally contribute to the development of nutritional deficiencies [57].

With the exception of the ECCO/ESPGHAN recommendations to use exclusive enteral nutrition as a first-line therapeutic approach in children with active CD [58], the strict guidelines for nutritional intervention in IBD does not exist. However, many different dietary approaches have been developed and studied, with intention to alleviate patients' symptoms or even treat the disease.

4.1. Exclusive and partial enteral nutrition

Exclusive enteral nutrition (EEN) means that 100% of a person's nutritional requirements is provided by a liquid nutritional formula either orally or via a feeding tube. Numerous studies have shown that the treatment of active CD with exclusive enteral nutrition (EEN), especially in children, is as effective as corticosteroids in inducing remission. EEN, used as monotherapy, can induce remission in up to 80% of patients with active CD [59, 60]. It is well established that treatment with EEN is capable of achieving mucosal healing. On the contrary, corticosteroids have poor ability to induce mucosal healing [61]. In comparison to therapy with drugs, EEN has no adverse effects and, even more importantly, improves growth, and reverses malnutrition [58]. Therefore, according to the ECCO/ESPGHAN guidelines for treatment of pediatric CD patients, EEN is recommended as a first-line treatment in children and adolescents with active CD [58]. Meta-analysis of the results of the studies using ENN for the therapy of active CD in adult CD patients indicated that it was less effective than steroids in inducing remission; however, this conclusion was based on intention-to-treat analysis [62]. However, when only the results of the patients who completed the course of EEN were analyzed, the remission rates were comparable to those achieved by steroids [63].

EEN is usually provided for 6–8 week, and then a normal diet is gradually reintroduced. Enteral formulas are differentiated by the structure of their protein content. Elemental diets contain no intact protein, but only amino acids. Semielemental diets are based on peptides of varying lengths. Polymeric formulas contain whole proteins and are therefore more palatable in comparison with elemental diets [64]. Protocols of EEN may be different regarding the composition of the enteral formula and route of administration. Elemental diets often require a feeding tube to administer due to their poor palatability. In addition, polymeric formulas are reported to cost less. Various studies and a large meta-analysis later demonstrated that polymeric formulas were as effective as elemental formulas [65].

Although EEN has been shown to be efficacious, its mechanism of action remains unknown. Possible mechanisms include a change in gut microbiota, bowel rest, dietary antigen elimination, improvement in the nutritional status, and potential anti-inflammatory properties of specific ingredients of enteral formulas. Currently, the modification of gut microbiota seems to be the most probable proposed mechanism for ENN efficacy. The next very important mechanism may be associated with exclusion of potentially harmful food ingredients [60].

One of the proposed challenges influencing acceptance of EEN is the restriction of other oral food intake, which may seriously limit compliance with the EEN protocol [66]. Therefore, studies on partial enteral nutrition (PEN), which allows patients with active CD to consume a part of their daily caloric needs from a normal diet, have been conducted.

The results reported from the first study on the efficacy of PEN did not indicate that PEN providing 50% of caloric needs by formula was effective for induction of remission in pediatric CD [67]. However, the results of some recently published studies are more promising. Israeli authors combined PEN with Crohn's Disease Exclusion Diet (CDED) [68]. CDED is a structured diet, which excludes animal fats, milk and dairy, gluten, and all processed and canned foods, which contain additives, especially emulsifiers and maltodextrin. The authors hypothesize that the major mechanism leading to response to EEN used in children with active CD is exclusion of specific dietary factors, which may have a negative impact on mucous layer, intestinal permeability, and colonization with adherent-invasive E coli (AIEC). The study protocol allowed patients to consume up to 50% daily calories from CDED. Response and remission were obtained in 78.7 and 70.2% patients, respectively. Different approaches using PEN was developed at the Children's Hospital of Philadelphia [69]. The patients receive 80–90% of their energy input from EN, but they were allowed to consume remaining calories from a normal diet. Retrospective analysis revealed remission rate of 65% and response rate of 87%, which is comparable with the remission rates from the studies using EEN. Further studies are needed to elucidate the efficacy of this treatment approach.

One of the problems of CD therapy with EEN is that disease relapses relatively frequently soon after stopping EN when the patients are not receiving maintenance therapy. Several studies using PEP as a maintenance therapy either alone or in combination with drugs were performed in both pediatric and adult patients with CD. The results of the majority of these studies, as well as their systematic reviews [70–72], showed that the relapse rate during observational period was significantly lower in patients using PEP compared with those consuming regular unrestricted diet and that efficacy of maintenance therapy with PEP might be comparable to standard therapy with drugs. In addition, nutritional status as well as linear growth of children with CD was found to be better in those using PEP during remission in comparison with patients on regular diet [73].

4.2. Total parenteral nutrition

In the 1980s, total parenteral nutrition (TPN) was used to treat patients with moderate to severe CD. The aim of TPN as primary therapy for IBD was to achieve bowel rest, to correct nutritional deficits, and to remove antigenic mucosal stimuli [74, 75]. In the 1990s, treatment with exclusive enteral nutrition (EEN) was shown to have similar or even better results in terms of remission rate in active CD disease. When TPN and ENN are compared, TPN is associated with higher costs and significant risk of serious adverse events including sepsis. Therefore, TPN should be restricted to patients who cannot be adequately fed by enteral route, mainly those with gut failure and short-bowel syndrome [76].

According to recent ESPEN guidelines on clinical nutrition in IBD, TPN is indicated only when EN has failed or it is impossible to be administered [77].

4.3. Diets based on carbohydrate modifications

Low-fiber or even so-called low-residue diets are frequently recommended during acute exacerbations of IBD [78]. While a low-fiber diet excludes only insoluble fiber, a low-residue diet requires exclusion of not only all vegetables, fruits, whole grains, legumes, but also dairy products and fibrous meat [79]. A basic idea behind these diets is that they reduce the volume and frequency of stools as well as the risk of intestinal obstruction. Although these diets are usually prescribed for a short-term use, many patients continue with them for a long period of time. Objective studies failed to find any difference in severity of symptoms, number of complications, and needs for hospitalization or surgery between patients using such diets and those consuming unrestricted diet [80]. As already mentioned, indigestible carbohydrates, especially the fermentable ones may play an important protective role in IBD, as they represent the main substrate for production of SCFAs by intestinal bacteria. The only patients that may benefit from fiber restriction are those with strictures and obstructive symptoms.

Significant proportion of IBD patients also suffers from functional irritable bowel syndrome-like symptoms even in remission independently of actual level of the inflammation [81]. Low fermentable oligosaccharide, disaccharide, monosaccharide, and polyol (FODMAP) diet results in symptom relief in many of such patients [82]. However, low-FODMAP diet is very restrictive, so it should be carefully planned by professional dietetics to prevent development of specific nutritional deficiencies. In addition, the influence of low-FODMAP diet on the microbiome, metabolism, and inflammation in patients with IBD is still unclear.

On the other side, several studies using fiber-rich supplements such as wheat or oat bran [83, 84], psyllium [85, 86], and germinated barley foodstuff [87, 88] revealed their efficacy in symptomatic improvement and in decreasing disease activity indices either in CD or UC patients. Moreover, reduced concentrations of inflammatory cytokines, such as TNF-α, IL-6, and IL-8, pointed to the possible anti-inflammatory effect of dietary fiber, probably through their influence on microbiota and SCFA production [89].

Another diet, based mainly not only on restriction of specific carbohydrates but also on some other foods, called the specific carbohydrate diet (SCD) was developed in the 1920s [90]. Since then, this diet has been used in a variety of different conditions, including IBD, irritable bowel syndrome, celiac disease, and autism [91]. The SCD restricts all carbohydrates except monosaccharides: glucose, fructose, and galactose. This diet is based on a hypothesis that complex carbohydrates may induce intestinal dysbiosis resulting in the development of inflammation [92]. While fresh or cooked fruits, vegetables, and legumes are in general acceptable, all grains as well as potatoes should be omitted. In more restrictive versions of SCD, even milk and dairy products, refined sugar and artificial sweeteners, corn, and maple syrup are prohibited. In addition, all-otherwise permitted food should not be processed (canned, smoked, etc.) and should not contain potentially harmful additives [91]. Several relatively small studies found out that SCD alone without taking medications may lead to clinical improvement, reflected by symptom disappearance and significant reduction of laboratory markers of inflammation, in some patient with active CD [91, 93]. However, recently published study using endoscopic evaluation before and after the treatment with SCD revealed that despite some clinical effect, complete mucosal healing was never achieved [94].

4.4. IBD-anti-inflammatory diet

Recently, an investigator group from USA developed the IBD-anti-inflammatory diet (IBD-AID) to be offered to IBD patients who are refractory to pharmacological therapy, or for whom the treatment is not as effective as desired [95]. The IBD-AID has five basic components. The first is the restriction of certain carbohydrates, including lactose, and refined or processed complex carbohydrates. The second is the use of pre- and probiotics and foods rich in the components that help to restore the balance of the intestinal microbiota (e.g., soluble fiber, leeks, onions, and fermented foods). The third is distinctive use of saturated, trans-, mono-, and polyunsaturated fats. The fourth principle is to review the overall dietary pattern, detect missing nutrients, and identify specific food intolerances. The last component is a modification of food textures to improve absorption of nutrients and to minimize the adverse effect of intact fiber. In practice, the IBD-AID consists of lean meats, poultry, fish, omega-3 eggs, particular sources of carbohydrates, select fruits and vegetables, nuts, and legume flours, but restricts the consumption of wheat, rye, and barley products as well as milk and dairy products other than yogurt, kefir, and limited aged cheeses. A retrospective review of their case series including both patients with CD and UC revealed that approximately one-third of the patients chose not to attempt this diet, while the vast majority of those who followed the diet for 4 weeks or more reported symptom reduction and were able to discontinue at least one of their prior IBD medications [95]. However, randomized clinical trials are needed to properly elucidate the efficacy of this treatment regimen.

4.5. Pharmaconutrition

Several studies have shown that specific nutrients when supplemented in quantities exceeding their nutritional role may affect the immune system, metabolism, and gastrointestinal structure and function. Such examples are some amino acids like glutamine, arginine and tryptophan [96], omega-3 PUFA [97], vitamin D [98], and curcumin [99].

Glutamine and arginine are thought to be immunomodulatory and could be involved in mediating responses to metabolic stress. Studies on animal models revealed that they improved biochemical and clinical parameters of chemical-induced colitis [100]. Histamine, a biogenic amine derived from the amino acid histidine, reduced symptoms of experimental immune-mediated colitis [101]. Similarly, threonine reduced features of colitis and enhanced intestinal mucus production, which in turn leads to better barrier function [102, 103]. Tryptophan, another essential amino acid, also possesses strong anti-inflammatory effect both by direct action on intestinal and immune system cells and indirectly serves as a precursor for serotonin and melatonin [103]. A detailed review on the effects of specific amino acids on intestinal inflammation can be found elsewhere [96]. Although these amino acids may have some positive effect in IBD patients, their efficacy has not been adequately studied yet.

Omega-3 PUFA negatively affects intestinal inflammation through several mechanisms. [97]. They can act as a substrate for anti-inflammatory eicosanoid production, as well as a substrate for the synthesis of resolvins, maresins, and protectins, engaged in resolution of inflammatory process. On the other hand, they reduce production of pro-inflammatory cytokines such as TNF-α, decrease expression of adhesion molecules and possess antioxidative and chemoprotective properties. The results of clinical trials using omega-3 PUFA in patients with either CD or UC were inconsistent. Cochrane review, considering the use of omega-3 PUFA for maintenance treatment published in 2011, revealed a small but significant benefit in CD, but not in UC patients [104].

Besides its role in calcium metabolism and bone mineralization, vitamin D is regarded as an important anti-inflammatory agent. It regulates immune cells trafficking and differentiation, intestinal permeability, and antimicrobial peptide synthesis [98]. Several studies revealed an inverse association between serum concentration of 25-hydroxy-vitamin D and mucosal inflammation in IBD patients [105, 106]. Therefore, supplementation in IBD patients with low serum level of vitamin D seems mandatory. In a randomized controlled trial, a maintenance dose of 1200 IU/day, regardless of vitamin D status at entry, reduced a relapse rate in patients with CD [107].

Curcumin is the active compound found in turmeric. It possesses anti-inflammatory, anti-oxidant, anticancer, and neuroprotective properties [99]. Several studies and systematic reviews reveal that supplementation with curcumin when provided simultaneously with medications is both effective and a safe option for maintenance treatment of UC [108, 109].

5. Conclusion

Nutritional intervention is an important part of the treatment in IBD patients. Goals of nutritional intervention exceed provision of energy, macronutrients, and micronutrients to ensure adequate nutritional status of the patients. Recognition of the ability of specific food ingredients to interfere with the disease mechanisms has led to the development of several therapeutic approaches based on a diet modification. However, only the effectiveness of exclusive enteral nutrition in active CD has been proven enough to find place in different international therapeutic guidelines. As this kind of diet is difficult to keep for a prolonged period of time, other potential options such as partial enteral nutrition and restriction or even exclusion of potentially harmful foods with simultaneous increased intake of food ingredients that potentially interfere with different pathologic mechanisms seem extremely promising. However, we need to confirm the efficacy and safety of these novel dietary approaches more firmly before recommending their routine use in an everyday clinical practice.

Author details

Rok Orel[1*], Evgen Benedik[1], Janez Eržen[1], Anija Orel[2] and Darja Urlep[1]

*Address all correspondence to: rok.orel@kclj.si

1 University Children's Hospital, University Medical Centre Ljubljana, Ljubljana, Slovenia

2 Clinical Nutrition Unit, Institute of Oncology Ljubljana, Ljubljana, Slovenia

References

[1] Bernstein CN. Review article: Changes in the epidemiology of inflammatory bowel disease—Clues for aetiology. Alimentary Pharmacology & Therapeutics. 2017;**46**:911-919. DOI: 10.1111/apt.14338

[2] Walker DG, Williams HRT, Kane SP, Mawdsley JE, Arnold J, McNeil I, et al. Differences in inflammatory bowel disease phenotype between south Asians and northern Europeans living in north West London, UK. The American Journal of Gastroenterology. 2011;**106**:1281-1289. DOI: 10.1038/ajg.2011.85

[3] Li X, Sundquist J, Hemminki K, Sundquist K. Risk of inflammatory bowel disease in first- and second-generation immigrants in Sweden: A nationwide follow-up study. Inflammatory Bowel Diseases. 2011;**17**:1784-1791. DOI: 10.1002/ibd.21535

[4] Dutta AK, Chacko A. Inflammatory Bowel Disease: Global view influence of environmental factors on the onset and course of inflammatory bowel disease. World Journal of Gastroenterology. 2016;**22**:1088-1100. DOI: 10.3748/wjg.v22.i3.1088

[5] Abegunde AT, Muhammad BH, Bhatti O, Ali T. Environmental risk factors for inflammatory bowel diseases: Evidence based literature review. World Journal of Gastroenterology. 2016;**22**:6296-6317. DOI: 10.3748/wjg.v22.i27.6296

[6] De Filippo C, Cavalieri D, Di Paola M, Ramazzotti M, Poullet JB, Massart S, et al. Impact of diet in shaping gut microbiota revealed by a comparative study in children from Europe and rural Africa. Proceedings of the National Academy of Sciences. 2010;**107**:14691-14696. DOI: 10.1073/pnas.1005963107

[7] Turnbaugh PJ, Ridaura VK, Faith JJ, Rey FE, Knight R, Gordon JI. The effect of diet on the human gut Microbiom: A metagenomic analysis in humanized Gnotobiotic mice. Science Translational Medicine. 2009;**1**:1-19. DOI: 10.1126/scitranslmed.3000322.The

[8] Leone, VA Cham, CM Chang E. Diet, gut microbes, and genetics in immune function: Can we leverage our current knowledge to achieve better outcomes in inflammatory bowel diseases? Current Opinion in Immunology. 2014:16-23. DOI:10.1016/j.jnutbio.2013.01.006. Nutritional

[9] Benno Y, Suzuki K, Suzuki K, Narisawa K, Bruce WR, Mitsuoka T. Comparison of the fecal microflora in rural Japanese and urban Canadians. Microbiology and Immunology. 1986;**30**:521-532. DOI: 10.1111/j.1348-0421.1986.tb02978.x

[10] David LA, Maurice CF, Carmody RN, Gootenberg DB, Button JE, Wolfe BE, et al. Diet rapidly and reproducibly alters the human gut microbiome. Nature. 2014;**505**:559-563. DOI: 10.1038/nature12820.Diet

[11] Tjonneland A, Overvad K, Bergmann M, Nagel G, Linseisen J, Hallmans G, et al. Linoleic acid, a dietary n-6 polyunsaturated fatty acid, and the aetiology of ulcerative colitis: A nested case-control study within a European prospective cohort study. Gut. 2009;**58**:1606-1611. DOI: 10.1136/gut.2008.169078

[12] Ananthakrishnan AN, Khalili H, Konijeti GG, Higuchi LM, de Silva P, Fuchs CS, et al. Long-term intake of dietary fat and risk of ulcerative colitis and Crohn's disease. Gut. 2014;**63**:776-784. DOI:10.1136/gutjnl-2013-305304

[13] Hou JK, Abraham B, El-Serag H. Dietary intake and risk of developing inflammatory bowel disease: A systematic review of the literature. The American Journal of Gastroenterology. 2011;**106**:563-573. DOI: 10.1038/ajg.2011.44

[14] Amre DK, D'Souza S, Morgan K, Seidman G, Lambrette P, Grimard G, et al. Imbalances in dietary consumption of fatty acids, vegetables, and fruits are associated with risk for Crohn's disease in children. The American Journal of Gastroenterology. 2007;**102**:2016-2025. DOI: 10.1111/j.1572-0241.2007.01411.x

[15] Akabas SR, Deckelbaum RJ. Summary of a workshop on n-3 fatty acids: Current status of recommendations and future directions. The American Journal of Clinical Nutrition. 2006;**83**:1536S-1538S

[16] Jantchou P, Morois S, Clavel-Chapelon F, Boutron-Ruault M-C, Carbonnel F. Animal protein intake and risk of inflammatory bowel disease: The E3N prospective study. The American Journal of Gastroenterology. 2010;**105**:2195-2201. DOI: 10.1038/ajg.2010.192

[17] Wagner SJ, Schmidt A, Effenberger MJP, Gruber L, Danier J, Haller D. Semisynthetic diet ameliorates Crohn's disease-like ileitis in TNFDeltaARE/WT mice through antigen-independent mechanisms of gluten. Inflammatory Bowel Diseases. 2013;**19**:1285-1294. DOI: 10.1097/MIB.0b013e318281f573

[18] Lammers KM. Lu R, Brownley J, Lu B, Gerard C, Rallabhandi P, et al. gliadin induces an increase in intestinal permeability and zonulin release by binding to the chemokine receptor CXCR3. Gastroenterology. 2009;**135**:194-204. DOI: 10.1053/j.gastro.2008.03.023. Gliadin

[19] Fasano A. Zonulin, regulation of tight junctions, and autoimmune diseases. Annals of the New York Academy of Sciences. 2012;**1258**:25-33. DOI: 10.1111/j.1749-6632.2012.06538.x

[20] Hollon J, Puppa EL, Greenwald B, Goldberg E, Guerrerio A, Fasano A. Effect of gliadin on permeability of intestinal biopsy explants from celiac disease patients and patients with non-celiac gluten sensitivity. Nutrients. 2015;**7**:1565-1576. DOI: 10.3390/nu7031565

[21] Spooren CEGM, Pierik MJ, Zeegers MP, Feskens EJM, Masclee AAM, Jonkers DMAE. Review article: The association of diet with onset and relapse in patients with inflammatory bowel disease. Alimentary Pharmacology & Therapeutics. 2013;**38**:1172-1187. DOI: 10.1111/apt.12501

[22] Lee D, Baldassano RN, Otley AR, Albenberg L, Griffiths AM, Compher C, et al. Comparative effectiveness of nutritional and biological therapy in north American children with active Crohn's disease. Inflammatory Bowel Diseases. 2015;**21**:1786-1793. DOI: 10.1097/MIB.0000000000000426

[23] Ananthakrishnan AN, Khalili H, Konijeti GG, Higuchi LM, de Silva P, Korzenik JR, et al. A prospective study of long-term intake of dietary fiber and risk of Crohn's disease and ulcerative colitis. Gastroenterology. 2013;**145**:970-977. DOI:10.1053/j.gastro.2013.07.050

[24] D'Souza S, Levy E, Mack D, Israel D, Lambrette P, Ghadirian P, et al. Dietary patterns and risk for Crohn's disease in children. Inflammatory Bowel Diseases. 2008;**14**:367-373. DOI: 10.1002/ibd.20333

[25] Nanau RM, Neuman MG. Nutritional and probiotic supplementation in colitis models. Digestive Diseases and Sciences. 2012;**57**:2786-2810. DOI: 10.1007/s10620-012-2284-3

[26] Galvez J, Rodriguez-Cabezas ME, Zarzuelo A. Effects of dietary fiber on inflammatory bowel disease. Molecular Nutrition & Food Research. 2005;**49**:601-608. DOI: 10.1002/mnfr.200500013

[27] Andoh A, Tsujikawa T, Fujiyama Y. Role of dietary fiber and short-chain fatty acids in the colon. Current Pharmaceutical Design. 2003;**9**:347-358

[28] Monteleone I, Pallone F, Monteleone G. Aryl hydrocarbon receptor and colitis. Seminars in Immunopathology. 2013;**35**:671-675. DOI: 10.1007/s00281-013-0396-2

[29] Sarbagili-Shabat C, Sigall-Boneh R, Levine A. Nutritional therapy in inflammatory bowel disease. Current Opinion in Gastroenterology. 2015;**31**:303-308. DOI: 10.1097/MOG.0000000000000178

[30] Chassaing B, Koren O, Goodrich JK, Poole AC, Srinivasan S, Ley RE, et al. Dietary emulsifiers impact the mouse gut microbiota promoting colitis and metabolic syndrome. Nature. 2015;**519**:92-96

[31] Nickerson KP, McDonald C. Crohn's disease-associated adherent-invasive Escherichia Coli adhesion is enhanced by exposure to the ubiquitous dietary polysaccharide maltodextrin. PLoS One. 2012;**7**:e52132

[32] Rahman K, Sasaki M, Nusrat A, Klapproth J-MA. Crohn's disease–associated Escherichia Coli survive in macrophages by suppressing NFκB signaling. Inflammatory Bowel Diseases. 2014;**20**:1419-1425. DOI: 10.1097/MIB.0000000000000096

[33] Tawfik A, Flanagan PK, Escherichia CBJ. Coli-host macrophage interactions in the pathogenesis of inflammatory bowel disease. World Journal of Gastroenterology. 2014;**20**:8751-8763. DOI: 10.3748/wjg.v20.i27.8751

[34] Weisshof R, Chermesh I. Micronutrient deficiencies in inflammatory bowel disease. Current Opinion in Clinical Nutrition and Metabolic Care. 2015;**18**:576-581. DOI: 10.1097/MCO.0000000000000226

[35] Rocha R, Santana GO, Almeida N, Lyra AC. Analysis of fat and muscle mass in patients with inflammatory bowel disease during remission and active phase. The British Journal of Nutrition. 2009;**101**:676-679. DOI: 10.1017/S0007114508032224

[36] Wiskin AE, Wootton SA, Hunt TM, Cornelius VR, Afzal NA, Jackson AA, et al. Body composition in childhood inflammatory bowel disease. Clinical Nutrition. 2011;**30**:112-115. DOI: 10.1016/j.clnu.2010.07.014

[37] Scaldaferri F, Pizzoferrato M, Lopetuso LR, Musca T, Ingravalle F, Sicignano LL, et al. Nutrition and IBD: Malnutrition and/or sarcopenia? A practical guide. Gastroenterology Research and Practice. 2017;**2017**. DOI: 10.1155/2017/8646495

[38] Hebuterne X, Filippi J, Al-Jaouni R, Nutritional SS. Consequences and nutrition therapy in Crohn's disease. Gastroentérologie Clinique et Biologique. 2009;**33**(Suppl 3):S235-S244. DOI: 10.1016/S0399-8320(09)73159-8

[39] Lucendo AJ, De Rezende LC. Importance of nutrition in inflammatory bowel disease. World Journal of Gastroenterology. 2009;**15**:2081-2088. DOI: 10.3748/wjg.15.2081

[40] Urbano APS, Sassaki LY, Dorna MS, Carvalhaes MA de BL, Martini LA, Ferreira ALA. Nutritional intake according to injury extent in ulcerative colitis patients. Journal of Human Nutrition and Dietetics. 2013;**26**:445-451. DOI: 10.1111/jhn.12064

[41] Ghishan FK, Epithelial KPR. Transport in inflammatory bowel diseases. Inflammatory Bowel Diseases. 2014;**20**:1099-1109. DOI: 10.1097/MIB.0000000000000029

[42] Hwang C, Ross V, Mahadevan U. Micronutrient deficiencies in inflammatory bowel disease: From a to zinc. Inflammatory Bowel Diseases. 2012;**18**:1961-1981. DOI: 10.1002/ibd.22906

[43] Capristo E, Addolorato G, Mingrone G, Greco AV, Gasbarrini G. Effect of disease localization on the anthropometric and metabolic features of Crohn's disease. The American Journal of Gastroenterology. 1998;**93**:2411-2419. DOI: 10.1111/j.1572-0241.1998.00696.x

[44] Santilli V, Bernetti A, Mangone M, Clinical PM. Definition of sarcopenia. Clinical Cases in Mineral and Bone Metabolism. 2014;**11**:177-180

[45] Bryant RV, Trott MJ, Bartholomeusz FD, Andrews JM. Systematic review: Body composition in adults with inflammatory bowel disease. Alimentary Pharmacology & Therapeutics. 2013;**38**:213-225. DOI: 10.1111/apt.12372

[46] Flores A, Burstein E, Cipher DJ, Feagins LA. Obesity in inflammatory bowel disease: A marker of less severe disease. Digestive Diseases and Sciences. 2015;**60**:2436-2445. DOI: 10.1007/s10620-015-3629-5

[47] Seminerio JL, Koutroubakis IE, Ramos-Rivers C, Hashash JG, Dudekula A, Regueiro M, et al. Impact of obesity on the management and clinical course of patients with inflammatory bowel disease. Inflammatory Bowel Diseases. 2015;**21**:2857-2863. DOI: 10.1097/MIB.0000000000000560

[48] Dignass AU, Gasche C, Bettenworth D, Birgegard G, Danese S, Gisbert JP, et al. European consensus on the diagnosis and management of iron deficiency and anaemia in inflammatory bowel diseases. Journal of Crohn's & Colitis. 2015;**9**:211-222. DOI: 10.1093/ecco-jcc/jju009

[49] Bermejo F, Algaba A, Guerra I, Chaparro M, De-La-Poza G, Valer P, et al. Should we monitor vitamin B12 and folate levels in Crohn's disease patients? Scandinavian Journal of Gastroenterology. 2013;**48**:1272-1277. DOI: 10.3109/00365521.2013.836752

[50] Yakut M, Ustun Y, Kabacam G, Soykan I. Serum vitamin B12 and folate status in patients with inflammatory bowel diseases. European Journal of Internal Medicine. 2010;**21**:320-323. DOI: 10.1016/j.ejim.2010.05.007

[51] Alves RA, Miszputen SJ, Figueiredo MS. Anemia in inflammatory bowel disease: Prevalence, differential diagnosis and association with clinical and laboratory variables. São Paulo Medical Journal. 2014;**132**:140-146

[52] Ananthakrishnan AN, Khalili H, Higuchi LM, Bao Y, Korzenik JR, Giovannucci EL, et al. Higher predicted vitamin D status is associated with reduced risk of Crohn's disease. Gastroenterology. 2012;**142**:482-489. DOI: 10.1053/j.gastro.2011.11.040

[53] Kong J, Zhang Z, Musch MW, Ning G, Sun J, Hart J, et al. Novel role of the vitamin D receptor in maintaining the integrity of the intestinal mucosal barrier. American Journal of Physiology. Gastrointestinal and Liver Physiology. 2008;**294**:G208-G216. DOI: 10.1152/ajpgi.00398.2007

[54] Levine A, Turner D, Pfeffer Gik T, Amil Dias J, Veres G, Shaoul R, et al. Comparison of outcomes parameters for induction of remission in new onset pediatric Crohn's disease. Inflammatory Bowel Diseases. 2014;**20**:278-285. DOI: 10.1097/01.MIB.0000437735.11953.68

[55] Lochs H, Forbes A. Nutritional Support in inflammatory bowel disease. In: Sobotka L, editor. Basics of Clinical Nutrition. 4th Ed., Prague: ESPEN. Publishing House Galen; 2011, p. 458-466

[56] Royall D, Greenberg GR, Allard JP, Baker JP, Harrison JE, Jeejeebhoy KN. Critical assessment of body-composition measurements in malnourished subjects with Crohn's disease: The role of bioelectric impedance analysis. The American Journal of Clinical Nutrition. 1994;**59**:325-330

[57] Vidarsdottir JB, Johannsdottir SE, Thorsdottir I, Bjornsson E, Ramel AA. Cross-sectional study on nutrient intake and -status in inflammatory bowel disease patients. Nutrition Journal. 2016;**15**:61. DOI: 10.1186/s12937-016-0178-5

[58] Ruemmele FMM, Veres G, Kolho KLL, Griffiths A, Levine A, Escher JCC, et al. Consensus guidelines of ECCO/ESPGHAN on the medical management of pediatric Crohn's disease. Journal of Crohn's & Colitis. 2014;**8**:1179-1207. DOI: 10.1016/j.crohns.2014.04.005

[59] Day AS, Lopez RN. Exclusive enteral nutrition in children with Crohn's disease. World Journal of Gastroenterology. 2015;**21**:6809-6816. DOI: 10.3748/wjg.v21.i22.6809

[60] Otley AR, Russell RK, Day AS. Nutritional therapy for the treatment of pediatric Crohn's disease. Expert Review of Clinical Immunology. 2010;**6**:667-676. DOI: 10.1586/eci.10.37

[61] Borrelli O, Cordischi L, Cirulli M, Paganelli M, Labalestra V, Uccini S, et al. Polymeric diet alone versus corticosteroids in the treatment of active pediatric Crohn's disease: A randomized controlled open-label trial. Clinical Gastroenterology and Hepatology. 2006;**4**:744-753. DOI: 10.1016/j.cgh.2006.03.010

[62] Zachos M, Tondeur M, Griffiths AM. Enteral nutritional therapy for induction of remission in Crohn's disease. In: Zachos M, editor. Cochrane Database of Systematic Reviews, Chichester, UK: John Wiley & Sons, Ltd; 2007, p. CD000542. DOI:10.1002/14651858.CD000542.pub2

[63] Yamamoto T, Nakahigashi M, Saniabadi AR. Review article : Diet and inflammatory bowel disease – Epidemiology and treatment. Alimentary Pharmacology & Therapeutics. 2009;**30**:99-112. DOI: 10.1111/j.1365-2036.2009.04035.x

[64] Malchow H, Steinhardt HJ, Lorenz-Meyer H, Strohm WD, Rasmussen S, Sommer H, et al. Feasibility and effectiveness of a defined-formula diet regimen in treating active Crohn's disease. European cooperative Crohn's disease study III. Scandinavian Journal of Gastroenterology. 1990;**25**:235-244

[65] Griffiths AM, Ohlsson A, Sherman PM, Sutherland LR. Meta-analysis of enteral nutrition as a primary treatment of active Crohn's disease. Gastroenterology. 1995;**108**:1056-1067

[66] Jackson CA, Clatworthy J, Robinson A, Horne R. Factors associated with non-adherence to oral medication for inflammatory bowel disease: A systematic review. The American Journal of Gastroenterology. 2010;**105**:525-539. DOI: 10.1038/ajg.2009.685

[67] Johnson T, Macdonald S, Hill SM, Thomas A, Murphy MS. Treatment of active Crohn's disease in children using partial enteral nutrition with liquid formula: A randomised controlled trial. Gut. 2006;**55**:356-361. DOI: 10.1136/gut.2004.062554

[68] Sigall-Boneh R, Pfeffer-Gik T, Segal I, Zangen T, Boaz M, Levine A. Partial enteral nutrition with a Crohn's disease exclusion diet is effective for induction of remission in children and young adults with Crohn's disease. Inflammatory Bowel Diseases. 2014;**20**:1353-1360. DOI: 10.1097/MIB.0000000000000110

[69] Gupta K, Noble A, Kachelries KE, Albenberg L, Kelsen JR, Grossman AB, et al. A novel enteral nutrition protocol for the treatment of pediatric Crohn's disease. Inflammatory Bowel Diseases. 2013;**19**:1374-1378

[70] Akobeng AK, Thomas AG. Enteral nutrition for maintenance of remission in Crohn's disease. In: Akobeng AK, editor. Cochrane Database of Systematic Reviews, Chichester, UK: John Wiley & Sons, Ltd; 2007, p. CD005984. DOI:10.1002/14651858.CD005984.pub2

[71] Nakahigashi M, Yamamoto T, Sacco R, Hanai H, Enteral KF. Nutrition for maintaining remission in patients with quiescent Crohn's disease: Current status and future perspectives. International Journal of Colorectal Disease. 2016;**31**:1-7. DOI: 10.1007/s00384-015-2348-x

[72] El-Matary W, Otley A, Critch J, Abou-Setta AM. Enteral feeding therapy for maintaining remission in Crohn's disease: A systematic review. Journal of Parenteral and Enteral Nutrition. 2017;**41**:550-561. DOI: 10.1177/0148607115621051

[73] Wilschanski M, Sherman P, Pencharz P, Davis L, Corey M, Griffiths A. Supplementary enteral nutrition maintains remission in paediatric Crohn's disease. Gut. 1996;**38**:543-548

[74] Scolapio JS. The role of total parenteral nutrition in the management of patients with acute attacks of inflammatory bowel disease. Journal of Clinical Gastroenterology. 1999;**29**:223-224

[75] Goh J, C a O'M. Nutrition and adult inflammatory bowel disease. Alimentary Pharmacology & Therapeutics. 2003;**17**:307-320. DOI: 10.1046/j.1365-2036.2003.01482.x

[76] Richman E, Rhodes JM. Review article: Evidence-based dietary advice for patients with inflammatory bowel disease. Alimentary Pharmacology & Therapeutics. 2013;**38**:1156-1171. DOI: 10.1111/apt.12500

[77] Forbes A, Escher J, Hebuterne X, Klek S, Krznaric Z, Schneider S, et al. ESPEN guideline: Clinical nutrition in inflammatory bowel disease. Clinical Nutrition. 2017;**36**:321-347. DOI: 10.1016/j.clnu.2016.12.027

[78] Owczarek D, Rodacki T, Domagała-rodacka R, Cibor D, Mach T, Owczarek D, et al. Diet and nutritional factors in inflammatory bowel diseases. World Journal of Gastroenterology. 2016;**22**:895-905. DOI: 10.3748/wjg.v22.i3.895

[79] Vanhauwaert E, Matthys C, Verdonck L, De Preter V. Low-residue and low-fiber diets in gastrointestinal disease management. Advances in Nutrition: An International Review Journal. 2015;**6**:820-827. DOI: 10.3945/an.115.009688

[80] Levenstein S, Prantera C, Luzi C, D'Ubaldi A. Low residue or normal diet in Crohn's disease: A prospective controlled study in Italian patients. Gut. 1985;**26**:989-993. DOI: 10.1136/gut.26.10.989

[81] Hoekman DR, Zeevenhooven J, D'Haens GR, Benninga MA. The prevalence of irritable bowel syndrome-type symptoms in inflammatory bowel disease patients in remission. European Journal of Gastroenterology & Hepatology. 2017;**29**:1086-1090. DOI: 10.1097/MEG.0000000000000921

[82] Prince AC, Myers CE, Joyce T, Irving P, Lomer M, Whelan K. Fermentable carbohydrate restriction (low FODMAP diet) in clinical practice improves functional gastrointestinal symptoms in patients with inflammatory bowel disease. Inflammatory Bowel Diseases. 2016;**22**:1129-1136. DOI: 10.1097/MIB.0000000000000708

[83] Brotherton CS, Taylor AG, Bourguignon C, Anderson JG. A high-fiber diet may improve bowel function and health-related quality of life in patients with Crohn disease. Gastroenterology Nursing. 2014;**37**:206-216. DOI: 10.1097/SGA.0000000000000047

[84] Hallert C, Bjorck I, Nyman M, Pousette A, Granno C, Svensson H. Increasing fecal butyrate in ulcerative colitis patients by diet: Controlled pilot study. Inflammatory Bowel Diseases. 2003;**9**:116-121

[85] Hallert C, Kaldma M, Petersson BG. Ispaghula husk may relieve gastrointestinal symptoms in ulcerative colitis in remission. Scandinavian Journal of Gastroenterology. 1991;**26**:747-750. DOI: 10.3109/00365529108998594

[86] Fernandez-Banares F, Hinojosa J, Sanchez-Lombrana JL, Navarro E, Martinez-Salmeron JF, Garcia-Puges A, et al. Randomized clinical trial of Plantago Ovata seeds (dietary fiber) as compared with mesalamine in maintaining remission in ulcerative colitis. Spanish Group for the Study of Crohn's Disease and Ulcerative Colitis (GETECCU). The American Journal of Gastroenterology. 1999;**94**:427-433. DOI: 10.1111/j.1572-0241.1999.872_a.x

[87] Hanai H, Kanauchi O, Mitsuyama K, Andoh A, Takeuchi K, Takayuki I, et al. Germinated barley foodstuff prolongs remission in patients with ulcerative colitis. International Journal of Molecular Medicine. 2004;**13**:643-647

[88] Faghfoori Z, Shakerhosseini R, Navai L, Somi MH, Nikniaz Z, Abadi A. Effects of an oral supplementation of germinated barley foodstuff on serum CRP level and clinical signs in patients with ulcerative colitis. Health Promotion Perspectives. 2014;**4**:116-121. DOI: 10.5681/hpp.2014.015

[89] Faghfoori Z, Navai L, Shakerhosseini R, Somi MH, Nikniaz Z, Norouzi MF. Effects of an oral supplementation of germinated barley foodstuff on serum tumour necrosis factor-alpha, interleukin-6 and -8 in patients with ulcerative colitis. Annals of Clinical Biochemistry. 2011;**48**:233-237. DOI: 10.1258/acb.2010.010093

[90] Haas S. The value of the banana in the treatment of celiac disease. American Journal of Diseases of Children. 1924;**28**:421-437

[91] Cohen SA, Gold BD, Oliva S, Lewis J, Stallworth A, Koch B, et al. Clinical and mucosal improvement with specific carbohydrate diet in pediatric Crohn disease. Journal of Pediatric Gastroenterology and Nutrition. 2014;**59**:516-521. DOI: 10.1097/MPG.0000000000000449

[92] Has S, Haas M. The treatment of celiac disease with the specific carbohydrate diet; report on 191 additional cases. The American Journal of Gastroenterology. 1955;**23**:344-360

[93] Suskind DL, Wahbeh G, Gregory N, Vendettuoli H, Christie D. Nutritional therapy in pediatric Crohn disease: The specific carbohydrate diet. Journal of Pediatric Gastroenterology and Nutrition. 2014;**58**:87-91. DOI: 10.1097/MPG.0000000000000103

[94] Wahbeh GT, Ward BT, Lee DY, Giefer MJ, Suskind DL. Lack of mucosal healing from modified specific carbohydrate diet in pediatric patients with Crohn disease. Journal of Pediatric Gastroenterology and Nutrition. 2017;**65**:289-292. DOI: 10.1097/MPG.0000000000001619

[95] Olendzki BC, Silverstein TD, Persuitte GM, Ma Y, Baldwin KR, An CD. Anti-inflammatory diet as treatment for inflammatory bowel disease: A case series report. Nutrition Journal. 2014;**13**:1-7. DOI: 10.1186/1475-2891-13-5

[96] Bao X, Feng Z, Yao J, Li T, Yin Y. Roles Of dietary amino acids and their metabolites in pathogenesis of inflammatory bowel disease. Mediators of Inflammation. 2017;2017:6869259. DOI:10.1155/2017/6869259

[97] Barbalho SM. Goulart R de a, Quesada K, Bechara MD, de Carvalho a de CA. Inflammatory bowel disease: Can omega-3 fatty acids really help? Ann Gastroenterol Q Publ Hell Soc Gastroenterol. 2016;**29**:37-43

[98] Meeker S, Seamons A, Maggio-Price L, Paik J. Protective links between vitamin D, inflammatory bowel disease and colon cancer. World Journal of Gastroenterology. 2016;**22**:933-948. DOI: 10.3748/wjg.v22.i3.933

[99] Vecchi Brumatti L, Marcuzzi A, Tricarico PM, Zanin V, Girardelli M, Bianco AM. Curcumin and inflammatory bowel disease: Potential and limits of innovative treatments. Molecules. 2014;**19**:21127-21153. DOI: 10.3390/molecules191221127

[100] Coëffier M, Marion-Letellier R, Potential DP. For amino acids supplementation during inflammatory bowel diseases. Inflammatory Bowel Diseases. 2010;**16**:518-524. DOI: 10.1002/ibd.21017

[101] Andou A, Hisamatsu T, Okamoto S, Chinen H, Kamada N, Kobayashi T, et al. Dietary histidine ameliorates murine colitis by inhibition of proinflammatory cytokine production from macrophages. Gastroenterology. 2009;**136**:564-74.e2. DOI:10.1053/j.gastro.2008.09.062

[102] Lee D, Albenberg L, Compher C, Baldassano R, Piccoli D, Lewis JD, et al. HHS public. Access. 2016;**148**:1087-1106. DOI: 10.1053/j.gastro.2015.01.007.Diet

[103] Kim CJ, Kovacs-Nolan JA, Yang C, Archbold T, Fan MZ, Mine Y. L-tryptophan exhibits therapeutic function in a porcine model of dextran sodium sulfate (DSS)-induced colitis. The Journal of Nutritional Biochemistry. 2010;**21**:468-475. DOI: 10.1016/j.jnutbio.2009.01.019

[104] Turner D, Zlotkin S, Shah P, Griffiths A. Omega 3 fatty acids (fish oil) for maintenance of remission in Crohn's disease. In: Turner D, editor. Cochrane Database of Systematic Reviews, Chichester, UK: John Wiley & Sons, Ltd; 2007, p. CD006320. DOI:10.1002/14651858.CD006320.pub2

[105] Meckel K, Li YC, Lim J, Kocherginsky M, Weber C, Almoghrabi A, et al. Serum 25-hydroxyvitamin D concentration is inversely associated with mucosal inflammation in patients with ulcerative colitis. The American Journal of Clinical Nutrition. 2016;**104**:113-120. DOI: 10.3945/ajcn.115.123786

[106] Raftery T, Merrick M, Healy M, Mahmud N, O'Morain C, Smith S, et al. Vitamin D status is associated with intestinal inflammation as measured by fecal calprotectin in Crohn's disease in clinical remission. Digestive Diseases and Sciences. 2015;**60**:2427-2435. DOI: 10.1007/s10620-015-3620-1

[107] Jorgensen SP, Agnholt J, Glerup H, Lyhne S, Villadsen GE, Hvas CL, et al. Clinical trial: Vitamin D3 treatment in Crohn's disease - A randomized double-blind placebo-controlled study. Alimentary Pharmacology & Therapeutics. 2010;**32**:377-383. DOI: 10.1111/j.1365-2036.2010.04355.x

[108] Kumar S, Ahuja V, Sankar MJ, Kumar A, Moss AC. Curcumin For maintenance of remission in ulcerative colitis. Cochrane Database of Systematic Reviews. 2012;**10**:CD008424. DOI:10.1002/14651858.CD008424.pub2

[109] Taylor RA, Curcumin LMC. For inflammatory bowel disease: A review of human studies. Alternative Medicine Review. 2011;**16**:152-156

14

Delayed Appendectomy is Safe in Patients with Acute Nonperforated Appendicitis

Sung Il Choi

Abstract

Objective: The present study examined whether acute nonperforated appendicitis is a surgical emergency requiring immediate intervention or a disease that can be treated with a semielective operation.

Summary of background data: Immediate appendectomy has been the gold standard in the treatment of acute appendicitis because of the risk of pathological progression. However, this time-honored practice has been recently challenged by studies suggesting that appendectomies can be elective in some cases and still result in positive outcomes.

Methods: This was a retrospective study using the charts of patients who underwent an appendectomy for acute appendicitis between January 2007 and February 2012. Patients were divided into two groups for comparison: an immediate group (those who were moved to an operating room within 12 hours after hospital arrival) and a delayed group (those who were moved to an operating room within 12 to 24 hours after hospital arrival). The end points were conversion rate, operative time, perforation rate, complication rate, readmission rate, length of hospital stay, and medical costs.

Results: of 1805 patients, 1342 (74.3%) underwent immediate operation within 12 hours after hospital arrival, whereas 463 (25.7%) underwent delayed operation within 12–24 hours. There were no significant differences in open conversion, operative time, perforation, postoperative complications, and readmission between the two groups. Length of hospital stay was significantly greater (3.7 ± 1.7 days) and medical costs were also greater (2346.3 ± 735.3 US dollar) in the delayed group than in the immediate group (3.1 ± 1.9 days, $p = 0.000$ and 2257.8 ± 723.8 US dollar, $p = 0.026$).

Conclusions: delayed appendectomy is safe for patients with acute nonperforated appendicitis.

Keywords: appendicitis, appendectomy, delay, complications, treatment outcome, safety

1. Introduction

Acute appendicitis is one of the most common acute diseases requiring an emergency operation. Immediate appendectomy is considered the gold-standard treatment for acute appendicitis. It is widely believed that delays in diagnosis and treatment significantly contribute to increased incidences of perforated appendicitis, which result in increased patient morbidity [1]. Nevertheless, in some cases, the appropriate operation has been delayed because of reasons such as lack of fasting time for general anesthesia, unavailability of operating rooms, and overscheduling of operating teams. Recently, some studies have challenged the impact of these delays and standard of care with appendectomy by suggesting that acute appendicitis can either be treated medically [2, 3] or operated on electively without increasing morbidity [4–7]. Given these considerations, we used electronic medical records to review 1805 cases of appendectomy for acute appendicitis between January 2007 and February 2012 to verify whether acute nonperforated appendicitis necessitates immediate intervention or can be treated with a semielective operation.

2. Methods

2.1. Patients

A retrospective review of the charts of all patients who underwent an appendectomy for acute appendicitis at Kyung Hee University Hospital at Gangdong from January 2007 to February 2012 was performed. Diagnosis of acute non-perforated appendicitis was based on a doctor's decision after considering clinical manifestation, physical examination, laboratory findings, and radiologic modalities. Patients who were preoperatively diagnosed with perforated appendicitis, underwent interval appendectomy or negative appendectomy, or underwent an operation after consulting with other departments were excluded from analysis. Antibiotics such as cephalosporin were administered as soon as possible after diagnosis and were continued until patient discharge. Nowadays, we just give one injection of antibiotics just before surgery. In the case of severe wound complications, we have used antibiotics even if it did not follow guidelines. The data for the following parameters were gathered from electronic medical records: demographic characteristics (age, sex), body mass index (BMI), American Society of Anesthesiologists (ASA) score, white blood cell (WBC) count at admission, body temperature at admission, time from onset of symptoms to hospital arrival (patient interval), time from hospital arrival to the operating room (hospital interval), radiologic findings according to diagnostic modalities, methods of surgery, operative time, and final pathology. The patients were divided into two comparison groups: immediate group (those with a hospital interval ≤12 hours) and delayed group (those with a hospital interval from 12 to 24 hours). The end points chosen for comparison were safety-related outcomes: laparoscopic to open conversion rate, operative time, perforation rate, complication rate, and readmission rate; economy-related outcomes: length of hospital stay and medical cost; and accuracy of diagnostic modalities for distinguishing the difference between nonperforated and perforated appendicitis.

2.2. Statistical analysis

Demographic and clinical characteristics were summarized as means (for continuous variables) or proportions (for categorical variables) and compared using *t* tests or χ^2 tests, respectively. A p value of less than 0.05 was considered statistically significant. All statistical analyses were performed using Statistical Package for Social Sciences (SPSS) software version 18.03 (SPSS Inc., Chicago, IL).

3. Results

3.1. Patient demographics

During the 5-year study period, 2093 patients underwent appendectomy for acute appendicitis. Of the 2093 patients, 288 patients were excluded from analysis because of perforated appendicitis in preoperative diagnosis, interval appendectomy, negative appendectomy, and operation after consultation from other departments. Among the 1805 patients included for analysis, 1342 (74.3%) underwent an appendectomy within 12 hours after hospital arrival

Variables	Immediate (n = 1342)	Delayed (n = 463)	p Value
Age (years ± SD)	31.4 ± 18.2	32.8 ± 16.9	0.144
Sex			0.440
Male	761 (56.7)	253 (54.6)	
Female	581 (43.3)	210 (45.4)	
BMI (kg/m^2)	22.1 ± 4.1	22.5 ± 4.1	0.074
ASA score			0.329
1	355 (27.3)	114 (25.1)	
2	922 (70.9)	331 (72.9)	
3	18 (1.4)	7 (1.5)	
4	2 (0.2)	0 (0)	
5	2 (0.2)	2 (0.4)	
Patient interval (hours)[a]	27.8 ± 33.4	27.2 ± 44.2	0.737
WBC (10^3/dL)	13.1 ± 4.6	12.9 ± 4.2	0.495
Body temperature (°C)	36.6 ± 0.6	36.7 ± 0.5	0.001

Values are presented as number (%) unless otherwise indicated.

SD, standard deviation; BMI, body mass index; ASA, American society of anesthesiologists; WBC, white blood cell; dL, deciliter; °C, centigrade.

[a]Time from onset of symptoms to arrival at hospital.

Table 1. Patient characteristics.

(immediate group) and 463 (25.7%) underwent an appendectomy from 12 to 24 hours after hospital arrival (delayed group). No patient underwent surgery more than 24 hours after hospital arrival. Patients were on average 31.7 ± 17.9 years old and predominantly male (1014/1805, 56.2%). On average, BMI (kg/m^2) was 22.2 ± 3.9, patient interval was 27.7 ± 36.4 hours, and WBC counts (10^3/dL) were 13.0 ± 4.5. No significant differences in age, sex, BMI, ASA score, patient interval, or WBC count were noted between the two groups. Body temperature was significantly different between the immediate group (36.6 ± 0.6°C) and delayed group (36.7 ± 0.5°C) ($p = 0.001$), but was considered clinically nonsignificant because body temperatures in both groups were within the normal range (**Table 1**).

3.2. Safety-related outcomes

There were no significant differences in the laparoscopic to open conversion rate (0.5% in the immediate group and 0.2% in the delayed group), operative time (45.8 ± 21.4 minutes in the immediate group and 46.0 ± 23.6 minutes in the delayed group), perforation rate based on final pathology (12.8% in the immediate group and 12.1% in the delayed group), postoperative complication rate (6.0% in the immediate group and 6.0% in the delayed group), and readmission rate (2.5% in the immediate group and 2.2% in the delayed group) between the two groups (**Table 2**).

Variables	Immediate (n = 1342)	Delayed (n = 463)	p Value
Operative procedure			
Laparoscopy	1266 (94.3)	443 (95.7)	0.267
Open	62 (4.6)	16 (3.5)	0.288
Open conversion	7 (0.5)	1 (0.2)	0.393
Cecectomy	7 (0.5)	3 (0.6)	0.752
Operative time (minute)	45.8 ± 21.4	46.0 ± 23.6	0.833
Postoperative diagnosis			0.687
Simple	1170 (87.2)	407 (87.9)	
Perforated	172 (12.8)	56 (12.1)	
Complications			
All	80 (6.0)	28 (6.0)	0.946
Wound infection	54 (4.0)	18 (3.9)	0.897
Intra-abdominal infection	23 (1.7)	7 (1.5)	0.769
Other[a]	3 (0.2)	3 (0.6)	0.180
Readmissions	33 (2.5)	10 (2.2)	0.716

Values are presented as number (%) unless otherwise indicated.
[a]Immediate; ileus (3), delayed; obstruction (2), mesenteric lymphadenitis (1).

Table 2. Safety-related outcomes.

3.3. Economy-related outcomes

Overall length of hospital stay was significantly greater in the delayed group (3.7 ± 1.7 days) than in the immediate group (3.1 ± 1.9 days) (p = 0.000). The difference in length of postoperative hospital stay, however, was nonsignificant between the two groups (3.0 ± 1.8 days in the immediate group and 2.9 ± 1.6 days in the delayed group) (**Table 3**). Total medical cost was 2346.3 ± 735.3 US dollar in the delayed group, slightly greater than the 2257.8 ± 723.8 US dollar in the immediate group (p = 0.000).

3.4. Accuracy of radiologic modalities

The sensitivity of computed tomography (CT) (probability of patients diagnosed with nonperforated appendicitis by CT among those diagnosed with nonperforated appendicitis by pathology) was 97.0% (879/906) and specificity of CT (probability of patients diagnosed with perforated appendicitis by CT among those diagnosed with perforated appendicitis by pathology) was 46.1% (125/271) in our data (**Table 4**). The false-positive rate of CT (probability of patients diagnosed

Variables	Immediate (n = 1342)	Delayed (n = 463)	p Value
LHS (days)[a]	3.1 ± 1.9	3.7 ± 1.7	0.000
Postoperative LHS (days)	3.0 ± 1.8	2.9 ± 1.6	0.622
Cost (US dollar)	2257.8 ± 723.8	2346.3 ± 735.3	0.000

[a]LHS, length of hospital stay.

Table 3. Economy-related outcomes.

Variables	Nonperforated in pathology	Perforated in pathology	All	
Nonperforated on CT	879	146	1025	85.8%[e] (879/1025)
	97.0%[a]	53.9%[c]		
Perforated on CT	27	125	152	82.2%[f] (125/152)
	3.0%[b]	46.1%[d]		
All	906	271	1117	

Values are presented as number unless otherwise indicated.

CT, computed tomography.

[a]Sensitivity; probability of patients diagnosed with nonperforated appendicitis by CT among those diagnosed with nonperforated appendicitis by pathology.

[b]False negative rate; 1-sensitivity.

[c]False positive rate; 1-specificity.

[d]Specificity; probability of patients diagnosed with perforated appendicitis by CT among those diagnosed with perforated appendicitis by pathology.

[e]Positive predictive value; probability of patients diagnosed with nonperforated appendicitis by pathology among those diagnosed with nonperforated appendicitis by CT.

[f]Negative predictive value; probability of patients diagnosed with perforated appendicitis by pathology among those diagnosed with perforated appendicitis by CT.

Table 4. Accuracy of computed tomography.

Variables	Nonperforated in pathology	Perforated in pathology	All	
Nonperforated on US	530	58	588	90.1%[e] (530/588)
	95.5%[a]	61.1%[c]		
Perforated on US	25	37	62	59.7%[f] (37/62)
	4.5%[b]	38.9%[d]		
All	555	95	650	

Values are presented as numbers unless otherwise indicated.

US, ultrasonography.

[a]Sensitivity; probability of patients diagnosed with nonperforated appendicitis by US among those diagnosed with nonperforated appendicitis by pathology.

[b]False negative rate; 1-sensitivity.

[c]False positive rate; 1-specificity.

[d]Specificity; probability of patients diagnosed with perforated appendicitis by US among those diagnosed with perforated appendicitis by pathology.

[e]Positive predictive value; probability of patients diagnosed with nonperforated appendicitis by pathology among those diagnosed with nonperforated appendicitis by US.

[f]Negative predictive value; probability of patients diagnosed with perforated appendicitis by pathology among those diagnosed with perforated appendicitis by US.

Table 5. Accuracy of ultrasonography.

with nonperforated appendicitis by CT among those diagnosed with perforated appendicitis by pathology) was as high as 53.9% (146/271). The sensitivity of ultrasonography (US) was 95.5% (530/555) and specificity of US was 38.9% (37/95) in our records (**Table 5**). The false-positive rate of US (probability of patients diagnosed with nonperforated appendicitis by US among those diagnosed with perforated appendicitis by pathology) was as high as 61.1% (58/95).

4. Discussion

The present study demonstrated that semielective appendectomies for patients with acute nonperforated appendicitis do not increase the morbidity (defined as open conversion rate, operative time, perforation rate, postoperative complication rate, and readmission rate) but do increase economic factors such as medical costs and length of hospital stay.

Our findings were consistent with those of several other studies that have not found increased rates of complications among patients with delayed appendectomy. In a study of 380 patients with acute appendicitis, Abou-Nukta et al. [5] demonstrated that an appendectomy delay of greater than 12 hours showed no significant increase in perforation rates, operative time, or length of hospital stay. In addition, Omundsen and Dennett [8] found that there were no differences in complication rates or length of postoperative hospital stay between patients who underwent appendectomy within 12 hours and from 12 to 24 hours after admission. Omundsen and Dennett's study of 345 appendectomies only showed an increase in morbidity when appendectomy was delayed more than 24 hours. Surana et al. [6] reported no difference in complication rates between patients undergoing appendectomy within 6 hours compared to 6 to 18 hours after admission in a study of 695 children with appendicitis. In a similar study of 126 pediatric patients with acute non-perforated appendicitis, Yardeni et al. [7] demonstrated that there were no significant increases in the complication rates or perforation rates when appendectomies were performed within 6, 6 to 12, or more than 12 hours after admission. In a population-based study that used a database of 32,782 patients and was the largest study supporting this semi-elective approach, Ingraham et al. [4] found that a delay in appendectomy was not associated with increased 30-day morbidity.

In contrast to these studies, several others continue to support the current standard of appendectomy as a standard emergency procedure. In 1081 adult patients with acute appendicitis, Ditillo et al. [9] found that the risk of developing advanced pathology and complications increased with time until appropriate treatments, suggesting that a delay in appendectomy was unsafe. Udgiri et al. [10] reported that the complication rates, lengths of hospital stay, and readmissions were greater in a delayed appendectomy group (performed more than 10 hours after admission) than in an immediate appendectomy group (performed less than 10 hours after admission) in a study of 211 patients with appendicitis. Recently, Teixeira et al. [11] showed that while an appendectomy delay of more than 6 hours did not increase the risk of perforation, it significantly increased the risk of surgical site infection in 4529 patients with nonperforated appendicitis. In contrast, the present study showed no difference in surgical site infection rate, which was approximately 5% in each group.

The safety of delayed appendectomy can be explained by the development of medical technologies, particularly the injection of antibiotics to halt the progression of appendicitis. A number of studies have shown the effectiveness of antibiotics in treating perforated appendicitis [12–14]. In most cases, antibiotic administration leads to resolution of the infectious and inflammatory processes of perforated appendicitis, which allows elective appendectomy to be performed 6–8 weeks after the initial presentation of disease. Moreover, two randomized controlled trials suggested that acute appendicitis could be successfully treated with antibiotics and that antibiotics might be a first-line therapy in acute appendicitis [2, 3].

Nowadays, we just give one injection of antibiotics just before surgery. In the case of severe wound complications, we have used antibiotics even if it did not follow guidelines.

Among a total of 1805 cases, we performed 190 appendectomies (10.5%) for acute appendicitis between the hours of 11 PM and 8 AM. When a patient was diagnosed with nonperforated appendicitis at these hours, we often had no choice but to delay an operation, offer antibiotic therapy, and schedule an operation for the following day. The unavailability of an emergency operating room or operating team members such as an anesthesiologist, nurse, or assistant prohibited the prompt operation. The results of this report may lessen surgeons' stress in this situation, as the increasing risk of perforation and subsequent morbidity in appendicitis progression may be less significant than previously thought. This optimistic finding could have a positive psychological effect on surgeons, resulting in a more meticulous operation the following day with enhanced care for patients. In addition, the current government policy that surgical specialists should care for their patients in the emergency room greatly increases the responsibility of surgeons. Our findings suggest that surgeons could delay operations for less critically ill patients, such as those with nonperforated appendicitis, in order to appropriately care for those requiring immediate attention, such as trauma patients and critical care patients, especially in situations with limited staff.

Accurate preoperative diagnosis to clarify whether the appendix is perforated or not must be a prerequisite to delayed appendectomy. CT is a main diagnostic tool with high sensitivity and specificity for acute appendicitis. The routine use of CT in patients with suspected acute appendicitis has been shown to shorten the time to operating room admission, reduce the number of negative appendectomies, and reduce medical costs [15]. Ultrasonography is another useful modality commonly used for children, pregnant patients, and outpatients, because it is noninvasive, does not require patient preparation, and avoids unnecessary exposure to ionizing radiation. Moreover, Peña et al. [16] demonstrated that an imaging protocol using US and CT was useful for distinguishing between nonperforated and perforated appendicitis, as shown by a marked decrease in the perforation and negative appendectomy rates in 1338 children with suspected appendicitis. However, this study showed that the false-positive rate of CT and US was as high as 53.9% (146/271) and 61.1% (58/95), respectively. As radiologic readings are not infallible, surgeons need to confirm the presence of perforation using symptoms, physical examinations, and laboratory findings. Radiologists must also pay close, critical attention to their radiologic interpretations. In our data, there were false positive and negative findings in CT and U/S. But there is no perfect diagnostic modality established of appendicitis before surgery. This was one of the limitations of our study.

At the beginning of this study, we predicted that there would be little difference in medical costs between the two groups because the additional hospitalization fees for the delayed group might be similar to the additional nighttime surgery fees for the immediate group. However, medical costs were significantly increased for the delayed group because the additional hospitalization fees were more expensive than the additional nighttime surgery fees in the immediate group. Surgeons should consider that increased medical costs can be a burden for patients and health insurance companies. In addition, the emotional and unanticipated economic cost of extended hospital stays in the delayed group should not be dismissed.

In conclusion, delayed appendectomy is safe for patients with acute nonperforated appendicitis. It can improve quality of provided care from surgeons, enhance quality of care for patients, and increase effective utilization of medical resources and operating rooms for life-threatening emergencies.

Author details

Sung Il Choi[1,2*]

*Address all correspondence to: drchoi@khu.ac.kr

1 Department of Surgery, Kyung Hee University School of Medicine, Kyung Hee University Hospital at Gangdong, Seoul, Korea

2 Department of Surgery, Kyung Hee University School of Medicine, Kyung Hee University Hospital, Seoul, Korea

References

[1] Berry Jr J, Malt RA. Appendicitis near its centenary. Annals of Surgery. Nov 1984;**200**(5): 567-575

[2] Hansson J, Körner U, Khorram-Manesh A, Solberg A, Lundholm K. Randomized clinical trial of antibiotic therapy versus appendicectomy as primary treatment of acute appendicitis in unselected patients. The British Journal of Surgery. May 2009;**96**(5):473-481. DOI: 10.1002/bjs.6482

[3] Styrud J, Eriksson S, Nilsson I, Ahlberg G, Haapaniemi S, Neovius G, et al. Appendectomy versus antibiotic treatment in acute appendicitis. A prospective multicenter randomized controlled trial. World Journal of Surgery. Jun 2006;**30**(6):1033-1037

[4] Ingraham AM, Cohen ME, Bilimoria KY, Ko CY, Hall BL, Russell TR, et al. Effect of delay to operation on outcomes in adults with acute appendicitis. Archives of Surgery. Sep 2010;**145**(9):886-892. DOI: 10.1001/archsurg.2010.184

[5] Abou-Nukta F, Bakhos C, Arroyo K, Koo Y, Martin J, Reinhold R, et al. Effects of delaying appendectomy for acute appendicitis for 12 to 24 hours. Archives of Surgery. May 2006;**141**(5):504-506. discussioin 506-7

[6] Surana R, Quinn F, Puri P. Is it necessary to perform appendicectomy in the middle of the night in children? British Medical Journal. May 1, 1993;**306**(6886):1168

[7] Yardeni D, Hirschl RB, Drongowski RA, Teitelbaum DH, Geiger JD, Coran AG. Delayed versus immediate surgery in acute appendicitis: Do we need to operate during the night? Journal of Pediatric Surgery. Mar 2004;**39**(3):464-469 (discussion 464-469)

[8] Omundsen M, Dennett E. Delay to appendicectomy and associated morbidity: A retrospective review. ANZ Journal of Surgery. Mar 2006;**76**(3):153-155

[9] Ditillo MF, Dziura JD, Rabinovici R. Is it safe to delay appendectomy in adults with acute appendicitis? Annals of Surgery. Nov 2006;**244**(5):656-660

[10] Udgiri N, Curras E, Kella VK, Nagpal K, Cosgrove J. Appendicitis, is it an emergency? The American Surgeon. Jul 2011;**77**(7):898-901

[11] Teixeira PG, Sivrikoz E, Inaba K, Talving P, Lam L, Demetriades D. Appendectomy timing: Waiting until the next morning increases the risk of surgical site infections. Annals of Surgery. Sep 2012;**256**(3):538-543. DOI: 10.1097/SLA.0b013e318265ea13

[12] Bufo AJ, Shah RS, Li MH, Cyr NA, Hollabaugh RS, Hixson SD, et al. Interval appendectomy for perforated appendicitis in children. Journal of Laparoendoscopic & Advanced Surgical Techniques. Part A. Aug 1998;**8**(4):209-214

[13] Weiner DJ, Katz A, Hirschl RB, Drongowski R, Coran AG. Interval appendectomy in perforated appendicitis. Pediatric Surgery International. Feb 1995;**10**(2-3):82-85

[14] Mazziotti M, Marley E, Winthrop A, Fitzgerald P, Walton M, Langer J. Histopathologic analysis of interval appendectomy specimens: Support for the role of interval appendectomy. Journal of Pediatric Surgery. Jun 1997;**32**(6):806-809

[15] Rao PM, Rhea JT, Novelline RA, Mostafavi AA, McCabe CJ. Effect of computed tomography of the appendix on treatment of patients and use of hospital resources. The New England Journal of Medicine. Jan 15, 1998;**338**(3):141-146

[16] Peña BMG, Taylor GA, Fishman SJ, Mandl KD. Effect of an imaging protocol on clinical outcomes among pediatric patients with appendicitis. Pediatrics. Dec 2002;**110**(6):1088-1093

15

Pregnancy and Delivery of Women with IBD

Kateřina Hokerová

Abstract

We provide a basic overview of inheritance, fertility and influence of IBD and pregnancy, therapy in pregnancy and childbirth options. A crucial factor for good results is the degree of inflammation at the time of conception and during pregnancy. If the disease is inactive, there is no decrease in fertility and no greater risk of deterioration of disease in pregnancy and pregnancy does not differ from the normal population. The opposite situation occurs if there is a pregnancy at the time of disease activity. Then, in up to 75% of pregnancy courses with big problems, fertility declines, inflammation also worsens and the risk of exacerbations increases during pregnancy. This aggravates the course of pregnancy and childbirth and has a negative effect on the fetus. Therefore, it is necessary to plan for a longer period of disease stabilization and continue chronic medication and not discontinue drugs for the fear of negative impact of medications on fetal development. Commonly used drugs such as aminosalicylates, corticosteroids, immunosuppressants and biological therapy appear to be safe and well tolerated during pregnancy. The method of delivery is different for each individual and depends on the form and location of the inflammation and the preceding operations.

Keywords: inflammatory bowel disease, Crohn's disease, ulcerative colitis, pregnancy, childbirth, breastfeeding

1. Introduction

Inflammatory bowel disease (IBD) is a chronic bowel inflammation of unknown origin, which includes Crohn's disease (CD) and ulcerative colitis (UC). The incidence in our population has increased, the incidence of UC is 10.4/100,000 and the incidence of CD is 5.6/100,000. IBD affects young adults in their fertile age, 50% of patients are diagnosed under the age of 35 and a quarter of patients get pregnant after they have been diagnosed with IBD. Young women are often concerned about the effect of IBD on their fertility, development of the fetus and as well about the effect of the pregnancy on their disease. They are interested in the effect of the chronic medication used during the pregnancy, management of the birth and possibility of breastfeeding. In the past, patients have been advised not to get pregnant, existing strategies of treating IBD makes the pregnancy possible and safe for the mother and the child.

2. Genetics and IBD

IBD is multifactorially determined. The risk for a child with a parent with an IBD is 2–13 times higher than the risk in the normal population [1]. A child of a parent with IBD has a 5% risk for CD and a 1.6% for UC. If both parents have IBD, the risk increases up to 37% [2, 3].

3. Fertility and IBD

Infertility of women with IBD ranges between 7 and 12%, which is in line with the normal population [4–7]. The fertility can decrease with the following conditions:

- An active inflammation (can affect the Fallopian tubes and the ovaries, in the perianal area it can cause dyspareunia)
- Surgery before the pregnancy (IPAA—ileo pouch anal anastomosis—is connected with lower fertility because of scarring in the area around the adnexae)
- Medication that affects men's fertility such as methotrexate, sulfasalazine [1, 9, 10]

4. The effects of IBD on pregnancy

Multiple studies on the effects of IBD on pregnancy, development and growth of the fetus, have come to a conflicting conclusions most likely due to disparate conditions of the individual studies. All the studies agree that the key factor for a successful pregnancy is a function of whether the disease is active at the time of conception. Patients with an inactive IBD (minimum 12 months without clinical, laboratory and endoscopic signs of an active inflammatory process) are not in a higher risk of bad perinatological results. On the other hand, if the disease is active, up to 75% of pregnancies are connected with a high number of problems and relatively high risk of abortion, preterm birth or hypotrophy of the fetus. Therefore, it is necessary to plan the pregnancy while the disease is in remission [1, 4–6, 8]. The activity of the disease at the time of conception leads to a higher risk of fetal loss and preterm deliveries. Also, activity of the disease during the pregnancy is associated with lower fetal weight and as well with a preterm delivery [1, 3, 8, 9, 10]. Pregnancy loss affects 12.2% of patients with IBD as compared to 9.9% in the normal population. Miscarriages are more common in cases where the patient has an intestinal resection before the pregnancy. The length of the resected tissue and activity of the disease are proportional to a higher risk of miscarriage [6]. The percentage of preterm deliveries (<g.h. 37) is around 8% in the Czech Republic in the normal population, studies describe higher risk of preterm deliveries in the group of people with IBD, the risk is 1.87 times higher, which is 11.5–16% [6]. The risk of low fetal weight (<2500 g) is two times higher, which is explained by undernourishment of the mother in the time of relapse, especially if there are repeated exacerbations in the course of the pregnancy. This occurs more often in diseased with the CD than the UC, Although some studies have found a connection between congenital malformations (especially a cleft palate and malformations of the urinary tract) and the mother's UC, this suspicion was not confirmed in extensive studies. Most of the studies show that IBD is not connected with a risk of congenital malformations. The rate of malformations ranges between 1 and 4.8% of newborns, which is the same range as in the normal population. More serious malformations were more often found in a group with a severe course of the disease during the pregnancy compared to the ones in relapse. After considering the grade of disease, no study was able to prove that any medication used (corticoids, azathioprine and mesalazine) affects the result of pregnancy [5].

5. The effect of pregnancy on IBD

There is no proof to suggest that pregnancy worsens the disease; therefore, there is no reason to end the pregnancy. On the contrary, there are studies that have demonstrated positive effects and long-term improvement of IBD (impact of the pregnancy on the immune system) shown decrease of relapses in the following 3 years [2]. Development of IBD during the pregnancy is correlated with the activity of disease at the time of conception. If the disease is inactive at the time of conception, then the pregnancy goes without bigger problems in the majority of the diseased, only around one-third of patients have a relapse during the pregnancy, which is the same number as in a group of nonpregnant women in the course of 9 months. In two-thirds of the patients, the disease stays in inactive state during the whole pregnancy [1, 4, 6, 8]. On the other hand, if the IBD is active at the time of conception, two-thirds of the patients have a persistent disease and even an aggravation of the disease. Therapy plays an important role in pregnancy by keeping the disease in remission; therefore, it is recommended that the therapy should not be stopped due to the fear of side effects to pregnancy.

6. Therapy in pregnancy

The majority of the drugs used for the treatment of IBD are considered to be safe during the pregnancy and breastfeeding [3]. Analysis of 19 retrospective studies has shown that the medication commonly used for therapy of IBD (aminosalicylates—ASA, corticoids, immunosuppressants and immunotherapy) does not significantly increase the incidence of stillborn, ectopic pregnancy, hypotrophy of the fetus or miscarriage. While using these drugs, the congenital anomalies were more often seen, which is probably connected to the activity of the disease and not to the therapy. Both methotrexate and thalidomide are clearly contraindicated [1].

If the therapy is able to keep the disease inactive, it is recommended not to stop and continue the therapy during the whole pregnancy because the benefits outweigh the risks of the conservative therapy and the danger of relapse after completing the therapy.

7. The mode of delivery

The percentage (44%) of the Cesarean section is higher in the group of patients with IBD than in normal population [3]. Recent population studies from Sweden have shown that women with the UC without any surgery in the past had two times higher risk of elective Cesarean section, even though vaginal birth is the safest way for the mother and the child. Additional studies have also shown that the Cesarean sections are mostly performed on the basis of patient's or the doctor's preference, but not from a real indication. Even though some doctors think that all the patients with IBD should have a Cesarean section, it seems reasonable to make the vaginal birth possible for the women with inactive or in the moderate stage of the disease. The decision about the mode of the delivery should be strictly individual and it should be an agreement among the mother, the obstetrician, the gastroenterologist and the surgeon [6].

Cesarean section is definitely indicated when there is an active perianal disease with abscesses and fistulas or active rectal disease (proctitis in UC and CD) with consideration of the protection of the anal sphincter. IPAA or ileorectal anastomosis is considered as a relative indication for the Cesarean section, the guidelines about the mode of delivery after IPAA are not uniform, and both ways are described. With a consideration of a protection of the anal sphincter and keeping the pouch continence, the Cesarean section is preferred. Patients with the IPAA have, due to the surgery, a border continence of stool and that is closely related to an intact sphincter and the function of the pelvic floor. The function of the pouch is affected already in the third trimester and it goes back to the original shape during 6 months after the delivery. In the vaginal birth, the pudendal nerves can be affected due to the pressure in the second stage of labor or in the forceps delivery, which can lead to more frequent stools. In the long-term observation (5 years), it is observed that after the vaginal birth, the function of the pouch worsens faster especially in the births with the higher risks of obstetric injuries (instrumental labor, episiotomy, the fetal weight above 4000 g, emergent Cesarean section, second stage of labor longer than 2 h) In the majority of the patients, the primary Cesarean section is chosen. Other reason for that is as well the emergency Cesarean section from the obstetrics indication can be very risky because of abdominal adhesions after previous surgeries [1, 3, 9, 10]. Vaginal birth should be allowed only to women without the signs of rectal and perianal forms of the disease [6]. Traumatic changes of the perianal area can be a cause of long-term festering complications or fistulas, preforming of episiotomy can induce the perianal lesions in the future course of the disease in 20% [5]. If the woman with IBD has a vaginal birth, it is appropriate to avoid episiotomy; however, it is better to perform an episiotomy than a spontaneous uncontrollable damage. Vaginal birth is also possible in the patients with colostomy or ileostomy and it is not associated with a higher risk of the complications with the stomies [1, 6].

8. Conclusion

IBD affects women in the fertile age with consequences to their fertility, pregnancy and breastfeeding. The disease and the pregnancy affect each other, and the development of the disease and the pregnancy is determined by the activity of inflammation at the time of conception. Patients who are in remission at the time of conception will most likely stay in the remission during the pregnancy. On the other hand, 70% of the patients with an active inflammation at the time of conception will stay in that shape or even get worse during the pregnancy. Women with an active IBD are at a higher risk of adverse results of the pregnancy, whereas the women with inactive disease can expect normal course and good results of the pregnancy. That is why it is crucial to plan their pregnancy during remission, and not to cut out the anti-inflammatory and immunosuppressant therapy put in place before the pregnancy. Most of the medication used in treatment of IBD is considered to be safe at the time of pregnancy and breastfeeding, but more studies are needed. Patients with IBD can have vaginal delivery, whereas patients with the perianal lesions, patients with affected rectum and patients after the reconstructive surgery with IPAA should deliver by the Cesarean section.

Author details

Kateřina Hokerová

Address all correspondence to: zavorova@nemocnice-horovice.cz

Nemocnice Hořovice, Hořovice, Czech Republic

References

[1] Van der Woude CJ. ECCO Guidelines/Consensus Paper. The second European evidenced-based consensus on reproduction and pregnancy in inflammatory bowel disease. Journal of Crohn's and Colitis. 2015;**9**(2):107-124. Available from: https://www.ecco-ibd.eu/images/6_Publication/6_3_ECCO%20Guidelines/FINAL_MASTER_JCC_Online_PulishedVersion_PregnancyGuidelines_2015_Doi101093_jju006.pdf

[2] Kment M. Idiopatické střevní záněty v graviditě. Interní medicína pro praxi. 2008;**10**(7a8):333-335

[3] Kwan LY, Mahadevan U. Inflammatory bowel disease and pregnancy: An update. Expert Review of Clinical Immunology. 2010;**6**(4):643-657

[4] Alstead EM, Nelson-Piercy C. Inflammatory bowel disease in pregnancy. 2013. Available from: http://www.ncbi.nlm.nih.gov/pmc/articles/PMC1774968/

[5] Kment M. Choroby gastrointestinálního traktu v graviditě. Triton. 2003:43-61

[6] Lukáš K, Pařízek A. Idiopatické střevní záněty a těhotenství. Časopis lékařů českých. 2010;**149**:163-172

[7] Pintérová Kolesárová M, Pintér M. Vliv idiopatického střevního zánětu na interval potřebný pro početí pacientek. Česká Gynekologie 2008;**732**:109-112

[8] Ferguson ChB. Inflammatory bowel disease in pregnancy. British Medical Journal. 2008;**337**(a427). Available from: http://dx.doi.org/10.1136/bmj.39566.681458.BE (Published July 2008); http://www.bmj.com/content/337/bmj.39566.681458.BE

[9] Peppercon MA, Mahadevan U. Fertility, pregnancy and nursing in inflammatory bowel disease. 2017. Available from: http://www.uptodate.com/contents/fertility-pregnancy and-nursing-in-inflammatory-bowel-disease

[10] Peppercon MA, Mahadevan U. Patient information: Inflammatory bowel disease and pregnancy. 2017. Available from: http://www.uptodate.com/contents/inflammatory-boweldisease-and-pregnancy-beyond-the-basics

Permissions

All chapters in this book were first published in IBSNCRT, by InTech Open; hereby published with permission under the Creative Commons Attribution License or equivalent. Every chapter published in this book has been scrutinized by our experts. Their significance has been extensively debated. The topics covered herein carry significant findings which will fuel the growth of the discipline. They may even be implemented as practical applications or may be referred to as a beginning point for another development.

The contributors of this book come from diverse backgrounds, making this book a truly international effort. This book will bring forth new frontiers with its revolutionizing research information and detailed analysis of the nascent developments around the world.

We would like to thank all the contributing authors for lending their expertise to make the book truly unique. They have played a crucial role in the development of this book. Without their invaluable contributions this book wouldn't have been possible. They have made vital efforts to compile up to date information on the varied aspects of this subject to make this book a valuable addition to the collection of many professionals and students.

This book was conceptualized with the vision of imparting up-to-date information and advanced data in this field. To ensure the same, a matchless editorial board was set up. Every individual on the board went through rigorous rounds of assessment to prove their worth. After which they invested a large part of their time researching and compiling the most relevant data for our readers.

The editorial board has been involved in producing this book since its inception. They have spent rigorous hours researching and exploring the diverse topics which have resulted in the successful publishing of this book. They have passed on their knowledge of decades through this book. To expedite this challenging task, the publisher supported the team at every step. A small team of assistant editors was also appointed to further simplify the editing procedure and attain best results for the readers.

Apart from the editorial board, the designing team has also invested a significant amount of their time in understanding the subject and creating the most relevant covers. They scrutinized every image to scout for the most suitable representation of the subject and create an appropriate cover for the book.

The publishing team has been an ardent support to the editorial, designing and production team. Their endless efforts to recruit the best for this project, has resulted in the accomplishment of this book. They are a veteran in the field of academics and their pool of knowledge is as vast as their experience in printing. Their expertise and guidance has proved useful at every step. Their uncompromising quality standards have made this book an exceptional effort. Their encouragement from time to time has been an inspiration for everyone.

The publisher and the editorial board hope that this book will prove to be a valuable piece of knowledge for researchers, students, practitioners and scholars across the globe.

List of Contributors

Julio Plata-Bello
Department of Neurosurgery, Hospital Universitario de Canarias, S/C de Tenerife, Spain

Silvia Acosta-López
Department of Gastroenterology and Hepatology, Hospital Universitario Nuestra Señora de La Candelaria, S/C de Tenerife, Spain

Mihaela Fadgyas Stanculete
Department of Neurosciences, Discipline of Psychiatry and Pediatric Psychiatry, University of Medicine and Pharmacy "Iuliu Hatieganu", Cluj-Napoca, Romania
Second Psychiatric Clinic, Emergency County Hospital Cluj, Cluj-Napoca, Romania

Samia Ali Gamie
Faculty of Medicine, Helwan University, Cairo, Egypt

Alfredo Alvarado
Alma Mater Universidad Nacional de Colombia, Bogotá, Colombia
Certified by the American Board of Surgeons and the American Board of Emergency Medicine, Miami, FL, USA
International College of Surgeons, Chicago, IL, USA
Society of Laparoscopic Surgeons, Chicago, USA
American College of Emergency Physicians, Irving TX, USA

Wei Kang, Jinglin Zhang and Ka Fai To
Department of Anatomical and Cellular Pathology, State Key Laboratory of Oncology in South China, State Key Laboratory of Digestive Diseases, The Chinese University of Hong Kong, Hong Kong SAR, PR China

Francesca Pasqui, Carolina Poli, Caterina Magrino and Davide Festi
Department of Medical and Surgical Sciences, University of Bologna, Bologna, Italy

Alexandra Chira and Dan Lucian Dumitrascu
Medical Clinic, Department of Internal Medicine, "Iuliu Hatieganu" University of Medicine and Pharmacy Cluj-Napoca, Romania

Romeo Ioan Chira
Medical Clinic, Department of Internal Medicine, Div. Gastroenterology, "Iuliu Hatieganu" University of Medicine and Pharmacy Cluj-Napoca, Romania

Volkan Sarper Erikci
Department of Pediatric Surgery, Saglık Bilimleri University, İzmir Tepecik Training Hospital, Izmir, Turkey

Victor V. Chaban
Department of Internal Medicine, Charles R. Drew University of Medicine and Science, Los Angeles, USA; Department of Medicine, University of California, Los Angeles, USA

Daryl Ramai
Department of Gastroenterology and Hepatology, The Brooklyn Hospital Center - Clinical Affiliate of The Mount Sinai Hospital, Brooklyn, New York, USA
Department of Anatomical Sciences, St George's University School of Medicine, True Blue, Grenada, West Indies

Sandar Linn and Madhavi Reddy
Department of Gastroenterology and Hepatology, The Brooklyn Hospital Center - Clinical Affiliate of The Mount Sinai Hospital, Brooklyn, New York, USA

Darja Urlep, Evgen Benedik and Rok Orel
University Children's Hospital, University Medical Centre Ljubljana, Ljubljana, Slovenia

Sabiu Saheed
Phytomedicine, Food Factors and Toxicology Research Laboratory, Biochemistry Department, School of Basic Medical Sciences, Kwara State University, Ilorin, Nigeria
Phytomedicine and Phytopharmacology Research Group, Plant Sciences Department, University of the Free State, Phuthaditjhaba, South Africa
Department of Microbial, Biochemical, and Food Biotechnology, University of the Free State, Bloemfontein, South Africa

Ajani Emmanuel Oladipo
Phytomedicine, Food Factors and Toxicology Research Laboratory, Biochemistry Department, School of Basic Medical Sciences, Kwara State University, Ilorin, Nigeria

Taofik Olatunde Sunmonu
Phytomedicine and Plant Biochemistry Research Laboratory, Biochemistry Unit, Department of Biological Sciences, Al-Hikmah University, Ilorin, Nigeria

Fatai Oladunni Balogun and Anofi Omotayo Tom Ashafa
Phytomedicine and Phytopharmacology Research Group, Plant Sciences Department, University of the Free State, Phuthaditjhaba, South Africa

Rok Orel, Evgen Benedik, Janez Eržen and Darja Urlep
University Children's Hospital, University Medical Centre Ljubljana, Ljubljana, Slovenia

Anija Orel
Clinical Nutrition Unit, Institute of Oncology Ljubljana, Ljubljana, Slovenia

Sung Il Choi
Department of Surgery, Kyung Hee University School of Medicine, Kyung Hee University Hospital at Gangdong, Seoul, Korea
Department of Surgery, Kyung Hee University School of Medicine, Kyung Hee University Hospital, Seoul, Korea

Kateřina Hokerová
Nemocnice Hořovice, Hořovice, Czech Republic

Index

www.ingramcontent.com/pod-product-compliance
Lightning Source LLC
LaVergne TN
LVHW060553210926
848485LV00005B/1306